PSYCHIATRY AND CHINESE HISTORY

Studies for the Society for the Social History of Medicine

Series Editors: David Cantor
Keir Waddington

Titles in this Series

1 Meat, Medicine and Human Health in the Twentieth Century
David Cantor, Christian Bonah and Matthias Dörries (eds)

2 Locating Health: Historical and Anthropological Investigations of Place and Health
Erika Dyck and Christopher Fletcher (eds)

3 Medicine in the Remote and Rural North, 1800–2000
J. T. H. Connor and Stephan Curtis (eds)

4 A Modern History of the Stomach: Gastric Illness, Medicine and British Society, 1800–1950
Ian Miller

5 War and the Militarization of British Army Medicine, 1793–1830
Catherine Kelly

6 Nervous Disease in Late Eighteenth-Century Britain: The Reality of a Fashionable Disorder
Heather R. Beatty

7 Desperate Housewives, Neuroses and the Domestic Environment, 1945–1970
Ali Haggett

8 Disabled Children: Contested Caring, 1850–1979
Anne Borsay and Pamela Dale (eds)

9 Toxicants, Health and Regulation since 1945
Soraya Boudia and Nathalie Jas (eds)

10 A Medical History of Skin: Scratching the Surface
Jonathan Reinarz and Kevin Patrick Siena (eds)

11 The Care of Older People: England and Japan, A Comparative Study
Mayumi Hayashi

12 Child Guidance in Britain, 1918–1955: The Dangerous Age of Childhood
John Stewart

13 Modern German Midwifery, 1885–1960
Lynne Fallwell

14 Western Maternity and Medicine, 1880–1990
Janet Greenlees and Linda Bryder (eds)

15 Human Heredity in the Twentieth Century
Bernd Gausemeier, Staffan Müller-Wille and Edmund Ramsden (eds)

16 Biologics, A History of Agents Made From Living Organisms
in the Twentieth Century
Alexander von Schwerin, Heiko Stoff and Bettina Wahrig (eds)

17 Bacteria in Britain, 1880–1939
Rosemary Wall

18 Health and Citizenship: Political Cultures of Health in Modern Europe
Frank Huisman and Harry Oosterhuis (eds)

19 Institutionalizing the Insane in Nineteenth-Century England
Anna Shepherd

20 The Politics of Hospital Provision in Early Twentieth-Century Britain
Barry M. Doyle

Forthcoming Titles

Stress in Post-War Britain
Mark Jackson (ed.)

PSYCHIATRY AND CHINESE HISTORY

EDITED BY

Howard Chiang

Routledge
Taylor & Francis Group
LONDON AND NEW YORK

First published in paperback 2024

First published 2014 by Pickering & Chatto (Publishers) Limited

Published 2016 by Routledge
4 Park Square, Milton Park, Abingdon, Oxon OX14 4RN

and by Routledge
605 Third Avenue, New York, NY 10158

Routledge is an imprint of the Taylor & Francis Group, an informa business

BRITISH LIBRARY CATALOGUING IN PUBLICATION DATA

Psychiatry and Chinese history. – (Studies for the Society for the Social History of Medicine)
1. Psychiatry – China – History. 2. Mental illness – China – History.
I. Series II. Chiang, Howard, 1983 – editor.
616.8'9'00951-dc23

ISBN: 978-1-84893-438-2 (hbk)
ISBN: 978-1-03-292349-9 (pbk)
ISBN: 978-1-315-65437-9 (ebk)

DOI: 10.4324/9781315654379

Typeset by Pickering & Chatto (Publishers) Limited

CONTENTS

List of Contributors ix
List of Figures xiii

Introduction: Historicizing Chinese Psychiatry – *Howard Chiang* 1
Part I: Historical Precedents
1 Exorcising Dreams and Nightmares in Late Ming China – *Brigid E. Vance* 17
2 Emotional Therapy and Talking Cures in Late Imperial China – *Hsiu-fen Chen* 37
3 Medicaments and Persuasion: Medical Therapies for Madness in Nineteenth-Century China – *Fabien Simonis* 55
Part II: Missionary Investments
4 Psychiatric Space and Design Antecedents: The John G. Kerr Refuge for the Insane – *Peter Szto* 71
5 An Iron Cage of Civilization? Missionary Psychiatry, the Chinese Family and a Colonial Dialect of Enlightenment – *Zhiying Ma* 91
6 Tropical Neurasthenia or Oriental Nerves? White Breakdowns in China – *Wen-Ji Wang* 111
Part III: Biomedical Modernity
7 Pathologizing Marriage: Neuropsychiatry and the Escape of Women in Early Twentieth-Century China – *Hugh Shapiro* 129
8 Gone with the *West Wind*: The Emergence and Disappearance of Psychotherapeutic Culture in China, 1936–68 – *Geoffrey Blowers and Shelley Wang Xuelai* 143
9 A Charted Epidemic of Trauma: Case Notes at the Psychiatric Department of National Taiwan University Hospital between 1946 and 1953 – *Harry Yi-Jui Wu* 161
Part IV: New Therapeutic Cultures
10 The Emergence of the Psycho-Boom in Contemporary Urban China – *Hsuan-Ying Huang* 183
Afterword: Reframing Psychiatry in China – *Nancy N. Chen* 205

Notes 213
Index 261

For Ari Larissa Heinrich

LIST OF CONTRIBUTORS

Geoffrey Blowers, formerly Associate Dean of Social Sciences and Professor of Psychology at the University of Hong Kong, is the Director of Graduate Studies at Hong Kong Shue Yan University. He is co-editor with Alison Turtle of *Psychology Moving East: The Status of Western Psychology in Asia and Oceania* (1987), co-author with Kieron O'Connor of *Personal Construct Psychology in the Clinical Context* (1996) and has published papers on the history of psychology and psychoanalysis in China and Japan. He was twice President of the Hong Kong Psychological Society and is currently its Registrar. He is also Founding President of the Hong Kong Institute of Analytical Psychology.

Hsiu-fen Chen is Associate Professor of History at National Chengchi University, Taiwan. After receiving her PhD from SOAS, University of London, she published several articles on the topics of madness, emotions and regimen in late imperial China. Her first book *Nourishing Life and Cultivating the Body: Writing the Literati's Body and Techniques for Preserving Health in the Late Ming* (2009) won a publication grant from National Science Council, Taiwan in 2010. She is writing her second book entitled *Empire of the Mind: Emotions, Madness and Mental Healings in Ming-Qing China.* In addition to the history of body and mind, Chen is also interested in cultural history, visual history and religious studies.

Nancy N. Chen is Professor of Anthropology at the University of California, Santa Cruz. A medical anthropologist, she is the author of *Breathing Spaces: Qigong, Psychiatry, and Healing in China* (2003) and *Food, Medicine, and the Quest for Good Health* (2009).

Howard Chiang is Assistant Professor of Modern Chinese History at the University of Warwick, UK. He received his PhD and MA in History of Science from Princeton University, after completing his MA in Quantitative Methods in the Social Sciences at Columbia University and his BS in Biochemistry and BA in Psychology at the University of Southern California. He is the editor of *Transgender China* (2012), *Queer Sinophone Cultures* (2013, with Ari Larissa Heinrich), and *Historical Epistemology and the Making of Modern Chinese*

Medicine (2015). He sits on the editorial boards of *Cultural History*, *Spontaneous Generations: A Journal for the History and Philosophy of Science*, and *TSQ: Transgender Studies Quarterly*.

Hsuan-Ying Huang is a Postdoctoral Fellow at the Australian Centre on China in the World, Australian National University. He received his MD and psychiatric residency training from National Taiwan University and his PhD in medical anthropology from Harvard University. His research, mainly based in Beijing and Shanghai, examines urban China's recent 'psycho-boom', a popular movement centered on psychotherapy training, with an emphasis on its broadly conceived psychoanalytic branch. He is particularly interested in how this psycho-boom may reveal or shape subjectivity in urban China and how a new mental health profession may have emerged from it.

Zhiying Ma is a PhD candidate of the Department of Comparative Human Development and the Department of Anthropology, University of Chicago. She received her bachelor degrees in Psychology and Philosophy at Peking University, China. In graduate school, Ma specializes in Cultural and Medical Anthropology. Since 2008, she has been conducting ethnographic and historical research on the development of psychiatry in China, particularly focusing on the role of the family and the emergence of community mental health. In 2011, she received the Andrew W. Mellon Foundation Research Fellowship to visit the Needham Research Institute. Her research has also been supported by various other organizations, including the Ford Foundation, the Henry Luce Foundation, and the Association for Asian Studies. Based on her ongoing research on psychiatry, she has published several peer-reviewed journal articles and book chapters. Besides psychiatry, Ma has started to examine the disability rights movement in China and the US–China dialogue on medical ethics reform. She currently serves as the book review editor of *Student Anthropologist*.

Hugh Shapiro is Associate Professor of Modern Chinese History at the University of Nevada. He earned his BA from Stanford and his PhD from Harvard. He has enjoyed visiting appointments at Princeton University, Nichibunken in Kyoto, National Taiwan Normal University in Taipei, and the Institute for Advanced Study in Princeton. He co-edited *Medicine Across Cultures: History and Practice of Medicine in Non-Western Cultures* (2003). He received the Li-Qing Prize for the History of Chinese Science and won his university's highest teaching award.

Fabien Simonis received his PhD in East Asian Studies from Princeton University in 2010. The title of his dissertation is 'Mad Acts, Mad Speech, and Mad People in Late Imperial Chinese Law and Medicine'. He is now working on two books, one on the history of Chinese medical thinking and another on the multiple practices surrounding madness in Qing China.

Peter Szto was born and raised in New York City. His parents emigrated from south China and instilled in him a passion for things Chinese. In his pursuit of Chinese knowledge he earned degrees from Calvin College, Michigan State University, Westminster Theological Seminary, and the University of Pennsylvania. His research interest is on social welfare development in China and the use of photography as a tool of social research. Dr. Szto is an Associate Professor at the Grace Abbott School of Social Work, University of Nebraska at Omaha.

Brigid E. Vance received her PhD in History from Princeton University, after completing her MA in East Asian Studies at Stanford and her BA in Psychology at Carleton College. Currently, Vance is an Assistant Professor at Colorado State University-Pueblo. Her research interests broadly lie in Ming-Qing history, Tokugawa Japan, and the history of medicine and science, with an emphasis on psychology.

Wen-Ji Wang is an Associate Professor in the Graduate Institute of Science, Technology and Society at the National Yang-Ming University, Taiwan. After doctoral work in the early history of psychoanalysis in Europe at the University of Cambridge, he has published on leprosy and colonial medicine in Taiwan, and the mental hygiene movement in the first half of the 20th century in China. He is now working on a book that traces the history of neurotic disorders with their relationship to the rise of psy disciplines in Republican China.

Shelley Wang Xuelai is a cardiologist who holds a doctorate in Community Medicine from the University of Hong Kong. She has published papers on risk factors associated with heart disease including psychological disorders such as depression and anxiety. She was formerly a Postdoctoral Fellow in the Faculty of Medicine and is currently Research Associate in the Department of Biochemistry at the University of Hong Kong.

Harry Yi-Jui Wu received his DPhil in History from the University of Oxford in 2012. Prior to his career as a historian, he studied Medicine in Taiwan with further training experiences in Psychiatry and Psychoanalytic Studies in England. He is currently Assistant Professor in Medical Humanities at the School of Humanities and Social Sciences and Lee Kong Chian School of Medicine, Nanyang Technological University, Singapore.

LIST OF FIGURES AND TABLES

Figure 1.1: Suppress Inauspicious Dreams about the Sky, Sun, Wind or Rain 26
Figure 1.2: Rat Day 27
Figure 1.3: Talisman for Breaking the Three Worms in the Upper Corpse-God 28
Figure 4.1: From Cruciform Plan to Radial Plan 76
Figure 4.2: The Main Routes of the Old Silk Road 83
Figure 4.3: The John G. Kerr Hospital in Canton, China 85
Figure 4.4: One of the First Two Buildings of the Kerr Asylum 86
Figure 4.5: A Schematic Rendering of the Kerr Asylum 89
Figure 5.1: Patient Tied to a Pig's Feeding Trough 102
Figure 5.2: Wire Restraining Frame 103
Figure 5.3: Patient Transported in Pig Baskets 103
Figure 9.1: Note of Present Illness from National Taiwan University Hospital Psychiatric Department Case Notes (1946) 171
Figure 9.2: Numbers of Outpatient Visits and Admissions 172
Figure 9.3: Numbers of Admitted Patients with Racial Distribution 173
Figure 9.4: Statistics of Taiwanese and Chinese Immigrants (Mainlanders) among Outpatients 173

Table 2.1: The 'Principle of Mutual Conquest of the Five Phases' 39

INTRODUCTION: HISTORICIZING CHINESE PSYCHIATRY

Howard Chiang

This collection of essays responds to the paucity of scholarship on the history of psychiatry and mental health in China.[1] Looking across developments in the early modern and modern periods, the essays focus on the diagnosis, treatment and broader socio-cultural implications of madness and mental illness. This volume brings together for the first time a cohort of scholars who have worked on this topic independently but have not had the opportunity to come together as a group to formulate a synthesis of their respective expertise. The coverage is not intended to be exhaustive, but its aim is to inspire further scholarly dialogue in this underexplored area of medical history and Chinese studies. Whereas the existing literature on the history of medicine in China tends to center on the health and diseased conditions of the body, this book offers a concise integration of recent works that, together, delineate a historical trajectory of the medicalization of the mind in China's shifting cultural and political contexts.[2]

This trajectory is neither linear nor unidirectional. As we will see, it is layered with competing meanings of key concepts such as madness, disorder, treatment and healing at different historical junctures; it has been shaped by various discourses as documented in a wide array of sources, from dream encyclopedias to case histories to missionary archives and from the patient records of neuropsychiatric wards to popular magazines to TV talk shows; above all, it has involved a diverse group of historical actors over time, including the literati elites and various classes of physicians in the late imperial period, missionary doctors and psychoanalysts in the late Qing–early Republican transition and Western psychiatrists, indigenous pioneers and licensed psychotherapists over the course of the twentieth century, not to mention the always changing profile of the sufferers of mental health problems. *Psychiatry and Chinese History* advances an integrative narrative about the convergences and competitions among these meanings, discourses and agents in the cultural history of China's psychiatric care.

Historical Precedents

The first part of the book explores historical precedents of medical knowledge about human psychology in late imperial China. In the twentieth century, Sigmund Freud championed the idea that dreams provided 'the "royal road" into the unconscious'.[3] The systematic study of dream and dreaming has since taken on a prominent role in the human sciences. At the dawn of the twenty-first century, psychiatrists have begun to promote a more collaborative framework that integrates neurobiological, cognitive scientific and psychoanalytic approaches to the medical understanding of dreams.[4] Given that such modern scientific interest owes significant intellectual debt to Western psychodynamic ideas, what can be said of dreams in non-Western and pre-modern societies? To address this question from a Chinese historical perspective, Chapter One turns to a 1636 compendium, *Meng lin xuan jie* 夢林玄解 [An Explication of the Profundities in the Forest of Dreams; hereafter *Forest of Dreams*], published in the late Ming dynasty (1368–1644). Brigid Vance argues that this 34-volume (1,278-page) tome, though not a 'psychiatric' text in the strictest sense of the term, can nonetheless be considered as an encyclopaedia of dream-related knowledge that predated the introduction of Western psychoanalysis in early twentieth-century China.[5] Indeed, *Forest of Dreams* not only catalogued nearly 5,000 dream-interpretation examples, it also offered its readers practical solutions for self-healing. Focusing on 'Dream Exorcism' (夢禳), the second of the four sections of the compendium, Vance analyzes the various treatment methods covered in *Forest of Dreams*, which differed in degree of complexity corresponding to the perceived degree of severity of the dreams and nightmares. The other sections are 'Dream Prognostication' (夢占), 'Dream Origins' (夢原) and 'Manifestation of Dreams' (夢徵). Presenting twenty five images of talismans (three of which are reproduced in this book) and accompanying incantations and advice, 'Dream Exorcism', according to Vance, 'provided the vocabulary and tools to educate readers on how to view and treat dreams and nightmares; moreover, it disciplined readers, not only offering them a means to comprehend the world of dreams, but also the methods necessary to escape a world of nightmares'.[6] The section begins with general advice on sleeping and dreaming proscriptions, for which even the timing of the manufacture of a certain kind of pillow was crucial and it ends with the social therapeutic functions of talismanic image-templates. Therefore, while it might be inaccurate to approach *Forest of Dreams* as a pre-modern example of psychiatric knowledge about human dreaming behaviour, what the encyclopaedia ultimately resembles is a how-to medical text and a compilation of empirical knowledge on dreams. By establishing a sophisticated connection between the social sphere and the realm of human cognition, the compilers of this text drew on examples of social anxiety as experienced by emperors, civil service exam candidates and even the authors themselves (who often felt anxious about the political situation of their countries). Based on these examples, the system of meaning that developed around invisible desires, anxieties, fears and nightmares made *Forest of Dreams* a unique precedent in exploring the correlation between dreams and health in Chinese history.

Whereas Vance focuses on dream-related knowledge and health practices, Hsiu-fen Chen looks at non-drug-based interventions in Chinese medicine. Despite the fact that herbal and pharmaceutical prescriptions prevailed in the history of Chinese medicine, Chapter Two presents a series of medical cases of emotional therapy, or 'talking cures', from late medieval to the Ming-Qing periods. In fact, documentations of the relationship between human emotions and illness could be found as early as in the classic *Huangdi neijing* 黃帝內經 [Inner Canon of the Yellow Emperor; hereafter *Inner Canon*] (*c.* 1st century BC), which singled out anger (怒), joy (喜), pensiveness (思), worry (憂) and fear (恐) as the five major human emotions. Throughout the imperial period, the predominant medical worldview assigned a manipulative effect on the physical body to the imbalance of these five emotional states, primarily through the movements of *qi* (氣) in the viscera. The various illnesses resulting from an irregular emotional condition thus could be treated by following the principle of the mutual constraint/restraint of the emotions: 'anger makes *qi* ascend; joy relaxes it; grief (悲) dissipates it; fear makes it descend; cold contracts it; heat makes it leak out; fright (驚) makes it chaotic; exhaustion consumes it; and pensiveness congeals it'.[7] This statement from the *Inner Canon* clearly indicates that the cause of sickness was never considered to be the emotions themselves, but the various abnormal configurations of *qi* induced by the emotional imbalance. By the late imperial period, Chinese physicians broadened the original 'five intent' (五志) concept to include two additional emotions – grief and fright – and referred to them as 'seven emotions' (七情).

Chen sheds light on the practical relevance of Chinese medical theories of emotion and how they were implemented in fifteen cases of emotional therapy from the Jin to the Qing dynasties. The physician Zhang Congzheng (張從正, 1156–1228) was not only the leading authority on the subject of his time, but also made a lasting impact on the ways in which subsequent doctors (including, most famously, the neo-Confucian scholar-physician Zhu Zhenheng 朱震亨) carried forward therapeutic approaches to emotional disorders that did not involve the more invasive method of drug intervention. Some physicians cured their patients without any emotional manipulation, as exemplified by the case in the *Shishan yian* 石山醫案 [Stone Mountain Medical Case Histories; 1519] where a governor of nobility was relieved of his distressed condition simply by being told that one day it would rain (his sickness was diagnosed as the result of his worry about the ongoing drought). More often, doctors went beyond a simple reliance on the medical doctrine of the mutual effect of emotions and treated their patients by inducing certain emotions that would counteract their irregular emotional (and physical) state. Above all, Chen's chapter shows that a successful emotional therapy always depended on a close relationship between the healer, the patient and the patient's family. After all, attending to the patient's family background, immediate surroundings and recent history has always been a crucial aspect of clinical encounter. The relative success of 'talking cures' among emotionally disturbed patients contributed to their minor popularity in early modern China. Although the preferred method of treatment throughout imperial Chinese medicine was drug therapy, scattered accounts in the historical record indicate that some physicians were more willing than others to entertain therapeutic approaches aimed at altering one's psychological character.

Yet even in the more invasive therapies that involved drug treatment, as Chapter Three on medical therapies for madness in nineteenth-century China suggests, communication with the insane patient and the patient's relatives remained a central element of clinical care. To tap into the broader history of psycho-behavioral pathology in Chinese medicine, Fabien Simonis draws on the case of Mr. Bao as recorded under the section on *diankuang* (癲狂) in *Wu Jutong yi'an* [Wu Jutong's Medical Case Files], which was published posthumously in 1916. Wu (1758–1836) was the last among a hundred or so doctors called in to cure Bao's madness. In line with the dominant approach of his contemporaries, Wu began by commenting on the association of emotions with insanity in Bao's case: namely, Bao 'had first become ill because his achievements did not follow his ambitions'. This attribution of insanity to social disappointments emerged in the sixteenth century among physicians of the Jiangnan region, the centre of late imperial Chinese culture where a large number of men were frustrated by the growing difficulty in securing a post in the central bureaucracy through the civil service exam system. The Chinese terms that bore the closest meaning to Western notions of madness and insanity were *dian* and *kuang* and their association with emotions (*dian* with joy and *kuang* with anger) appeared as early as in the eighth century. This formulation was later approved in the twelfth century by medical writers like Liu Wansu and relayed again by the notorious neo-Confucian scholar Zhu Zhenheng, whose writings made a lasting influence on Chinese doctors through the mid-sixteenth century. Upholders of Zhu's doctrines understood human emotions to be the products of inner Fire, which was in accordance with the depiction of emotions in the *Inner Canon*, but by the late Ming period, they began to address the need of distinguishing *dian* from *kuang* in light of the two concepts' epistemic affinity over the centuries.

Whereas most of the cases described in Chapter Two involve a type of therapeutic intervention that targeted mainly emotions without direct drug therapy, Wu's approach focused on the physical and organic bases of Bao's insanity. His diagnosis and treatment method often followed the theories of the Warm-factor school, of which he was an important proponent. Unlike Bao's earlier healers, most of whom had prescribed replenishing drugs, Wu gave Bao a potent purgative that eliminated the excess inner Fire caused by his career disappointments. However, the added persuasion and efficacy of Wu's treatment came from the fact he did not stop at the level of organic intervention; rather, similar to the doctors who subscribed to emotional therapy discussed in Chen's chapter, Wu Tang attended to the personal roots of his patient's suffering. Specifically, in Bao's case, Wu reinstated Bao into a meaningful social role after the purgative treatment, highlighting the importance of exhortation and persuasion in effecting a cure. As Simonis correctly points out, it would be ahistorical to identify Wu's approach as evidence of psychiatry in early nineteenth-century China. Despite their historically situated differences (most notably, the absence of institutional bodies like asylums for the insane in China), both Chinese medicine's clinical hybridity – as exemplified by Wu Tang's use of both purgative drugs and dialogues – and the various combinations of biological and psychodynamic approaches that characterize modern psychiatric care share a remarkable interest and approach in treating those acts and people that specialists of both disciplines considered mad. In late imperial China, Simonis concludes, physicians understood insanity as chiefly a behavioural disorder that was usually attributed to dysfunctions of the Heart, the command centre of mental activities.

Missionary Investments

Although indigenous Chinese doctors paid careful attention to emotional or mental disorders, the idea of developing an independent medical facility for the treatment (if not confinement) of mad people never gained footing in China until the late nineteenth century. As Peter Szto explains in Chapter Four, this is because Confucian morality placed the care of mad individuals within the realm of familial responsibility. This particular form of kinship-clan obligation made the social tolerance of the insane a community-based duty rather than a physician-centered obligation. The situation began to change with the influx of American Protestant missionaries, especially Dr. John Kerr who arrived in Canton in 1853 under the aegis of the American Presbyterian Board of Foreign Missions. Kerr brought with him new ideas of salvation, social order and insanity. He believed that the care of the insane went beyond the sphere of the family and fell within the proper role of social structures, such as the government, the economy and religion, which would in turn help support and sustain psychiatric practice.

Although nascent forms of psychiatric space first emerged in medieval Europe, the sources of Kerr's plans for developing an asylum in China came from three mental hospitals established in Philadelphia between the mid-eighteenth and the mid-nineteenth centuries. Kerr learned from the experience of the Pennsylvania Hospital, America's first private medical facility founded by Benjamin Franklin in 1755, the necessity to distinguish purely mental from medical cases and, by extension, the value of a separate space for mad patients. He shared a similar moral framework with the founder of the Friends Hospital, America's first private, non-profit and faith-based asylum built in 1817, in designing a small and intimate space that would be congenial for retreating from the exigencies and harshness of modern society. He also took from the experience of the Pennsylvania Hospital for the Insane, Philadelphia's second private insane asylum established in 1841, the significance of synthesizing architectural design with modern medicine so that the buildings themselves carried curative function.

In China, Kerr was initially alarmed by the number of insane patients who visited the Canton Medical Hospital (the Guangzhou Boji Hospital where he succeeded Peter Parker as the superintendent) for medical treatment. When he first presented the idea of building a separate space for this type of patients in 1872, the American Presbyterian Board of Foreign Missions unhesitatingly rejected him on the basis that lunatic care did not fit the overall aim of its work in China. But this did not deter Kerr. Instead, he devoted the next two decades to the planning and development of the first Chinese asylum, the John G. Kerr Refuge for the Insane, which was erected in the Fong Tsuen suburb of Canton in 1891. His vision clearly embodied the value-system that underpinned the earlier American asylums: 'With kind and careful attention, comfortable surroundings, good food and out-door exercise, the change from the treatment and influences of heathen relatives will have a beneficial effect and will be sufficient in some cases to result in cure'.[8] Due to its geocultural location on the southern border of Chinese society, Canton proved to be an enabling place for Kerr and eventually his successor Charles Selden, to inherit the legacy of American asylum designs and adapt them in a radically different cultural context.[9]

The legacy of Kerr's insane asylum came from beyond the American roots of its infrastructural designs. Drawing on missionary correspondences, the annual reports and staff memoirs of the Kerr Refuge and major medical publications such as *The China Medical Journal*, Chapter Five shows that 'the Chinese family' emerged in this period as a pivotal category for missionary doctors' understanding of the aetiologies of insanity, legitimation of psychiatric segregation and representation of the essence of Chinese culture. From the 1890s to the 1920s, when the Kerr Refuge was closed down due to a labour strike, missionary psychiatrists embarked on a humanitarian project that aimed to unchain the mad from domestic confinement. Their depiction of the Chinese family as the antithesis of modernity and a cultural indicator of China's lagging behindness squarely placed the suffering insane within a universal category of human nature hidden behind abnormality. Despite their demarcation of the humanitarian refuge from the superstitious household, turn-of-the-twentieth-century missionary physicians borrowed from at the same time that they criticized Chinese wisdoms. The most striking example is the resemblance between the pig basket that the natives used to transport patients to the Refuge and the wire restraining equipment that the Refuge staff devised as a tool of patient restraint.[10] In other words, the plasticity of the meaning of the Chinese family made it as much a resource for psychiatric innovation as a source of condemnation in Western missionary interventions.

By the 1920s, the critique of the Chinese family as 'an iron cage' became a dominant trope that reverberated across the country and circulated widely in the West. In 1913, the concept of heredity appeared for the first time in the publications from the Kerr Refuge, anchoring the development of a nascent eugenics discourse that, again, challenged Chinese family customs. Middle-class families, especially those wealthy enough for early marriage and polygamy, were construed as units of social reproduction that worsened the propagation of unfavourable hereditary conditions. Similarly, the mental hygiene campaigns promoted ideas about the correlation between feeblemindedness, on the one hand, and crime, prostitution and the spread of venereal diseases, on the other. Building on these visions, missionary psychiatrists subsequently used psychoanalysis to uncover the pathogenic dynamics of the Chinese family. Through and through, the Chinese concubinage system sat at the centre of psychiatric criticism, emanating from the proclaimed emancipatory rhetoric of saving the drowned concubine as well as the eugenics discourse that urged the patriarch to govern the concubine's sexual impurity. In this context, the analytically oriented physicians adopted new techniques of clinical intervention, such as therapeutic conversation and social service investigation, which would remain central to Chinese psychiatric practice throughout the twentieth century.

Meanwhile, missionary activities in China themselves turned into an area of medical anxiety and intervention. In the early twentieth century, psychiatrists in Europe and America paid increasing attention to a condition suffered by missionaries and other Westerners in China known as tropical neurasthenia. Chapter Six uses the writings of the American psychiatrist James Lincoln McCartney (1898–1969) to delineate the broader historical patterns of psychiatric thought on this disorder across chronological and colonial contexts. Whereas the medical views of tropical neurasthenia and other illnesses in the tropics of colonial Australia, Africa, Southeast Asia and Taiwan played an important role in reshaping colonial identity and reinforcing racial difference, Wen-Ji Wang suggests that psychiatric discussions of tropical neurasthenia in Republican China not only changed over time, but their infrequency and unevenness were indicative of China's unique informal colonial status.

In the 1910s and 1920s, Freudian psychoanalysis began to dominate colonial discourses of mental disorder.[11] Warwick Anderson has shown that around this time, a transformation occurred in colonial doctors' theoretical preference towards Freudian theory of sexuality and psychical conflict.[12] Wang observes a similar shift from climatic to psychogenic models of etiological explanation in China. McCartney, in particular, held psychoanalysis as the key to explain away the often presumed connection between climatic difference and tropical neurasthenia, especially given the vast size of the Chinese continent where climate differed by region but throughout which nervous conditions were present.

Unlike medical experts in other colonial contexts, McCartney's descriptions of China did not feature the Orientalist and derogatory overtones that permeated most Western understandings of tropical diseases. Rather than attributing the causes of tropical neurasthenia to China's climate, he explained this particular condition by way of the weak will and unstable personalities of the occidentals living in China: 'The foreign customs and habits may be the factors that bring on the neurosis, but they are not the *cause* of the neurosis – the *cause* lies within the individual, the difficult situation being at most a precipitating factor'.[13] He added that those who had commanded the native language seldom developed oriental nerves while living in China. Missionaries in China were 'morbid' due to their troubled internal psyche (not environmental pressure from the climate of the tropical regions); similarly, Chinese people's insatiable appetite for the classics fixed their libido at 'the level of narcissism'. Throughout the 1920s and 1930s, McCartney promoted the universal efficacy of psychoanalytic treatment as the key to understanding the psychopathology of everyday life. It was only during the Second World War, in 1943 more specifically, that McCartney began to retreat to a more general climate-based model for explaining tropical psychoneurosis, claiming that any blond American soldier (not just those with questionable characters) would be vulnerable to the diseases of the tropics.

Biomedical Modernity

The impact of missionary activities grew deeper into China's hinterland as the Qing dynasty began to lose its grip. Amidst the imperium's disintegration, public intellectuals and cultural critics often construed Confucian values as traditional, backward and out of time and place. The lagging 'behindness' of Chinese culture became a growing social concern that culminated in the May Fourth movement throughout the second half of the 1910s and 1920s. This was a period that some historians have dubbed the 'Chinese Enlightenment', a label that conveyed an overwhelming iconoclastic preoccupation with scientific modernity in overlapping corners of Chinese society.[14] Gender equality, meanwhile, acquired a national urgency for the first time, as powerfully manifested through the unprecedented anti-footbinding, feminist and education reform movements.[15] These socio-political transformations both initiated and captured the changing meanings of marriage, family and the relations between men and women.[16] Free love, psychoanalytic concepts and individual desire defined the new parameters of China's sexual landscape.[17] In the medical realm, the transmission of Western biomedicine now departed from its strict correlation with missionary activities, as was the case in the late Qing period and took considerable institutional roots in urban China under the aegis of American philanthropic organizations such as the Rockefeller Foundation.[18] Drawing on the patient records of the Shanghai Special Hospital for the Insane (*Shanghai fengdian zhuanmen yiyuan* 上海瘋癲專門醫院) and the Peking Union Medical College (*Xiehe yiyuan* 協和醫院; hereafter PUMC), Hugh Shapiro explores in Chapter Seven the parallel changes in cultural and biomedical modernity as revealed in the shifting etiological significance of women's madness in the early Republican period.

In providing women a new opportunity to escape from their marriages, psychiatric hospitals redefined the relation between gender and madness specifically, but also the broader cultural norms of the intimate sphere, including family life. In Shanghai, married women turned to psychiatric experts to relieve the various kinds of pressure that they endured in patrilineal households: marital discord, husband taking concubine, husband having an extramarital affair, conflict with family, lack of inheritance, husband disappearance and sense of failing in domestic role. In Beijing, the city's psychopathic asylum was integrated into the responsibility of the PUMC neuropsychiatric ward under the directorship of Richard S. Lyman in the 1930s. This enabled some patients to calibrate their responses to doctors' questions or modified their behaviour in order to prolong their stay in the ward and to avoid what awaited them outside. In Shapiro's words, 'during the 1930s, downwardly mobile patients, often detained or arrested by the police, some fleeing violence, others poverty, were transported from the asylum to the PUMC'. While Republican-era mental hospitals defined women as the cultural agents of a new era by offering them a distinct refuge from their natal and marital families, this was underpinned by a deeper transformation in the doctors' vision of female mental health problems: a new style of medical reasoning rooted in women's home environment, family life and socially compromised status, rather than menstrual disorders, phlegm accumulations, or emotional disturbances.[19]

Psychological health did not emerge only as a serious concern in the confines of psychiatric wards, but its very idea soon sunk into popular culture. Although well-funded mental hospitals in Shanghai and Beijing provided a concrete institutional basis for the development of Western psychiatry in China, it was the monthly magazine, *Xi Feng* 西風 [West Wind], that considerably enhanced the publicity surrounding psychotherapeutic theories and practices in the second third of the twentieth century. As Wen-Ji Wang has already demonstrated, the articles and editorials featured in *West Wind* and its supplement played a vital role in introducing foreign ideas about mental hygiene to Chinese readers in the 1930s.[20] In Chapter Eight, Geoffrey Blowers and Shelley Wang explore the emergence and abeyance of the popularity of psychotherapy through the prism of the biographies of major mental health experts associated with *West Wind*. Above all, their chapter highlights an important historical transition around the mid-century: the initial activities in the publishing industry that promoted a psychotherapeutic culture were concentrated in Beijing, Shanghai and Nanjing, but they were later disseminated to Chongqing, the centre of scientific research to which major institutions, universities and scholars migrated during the period of Japanese invasion (1937–45).

Between the mid-1930s and the late 1960s, the career trajectories of key affiliates of *West Wind* reflected the social patterns whereby psychology and psychotherapy underwent major transformations in mainland China. The chief editor and publisher of *West Wind*, Huang Jiayin (黄嘉音, 1913–61), for example, founded the magazine in 1936 and, from that point on, the serial joined an entire cast of monthly magazines that brought overseas intellectual trends to the forefront of Chinese mass culture, including *Oriental Magazine* (東方), *New Youth* (新青年) and *Psyche* (心理), the first Chinese journal devoted to psychological themes. In addition to publishing texts on abnormal psychology and developmental psychology throughout this period, Huang was the deputy director of the Shanghai Mental Health Promotion Association and a member of the Chinese Mental Hygiene Society.

The readership of *West Wind* attracted a new generation of medical doctors educated abroad or at the PUMC. Notable among them were the psychiatrists Su Zonghua (粟宗華, 1904–70), Ding Tsan (丁瓚, 1910–68) and Cheng Yu-lin (程玉麟, 1905–93). Su graduated from and then worked at Shanghai Medical College and followed Richard Lyman to PUMC. In 1935, he went to the United States to specialize in neuropsychiatry at Johns Hopkins University and later Harvard University. After returning to China, he opened the Hongqiao Psychiatric Rehabilitation Hospital in Shanghai in 1944 and ran it until 1954. Ding began working in the department of psychiatry and neurology at PUMC in 1936 and was trained in psychoanalysis by Bingham Dai (Dai Bingheung), the first psychoanalytically trained Chinese psychotherapist who was invited by Lyman to supervise psychotherapy at both the Peking Municipal Psychopathic Hospital and PUMC. Ding went on to set up an experimental lab and a mental health division in Central Health Experimental College (which became the Chinese Psychological Institute after 1949), relocated with the Nationalist government to carry out his work on children's behavioural disorders in Chongqing during WWII and turned into a pioneer of medical psychology by introducing the concept of psychosomatic medicine to China. Cheng set up in Nanjing the first public psychiatric hospital in China in 1947 and invited Ding to direct its psychological unit. This unprecedented public hospital was attached to the Nanjing Central Hospital, which was later funded by the World Health Organization and the United Nations Relief and Rehabilitation Administration. As loyal contributors to *West Wind*, this group of psychiatrists enhanced the magazine's prestige, according to Blowers and Wang, 'as it moved from being initially a vehicle showcasing in translation articles of mental health conceived and written abroad, to articles written by Chinese scholars and practitioners about a variety of problems confronting the population – as well as non-specialists with an interest in these problems to voice their concerns'.

By the early PRC period, these pioneers faced escalated difficulty in trying to sustain their activities. The political orthodox of the new communist regime defined mental health policy in ways that were in serious conflict with individualized psychotherapy. The ideological turn to Russia brought forth a condemnation of many of the assumptions upon which the interventions of these earlier advocates were predicated. Their effort in maintaining their vision and practice proved fatal in the case of Huang Jianyin, detrimental to the professional and disciplinary development of Ding Tsan and inoculative for a serious loss of prestige in the case of Su Zonghua and for forcing Cheng Yulin, along with many other intellectuals and professionals, to flee to Taiwan with Chiang Kai-shek's Nationalist regime. The Chinese Mental Hygiene Society, for instance, was originally founded in Shanghai in 1936, but was re-established in Taiwan in 1955.[21] It would be at least a few decades, as will be seen in Chapter Ten, before specialized psychological practices would emerge across mainland China in full force again with rapidly ascending popularity.

When people like Cheng relocated to Taiwan during the Nationalist government's retreat, psychiatric science on the island itself was caught in the turmoil of political decolonization and wholesale re-institutionalization, especially with respect to staffing, the kind of services provided, objectives, education and dominant theories. Focusing on the medical records from the Department of Psychiatry at National Taiwan University Hospital (hereafter NTUH), Chapter Nine provides a valuable and insightful analysis of the profession's major transformations between 1946 and 1953. After Japan handed Taiwan back to China in 1945, there was an initial wave of enthusiasm welcoming Chiang's territorial acquisition of the region. However, as the Nationalist government took over Japanese institutional properties, despite the shortage of labour and financial resources, it behaved more as yet another colonial regime. Local inhabitants became resentful of what they perceived as a high handed and frequently corrupt Guomingdang (hereafter GMD) authorities, inclined to the arbitrary seizure of private property and economic mismanagement. The tensions reached a crescendo during the infamous 228 Incident in 1947, which has often been considered as the turning point for GMD's white terror in Taiwan. In this politically volatile context, the content of psychiatric education and practice evolved from an orientation of the Japanese-German model to an Anglo-American system. Tsung-yi Lin (林宗義), who was the first Taiwanese native to purse the study of psychiatry (in Japan) before the Pacific War, returned in 1946 and led the establishment of a new psychiatric paradigm in Taiwan. Under his directorship, the Psychiatry Department at NTUH trained an entire generation of pioneering psychiatrists – including, most notably, Rin Hsien (林憲) and Tseng Wen-Shing (曾文星). Many of them visited the United States to further their professional experience and subsequently helped establish the medical profession in Taiwan as one of the leading centres in the field of cultural psychiatry.[22]

In the immediate postwar years, mental health practitioners at NTUH confronted a series of linguistic and cultural difficulty, but they adopted 'trauma' as a useful lens through which the complex conditions expressed by their patients could be understood (excluding psychotic and functional disorders such as schizophrenia, hebephrenia and other delusional disorders). The background of their patients reveals striking diversity, but they were mainly those suffering from immigration experiences and ethnic conflicts, including Chinese public servants who recently migrated from mainland China to Taiwan, Japanese salary men who remained on the island and local Taiwanese people who became increasingly anxious of the tidal-wave social change. Reflecting the gradual shift in the profile of their patients, NTUH psychiatrists transformed their language habit from the Japanese-German to the English-Chinese system. It is therefore not surprising to find German, Japanese, English, Chinese and Romanized Taiwanese-language characters used intermittently in the medical records. As a young community in Taiwan, psychiatrists learned to practice their newly acquired clinical skills and medical language in response to the external reality they concurrently encountered. The case notes filed by the Psychiatry Department show the complexity of 'psychological trauma' as it was conceived in the conflicting cultural context of the postcolonial period, detailing war termination depression, psychogenic reaction from the February 28 Incident, adjustment disorders among Chinese immigrants, traumatic neurosis preceded by physical injuries and even common suffering and unaccountable trauma. These wide-ranging examples help illustrate the broader development of the general concept of trauma during key transitions in the leading framework of psychiatric practice, the controversial and subjective nature of related medical diagnoses and the social origins of a non-Western society that witnessed unprecedented medicalization as psychiatric science in general was increasingly institutionalized and professionalized in the late 1940s and early 1950s.

New Therapeutic Cultures

Whereas Western behavioral sciences and psychological treatments had been repudiated as 'bourgeois' in the Maoist period (1949–76), psychotherapy and private counseling reemerged and enjoyed an unprecedented proliferation in the post-reform era especially in major cities like Shanghai and Beijing. While many have viewed the resurgence of psychotherapy in twenty-first century China as the natural outcome of economic prosperity (the logic being that economic development either leads to mounting stress and a number of new ailments such as anxiety and depression or makes people more willing to consume expensive treatments for their psychological well-being), Hsuan-Ying Huang in Chapter Ten offers a more systematic examination of the various historical conditions that paved the way for what he calls the recent 'psycho-boom'. Unlike in the United States and many other Western countries, the psycho-boom in urban China is dominated by people without professional backgrounds in medicine or academic psychology. Moreover, whereas psychoanalysis has been in decline in Europe and America since the rise of psychopharmacology in the 1960s, it has gained unmatched popularity in China.

In the aftermath of the Cultural Revolution, the early roots of the return of psychotherapy can be traced to the coinage of the idea of 'psychological counselling' (心理諮詢) around 1980. This was an innovative intervention to enhance the ability of patients to adapt to life after discharge by being informed by the physicians the details of their diagnosis, medications and possible coping strategies. It morphed into a model of outpatient clinical care in general hospitals, first in Xi'an in 1982 and then in Guangzhou in 1983. This model further won the state support in the late 1980s as the Ministry of Health stipulated that hospitals above the county level should set up 'psychological counseling' facilities. These requirements even found their way into the newly established hospital accreditation standards in the early 1990s.

Despite the importance of these facilities, the pivotal moment that set the stage for mental health reform came from the turn of the century, when China began to engage more seriously with international efforts that promoted mental health in developing countries. At the WHO/China awareness-raising conference in 1999, the Chinese government officially acknowledged mental health problems as a pressing public health issue and pledged to improve the existing system. In November 2001, the Third National Mental Health Care Conference was convened in Beijing and led to the compilation of *The National Mental Health Plan (2002–2012)* and *The Guiding Principles on Further Strengthening Mental Health Care* by leading experts from the psychiatric community. As the state became increasingly invested in public health measures in the post-SARS period, these two documents turned into the *de facto* national mental health policy. It was the first time that new problems such as suicide, depression, dementia and post-disaster conditions appeared in official discourses. In 2002, the Ministry of Health finally added 'psychotherapist' (心理治療師) as a new entity to its certification for health professionals.

Nonetheless, this new certification system was not only restricted to medical personnel, but it also had negligible impacts on the emerging psycho-boom. According to Huang, it was the Ministry of Labor and Social Security (which became the Ministry of Human Resources and Social Security in 2008), rather than the Ministry of Health, that played a role more central to the development of the psycho-boom: namely, by announcing a new occupation, 'psychological counselor' (心理諮詢師), in the *National Vocational Standards* in August 2001. As a result of the collaboration between state agency and the Chinese Association for Mental Health, the certification protocols for this occupation is commonly deemed as the only license-issuing route at the national level for psychological practitioners. Seizing the opportunity created by this critical moment, Huaxia Xinli (华夏心理) became the largest company specializing in psychotherapy training for the Ministry of Labor certification. Television programs, such as *Xinli fangtan* 心理访谈 (Psychological Interviews), produced a paradigmatic image of the counseling profession and made it more deeply ingrained in the popular imagination. And in the aftermath of the 2008 Sichuan earthquake, the spread of the idea of 'psychological aid' (心理援助) pushed the psycho-boom to enter a new phase of accelerated growth.

As Nancy Chen points out in her afterword, the year 2013 marked a crucial turning point in the development of psychiatry, in China and internationally. The first major event came in May with the coming into effect of China's mental health law, which was passed in October 2012 after 26 years of drafting.[23] The impact of this legislation will undoubtedly unfold in the coming years if not decades, but what is readily apparent by the second decade of the twenty-first century is that mental health has arisen sharply as a top priority in China's state focus on health care. The second major event was the publication of the fifth edition of the American Psychiatric Association's *Diagnostic and Statistical Manual of Mental Disorders* (DSM-V), superseding the DSM-IV-TR, which appeared in 2000. This was the result of more than a decade of debates, panels, forums and conferences concerning the revision process, but the overall goal of the production of the manual remained the synthesis of globally standardized diagnostic categories. As before, the broader influence of this definitive psychiatric text spans all relevant contexts of social and cultural life, now with a heightened awareness of its global and non-Western reach.

These two advancements can be understood in the recent historical context of China's mental health profession. Since the late twentieth century, psychiatrists in China have become increasingly adaptive to international standards of psychiatric categories and classification, such as the DSM and the *International*

Classification of Disease published by the World Health Organization. This openness culminated in the release of the *Chinese Classification of Mental Disorders* (CCMD-3) in 2001, which, as Sing Lee has shown, reflected Chinese mental health leaders' break from an earlier generation of experts who were mainly trained in the Russian system of psychiatry and extremely cautious about adopting Western science and technology.[24] The fact that the changes made in the CCMD-3 system renders it more attune with international usage speaks to the global dispersion of information technology and China's growing openness under economic reform. However, perhaps what is more at stake here is the ways in which the CCMD-3 system provides an unique opportunity to reflect on – and even critique – the nosological assumptions in Western psychiatry, especially neo-Kraepelinian taxonomy, by taking into account the changing reality of illness in contemporary China. Part of this reality concerns a parallel trend to Western psychiatry in which an increased usage of psychopharmacology has become an integral part of Chinese consumer life. Other aspects of this reality that set the mental health system in China apart from its Western counterparts can be seen in the rural-urban difference in access to medical care and, significantly, the on-going tensions between the country's one-party socialist political structure and the country's rapid pace in its embrace of global capitalist economy – a tension that continue to reorient the social and moral landscape of Chinese people's illness experience.[25]

To date, the flourishing literature on the history of psychiatry in non-Western societies tends to centre on colonial subjects and contexts. Even when localized and hybridized formations of mental health practice emerge from such settings, their innovativeness (sometimes dubbed 'resistance') is often routed through the shadow of colonial and imperial agendas. In the context of South/east Asia and Africa, for instance, historians have compared the alleged madness of formal colonialism with the madness of the mad and have shown the role of professional psychiatry in consolidating colonial authority and its attendant projects of social and political control.[26] These are themes notably absent in this volume, especially since China was never fully colonized by a single foreign imperial regime, including the Japanese.[27] Other critics have highlighted the politically abusive nature of forensic psychiatric custody since the Maoist period.[28] However, this volume shows that repressive politicization is not necessarily the cornerstone of the structural and intellectual development of psychiatry in China, which features instead the contribution of native medical and cultural elites in a historical setting where longstanding indigenous standards, norms and ideas about mental illness and the body continue to hold traction in their modern representations and transformations. From late Ming dream encyclopaedias to diagnostic classification systems in the twenty-first century, the history of psychiatric medicine in Chinese culture challenges those conventional narratives that place Euro-American hegemony in a privileged position in the development of modern medicine.

1 EXORCISING DREAMS AND NIGHTMARES IN LATE MING CHINA

Brigid E. Vance

In the twentieth century, dreams were demystified by focusing on the measurable neurobiological impact of dreaming, especially on memory processing and consolidation. Scientific studies attest to the role of REM sleep (when dreaming occurs) in memory processing and consolidation, particularly in emotionally charged memories. Behavioural studies of sleep and learning in both animals and humans attest to the neurobiological and neurophysiological basis of sleep-dependent memory processing. Chronic nightmare sufferers, sleepwalkers and narcoleptics today can turn to medical professionals for treatment such as nightmare imagery rehearsal therapy, diet changes, stimulants, anti-depressants, and more. But, how were dreams and nightmares treated in other historical times and places? How were dreams and nightmares defined and differentiated from one another? How were dreams and nightmares dealt with in late Ming China (1368–1644)?

Below, these questions will be addressed, viewed through the lens of '*meng rang*' 夢禳 [Dream Exorcism], one of four sections in the 1636 compendium *Meng lin xuan jie* 夢林玄解 [An Explication of the Profundities in the Forest of Dreams; hereafter *Forest of Dreams*]. In addition to cataloguing and organizing nearly 5,000 dream examples from the dynastic histories, *Forest of Dreams* also provided readers with practical solutions for self-healing. 'Dream Exorcism' presented twenty-five images of talismans, accompanying incantations and advice aimed either generally at ensuring a good night's sleep, or specifically at offering protection against the deleterious effects of inauspicious dreams or nightmares.

This chapter argues that 'Dream Exorcism' was a repository of dream-related knowledge, aimed at organizing and categorizing dreams for dream prognostication practitioners and readers alike. 'Dream Exorcism' set the parameters for what could and should be done with dreams and provided the vocabulary and tools to educate readers on how to view and treat dreams and nightmares; moreover, it disciplined readers, not only offering them a means to comprehend the world of dreams, but also the methods necessary to escape a world of nightmares. It can be read as much as a how-to medical text on dreams as a compilation of knowledge or general dream lore. This chapter explores two inter-related themes: the publicization of specific dream-related medical knowledge and the medicalization of dreams and nightmares. Here, the parameters of the term 'medicalize' encompass the somatic, psychological, moral and spiritual. As is apparent from the sleep-related advice and treatment techniques in 'Dream Exorcism', dreams were a barometer of health and well-being. Nightmare sufferers in the seventeenth-century Chinese context relied upon specific material, conceptual and spiritual means to heal themselves.

This reading of 'Dream Exorcism' underscores both the apparent physical and moralistic impacts of dreams and nightmares. 'Dream Exorcism' instructed nightmare sufferers to look inward and outward; inward to a corporeal realm populated with benevolent and innocuous spirits along with malevolent demons, and outward to a pantheon of spirits and gods who communicate with individuals through dreams. Individuals' dreams apparently connected these two realms. Nightmares were thus considered both a product of both internal and external factors. The preface and the contents of 'Dream Exorcism' reveal a moralistic overtone not simply to nightmare treatment and prevention, but to dreams and dreaming as well. Nightmare sufferers were conceived of as being at least partially responsible for bringing these nightly terrors upon themselves.

What were dreams and nightmares? Dreams purveyed messages from spirits, and thus offered the potential means to self-understanding or religious revelations. Contemporary and earlier texts strongly indicated that even positive or auspicious dreams were not desirable and that true sages and enlightened persons did not dream. Thus, the mental state of non-dreamers was perhaps deemed more settled or less disturbed. Nightmares indicated either a physical or spiritual imbalance or possession by demons. Texts were devoted to explaining ways of attracting auspicious dreams and repelling negative ones. Spells used against nightmares date from as early as the third century BC.

Forest of Dreams

Firstly, it is necessary to introduce the source, its compilers, and its audience. *Forest of Dreams* consists of thirty-four volumes and is 1,278 pages long. It is the largest extant dream compendium from the Ming dynasty (1368–1644). In addition to indexing and cataloguing nearly 5,000 dream interpretation examples, this tome also provided readers with practical solutions for self-healing. *Forest of Dreams* incorporated a broad spectrum of texts, genres and literary modes drawn from multiple sources. The compilers of *Forest of Dreams* chose which sources to include, then edited and organized the contents. The work represents a layering of multiple textual translations, taken from historical works and organized thematically.

An examination of this thirty-four-volume work highlights the complex ways in which dreams were used. To the compilers of *Forest of Dreams*, dreams offered the means to justify career and life choices, understand the present and predict the future, and gauge health. Dreams were credited as an integral and often determining factor in the quotidian choices made by the literati compilers. In other words, dreams were tied up as part of a belief system; dreams were inextricably linked to fate and inevitability, health and illness, and reflections of a certain anxious state of mind or a certain as yet uncovered truth. An examination might be failed and the promise of a glorious official career lost. An illness might worsen, leading to death. Life was uncertain and dreams were a means to address this uncertainty and alleviate the associated worry.

According to its prefaces and table of contents, *Forest of Dreams* comprises five previously published and subsequently revised dream encyclopaedias, two of which are extant. Chen Shiyuan's 陳士元 (1516–95) *Meng zhan yi zhi* 夢占逸旨 [Guidelines to Dreams and Dream Interpretation], first published in 1564, and Zhang Fengyi's 張鳳翼 (1527–1613) *Meng zhan lei kao* 夢占類考 [Classified Studies of Dream Interpretations], first published in 1585, are both quoted in *Forest of Dreams*, minus the commentary. The remaining titles date from the Tang and Song dynasties and do not exist separately from *Forest of Dreams*. In the title page and four general prefaces, primary compiler He Dongru 何棟如 (1572–1637) presented *Forest of Dreams* as the partial recovery of a heretofore secret dream prognostication manual, purportedly written by a Daoist sage in the third century, and re-discovered in the early seventeenth century, supposedly in He Dongru's family library.

The title page of *Forest of Dreams* asserted that the work represented the partial retrieval of knowledge on dreams and dream interpretation, crediting Daoist master Ge Hong 葛洪 (AD 284–364) as the author of portions of the text. Because He Dongru attributed partial authorial credit to Ge Hong, a claim which cannot be verified, *Forest of Dreams* was later dismissed as a partial forgery by the Qing editors of the *Siku quanshu* 四庫全書 [Four Treasuries Imperial Library]. Ge Hong was a well-known Daoist, who wrote *Bao pu zi* 抱朴子 [(Book of the) Master who Embraces Simplicity], which includes talismans and techniques for immortality elixirs. Due to his upright qualities and compassion for the poor and sick, Ge Hong was bestowed with the title 'Daoist Heavenly Master' (*Tian shi zhi zhi* 天師之職) and honored as a deity.[1] It is arguable that *Forest of Dreams* used Ge Hong's name to lend both authority and credibility to the late Ming compendium. The compilers promoted themselves and their editorial efforts as tied to a lineage of famous dream interpreters, beginning with Ge Hong.

The printing and publication of *Forest of Dreams* was a private venture, overseen by primary compiler He Dongru. Although compilation credit was also attributed to the aforementioned Chen Shiyuan and Zhang Fengyi based on the years in which *Forest of Dreams* was printed, the final textual intervention was He's. In the general prefaces, the literati compilers ascribed to dreams a motivating and important influence in their lives. Indeed, the compilers asserted that they had finally figured out how dreams fit into their lives and wished to share this knowledge with others who might also be capable of understanding the import of dreams. The compilers used dreams not only to justify their compiling, printing and publishing endeavour, but also apparently for previous major life decisions. Through the publication of *Forest of Dreams*, the compilers wrote that they sought to render public the so-called ancient and secret art of dream interpretation, reaching out in print to a new stratum of partly educated and uneducated readers. As described in its title page, general prefaces, and reader's guide, *Forest of Dreams* was not simply the restoration of a dream classic, but an edited improvement on earlier works on dreams, and therefore a culmination of dream lore and knowledge.

The compendium is divided into four sections. The first section, '*meng zhan*' 夢占 [Dream Prognostication], organized dream symbols and their corresponding interpretations from large- to small-scale categories, from manifestations of the heavens (*tian xiang* 天象) to geographical formations (*dili* 地理), from external appearances (*xing mao* 形貌) to precious baubles (*zhen wan* 珍玩). The second section, '*meng rang*' 夢禳 [Dream Exorcism], included images of talismans, accompanying incantations and sleep-related advice. '*meng yuan*' 夢原 [Dream Origins], offered explanations for the origin of dreams, taken from thirty-three separate sources. The fourth section, '*meng zheng*' 夢徵 [Manifestation of Dreams], offered examples from which dreamers and readers could extrapolate the tools necessary to interpret dreams.

Although it is difficult to determine the actual readership of *Forest of Dreams*, based on both the physical and textual characteristics of the work, it is relatively safe to assume the work was intended for the library collections of well-educated literati. It is impossible to reconstruct the late Ming reading experience; that said, it is possible to imagine how an imagined late Ming reader might have approached the text. Intensive, cover-to-cover reading was unlikely, given the truncated dream narratives contained within *Forest of Dreams*. That said, by including these dream fragments, *Forest of Dreams* might have appealed to readers who shared this world of reference. Readers familiar with the genre and with dream theory could navigate the work, searching in the table of contents for sections of interest. In that sense, the *Forest of Dreams* offered choices to readers. They could skim the contents, pausing to read more closely when the topic interested them.[2]

Defining Terms

But what were dreams in the late Ming? Here, *meng* 夢 has been translated into English as 'dream', which the *Concise Oxford English Dictionary* defines as a 'series of thoughts, images, and sensations occurring in the mind during sleep; a state of mind in which someone is not fully aware of their surroundings; a cherished hope or ideal; a fantasy; a wonderful or perfect person or thing'.[3] However, the Oxford definition oversimplifies and does not wholly reflect the late Ming understanding of dreams, in which the heart and other organs, rather than the brain alone, were also construed as the origins of dream activity. The *Kangxi zi dian* 康熙字典 [Kangxi Dictionary], first published in 1716, defined *meng* 夢 as follows: 'The things and forms seen while sleeping'.[4]

What exactly was a *meng* in the context of *Forest of Dreams*? Based on a reading of the four prefaces to the compendium *Forest of Dreams*, as well as an analysis of the contents of the compendium, *meng* in this particular context can be seen to have referred to a broad range of non-waking phenomena taking place during sleep.

In his general preface to the compendium, primary compiler He Dongru demonstrated that there is no straightforward definition of dreams. He wanted the reader to recognize that the term *meng* was not simple, but complicated. He wrote that dreams are both illusory and real, claiming that there was a fundamental and meaningful ambiguity between that which could be defined as 'illusory' and that which could be defined as 'real'. Although He conceded that what occurs in dreams is not the same as what occurs in the ordinary, experiential world, ultimately, He believed that a dream could and should be understood as potentially both illusory and real.[5] There were dreams that reflected the waking world and dreams that did not. Aside from He's logical analysis of dreams at the beginning of his preface to *Forest of Dreams*, there was no other attempt to define the term in the remainder of the compendium.

In *Forest of Dreams*, the frequent conjunction of the term *meng* with *zhan* 占 (alternately translated into English as 'to divine', 'to prognosticate', or more generally as 'to interpret'), indicates a strong connection between the two. Primary compiler He Dongru's preface to *Forest of Dreams* cites a claim in 'The Treatise of Literature' chapter *The Han History* that 'there are many interpretation techniques; that of dream interpretation is the most important'.[6] Here, the term *zhan* 占 is loosely translated as 'interpret'; based on the context in which the word is used, it is necessary to seek to understand the connotations of the accompanying interpretations. In the compendium, there often was an element of prognostication, of fortune telling with implications for the future, but the basic act was still one of general interpretation. That is, 'prognostication' can be seen as simply one type of interpretation. The late Ming dream was the private act that allowed for the possibility of interpretation, which was both public and shared. *Zhan* 占,

then, was not simply a personal interpretation, but rather a generalizable one in its public context.

One stated purpose of *Forest of Dreams* was to reveal techniques and methods of dream interpretation. Thus, the concept of *meng* by itself in this particular printed context, although similar to the modern English connotations implied by the term 'dream', also implied interpretation and divination. The term *meng* included the meaning of 'dream' as a series of thoughts or images occurring during sleep; additionally, it often implied a sense of the future, distant or near, real or imagined. Dream interpretations were not limited to the future. Some of the dream interpretations in *Forest of Dreams* also clarified the past or events unfolding in the then present.

In the context of *Forest of Dreams*, dreams were a means not only to understand past, present and future events, but also to understand the body and the way the body met the mind. The body was not conceived of as separate from emotions. Dreams, then, promised to illuminate hidden connections between emotions and the body, revealing latent illness or potential *qi* blockage, both physical and spiritual.

If dreams were not precisely defined in *Forest of Dreams*, neither were nightmares. The boundary between dreams and nightmares was left blurred and porous. 'Dream Exorcism' offered treatment and potential relief from dreams (*meng* 夢), inauspicious dreams (*bu xiang zhi meng* 不祥之夢), and nightmares (*e meng* 惡夢). Besides these three different names, no other specific textual distinction was made between dreams, inauspicious dreams and nightmares. That said, a reading of the language and information in 'Dream Exorcism' provides insights into the distinctions made between types of dreams and the ways in which those types were viewed by the compilers. Although not all dreams were equally nightmarish, the compilers nonetheless stressed that, subject matter notwithstanding, bad dreams and nightmares were detrimental to individual health and well-being and needed to be exorcized.

Dreams were differentiated according to their ill effects on the dreamer; *Forest of Dreams* reserved the term 'nightmare' (*e meng* 惡夢) for situations in which the physical health of the dreamer had deteriorated prior to the dream. This distinction is explored below, which reveals the ways in which compilers found hidden meanings in both dreams and nightmares. 'Dream Exorcism' contained incantations (*zhou shuo* 咒說), talismans (*fu shi* 符式) to be copied by readers, as well as related information and anecdotes (*za shuo* 雜說). The anti-nightmare talismans printed in *Forest of Dreams* – intended for ingestion or display during the day offered – protection for sleeping and dreaming at night. Daily actions were thus construed as affecting dreams. Conversely, improved sleep or dreams reflected a concomitant improvement in non-dreamed life.

The character '*rang*' 禳, translated as 'exorcism' in the section title, implies the avoidance of future misfortune by means of a specific action – such as prayers, general change in deportment, or incantations – which implies taking fate into one's own hands.[7] In my discussion below, the sleep-related techniques are separated according to the means by which they were to be followed. For example, some techniques suggested making basic life-style changes to aid in the prevention of dreams and nightmares. Other techniques included talismans, all to be visually reproduced, some then to be publicly displayed, and others still to be to be orally ingested after the first two steps. In this sense, the nightmare-expunging methods contained in 'Dream Exorcism' may be divided along a scale of external to internal, with some overlap between the methods. The degree of complexity of the treatment correlates directly to the perceived degree of severity of the dreams and nightmares. Below, the techniques will be considered from those that were applied externally to those that were intended to be internalized, moving from less complex treatment regimes to more complex and from bad dreams to nightmares.

General Advice: Sleeping and Dreaming Proscriptions

The general advice section of 'Dream Exorcism' is reminiscent of late Ming longevity texts and medical encyclopaedias. Scholars have written on the publication of advice for everyday life, including daily routine, diet and ways to avoid harmful excesses. In these texts as in 'Dream Exorcism', health was equated with purity and freedom from wrongdoing.[8] Longevity treatises such as Gao Lian's 高濂 (1573–1620) *Zunsheng bajian* 遵生八箋 [Eight Treatises on the Principles of Life], which addressed different aspects of longevity practices, and Wang Ji's 王畿 (1498–1582) *Tiaoxi fa* 調息法 [Methods for Regulating the Breath], which focused on a single method of prolonging life, were integrated into general medical literature. In both of these aforementioned texts as in others, a greater emphasis was placed on disease prevention, rather than its treatment per se. Contemporary encyclopaedias and compendia alike listed preventive techniques including: gymnastics (*daoyin* 導引), breathing exercizes (*tugu naxin* 吐古吶新, literally: expel the old and take in the new), abstention from grains (*quegu* 卻穀 or *bigu* 辟穀), talisman water (*fushui* 符水), sexual practices (*fangzhong* 房中), clenching the fists (*wogu* 握固) and clapping the teeth (*kouchi* 叩齒). In the third and fourth centuries, clapping the teeth was apparently an effective way of calling forth the gods or spirits and also provided protection against inauspicious *qi*.[9]

'Dream Exorcism' began by delineating proper sleeping habits, stressing the importance of body position, the placement of the pillow and more. Here, the compilers connected the importance of a good night's sleep with dream or nightmare avoidance. Following these proscriptions helped guarantee a sleeper a restful night, untroubled by bad dreams or nightmares. The first entry in 'Dream

Exorcism', titled '*Qin shi wo zhou shuo*' 寢室臥呪說 [An Incantation for Lying Down in the Bedroom], explained that bed placement and height were important; a low bed allowed harmful *qi* to invade people's bodies, leading to 'absurd desires' and affecting their sleep and health.[10] Later in the passage, the compilers suggested performing a nightly bedtime ritual to 'block evil and reduce inauspiciousness'.[11] The ritual included gently patting the heart, closing the eyes, knocking the teeth together and saying an incantation aloud.

The compilers next included a list of general sleep-related admonitions and proscriptions (*lin wo zhuji shuo* 臨臥諸忌說), along with some explanation as to why these particular admonitions and proscriptions ought to be followed. Not following the advice had physical effects on the body (such as *qi* desecration) and would lead to bad dreams or, worse, to nightmares. Following the physical guidelines for bed and body placement helped eliminate the possibility of bad dreams and nightmares. The proscriptions quoted below offer general advice about creating a healthy sleeping and dreaming environment.

> All people's pillows must be placed high and the body must lie at a slant. Do not lie on your back as a corpse does. Do not lie down for too long. While lying down, do not open your mouth, as that will desecrate the pure *qi*. Do not lie down when naked, as that will drain the three luminaries. Do not lie down when cold. Do not lie naked on the floor. Do not block the wind. Do not [sleep] in a place where wind can enter through cracks [in the walls] ... When lying down, do not speak much. When lying down, do not laugh ridiculously. Do not eat hot foods and then lie down immediately afterwards. If you awaken overheated, do not rush to get a drink of water right away. Do not quickly lie down after bathing when you are not yet dry ... Take care not to use your hand to block your heart and press your mouth as this will result in nightmares, just like people visited by demons. Do not casually enter into the bedroom of one who is having a nightmare. Do not quickly pull aside the bed-curtains and look at a person who has a nightmare or use light to look at this person as it will scare their *hun* [ethereal spirit] to the point of killing that person. Rather, you must shout from a distance and wait for the person to awaken slowly. If the person does not awaken, in the dark, use your fingernail and press the person's philtrum [an acupressure spot: the indentation just above the upper lip]. Or, use your mouth to squeeze your thumb and spit on the face of the person having the nightmare and shake that person's body until their spirit returns.
>
> Normally, when people are sleeping, it is not permissible to use a brush or ink to draw on their faces, even in jest. This causes the wandering *hun* to be unable to recognize its body and can even lead to not awakening and death. Therefore, it is important to be cautious. Some people snore while sleeping; do not use a lantern to look at them while they snore. This causes anxiety in the person who is sleeping. For all sleepers, each season has its suitable direction. In the spring, sleep with your head facing east. In the summer, sleep with your head facing south. In the autumn, sleep with your head facing west. Only in the eleventh month of the lunar year is it proper to sleep with your head facing north. In each of these positions, it is possible to welcome *qi* ... Do not casually tell your nighttime dreams to others in the morning. This is the gist of the taboos of heaven, earth and people. Shouldn't you be careful?[12]

The above quote illuminates late Ming cultural attitudes and assumptions about both sleeping and dreaming. For example, dreaming and sleeping were social in nature: dreamers' nightmares were observed and nightmare sufferers were acted upon by others. The passage also reveals certain ideas about the relationship between the body, *qi*, the *hun* (or ethereal spirit), and dreams.

In addition to the generalities about proper sleeping habits, the compilers also included some specifics, including instructions for making a tiger-shaped pillow (*huzhen* 虎枕), which purportedly prevented nightmares. Such pillows still exist today in China and Taiwan. According to its description in *Forest of Dreams*, the tiger shape protected sleepers from evil. The pillow was supposed to be constructed out of a thousand-year old cedar tree, carved into the shape of a tiger holding up its head and with its tail curled around its left thigh.[13]

In order for the pillow to be effective in dispelling nightmares, the timing of its manufacture was key. The year, month, day and hour of the pillow production all needed to contain the tiger (*yin* 寅) earthly branch.[14] Specifically, choosing the wood was to occur on a *jiayin* 甲寅 day. Twelve days later on a *bingyin* 丙寅 day, the pillow was to be carved. Twelve days later on a *wuyin* 戊寅 day, the herbs (cinnabar from Changzhou, realgar, amber, luminous stone, the forehead bone of a tiger, a dragon neck bone, pure gold and eaglewood) were to be divided into equal parts, inserted into a crimson-coloured bag and placed in the centre of the pillow. The pillow was to be sealed twelve days later on a *gengyin* 庚寅 day. Finally, twelve days later on a *renyin* 壬寅 day, the pillow was to be used for the first time. According to testimonials included in 'Dream Exorcism', the tiger pillow helped attract positive dreams and dispel nightmares. The entries on the tiger pillow did not mention who was to manufacture the pillow. It seems likely a pillow could be commissioned or purchased according to the specifications detailed in 'Dream Exorcism'.[15]

Written Talismans and Oral Incantations

This section turns away from general advice on attaining a good night's sleep to specific ways to counteract the ill effects of inauspicious dreams and nightmares, focusing on talismans and accompanying oral incantations. Images of twenty-five distinct talismans were included in 'Dream Exorcism'. These talismanic images were templates for action and offered the possibility to effect cosmic or other transformative changes through the very act of inscription by the nightmare sufferer. The images of talismans in 'Dream Exorcism' were presented in combination with accompanying text, which gave the reader instructions to make sense of the images. Each talismanic image was printed on a separate folio and was clear and copyable; three representational images of talismans from 'Dream Exorcism' are presented below.[16]

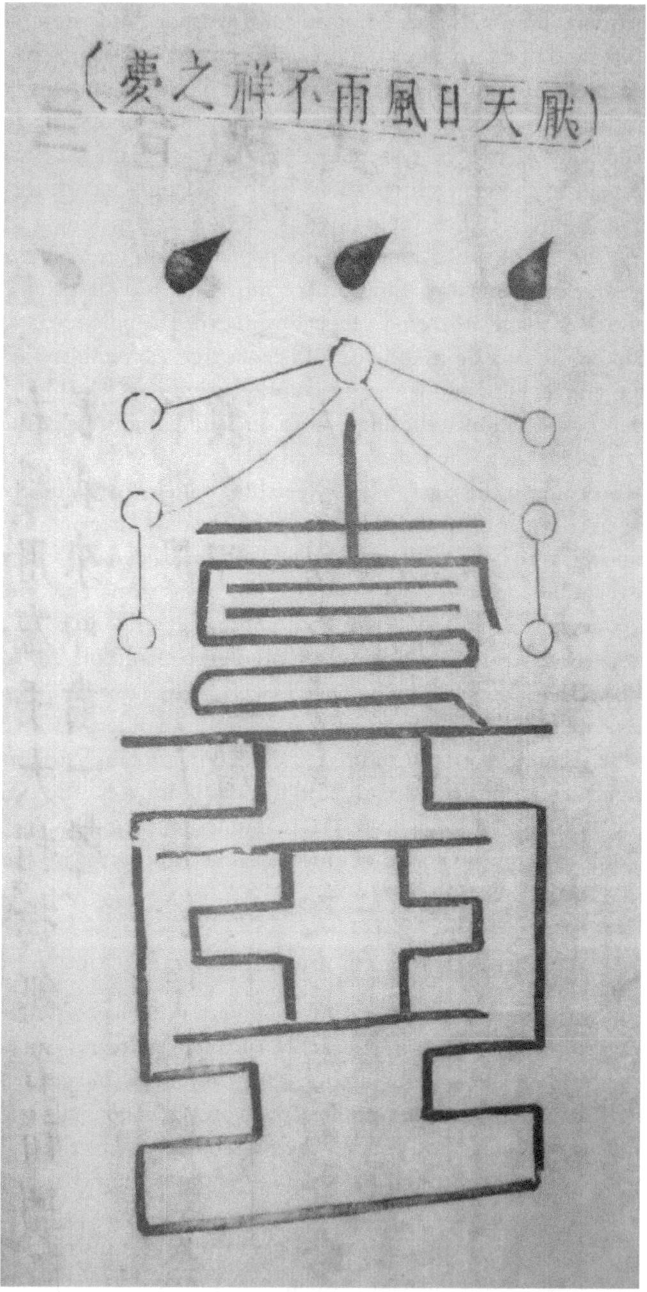

Figure 1.1: ***Yan tian ri feng yu bu xiang zhi meng*** **厭天日風雨不祥之夢［Suppress Inauspicious Dreams about the Sky, Sun, Wind or Rain］. Reproduced with permission from the Chinese Collection, Harvard Yenching Library Rare Book Collection**

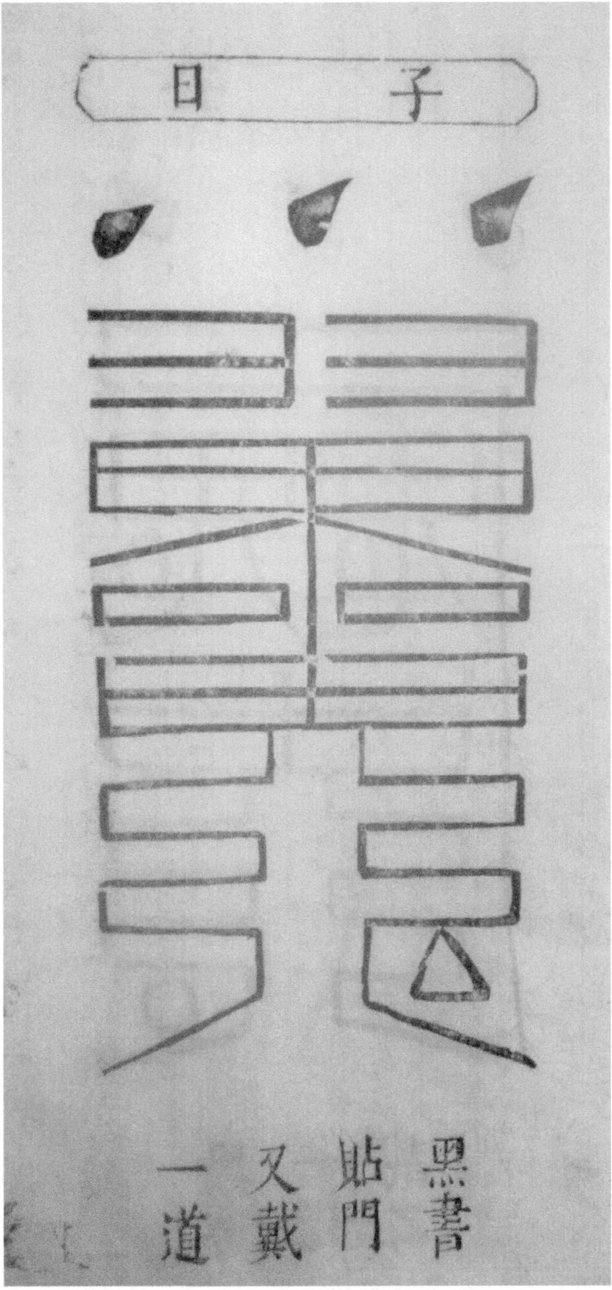

Figure 1.2: ***Zi ri*** **子日 [Rat Day]. Reproduced with permission from the Chinese Collection, Harvard Yenching Library Rare Book Collection**

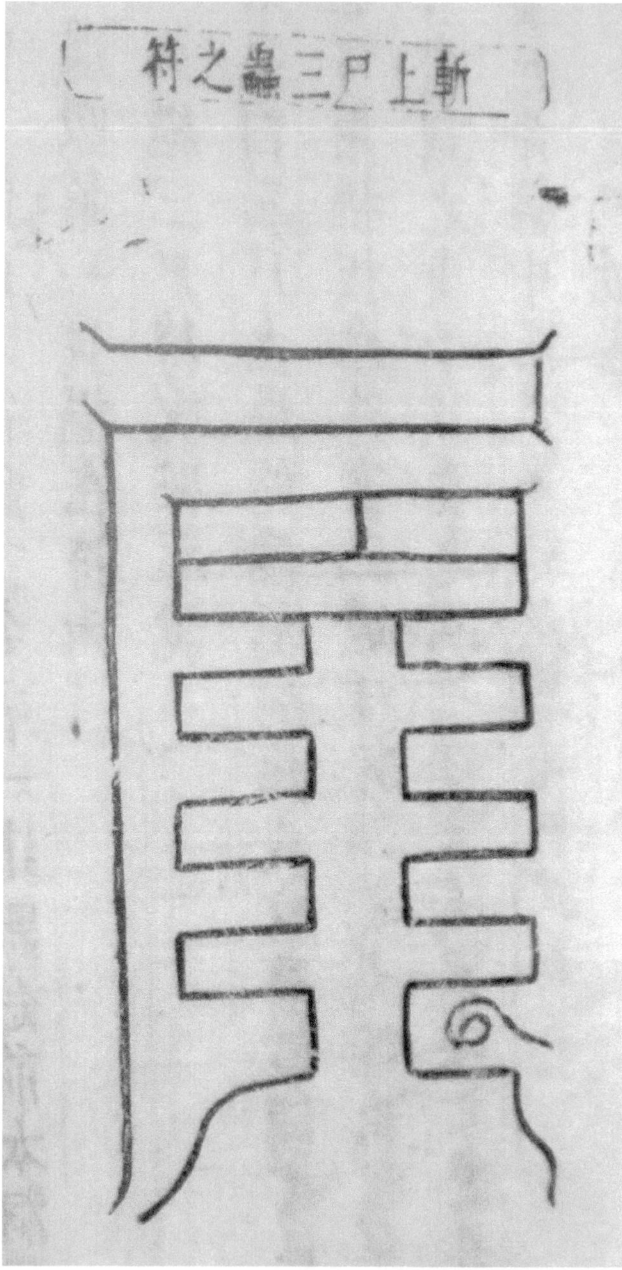

Figure 1.3: *Zhan shang shi san chong zhi fu* 斬上尸三蟲之符 [Talisman for Breaking the Three Worms in the Upper Corpse-God]. Reproduced with permission from the Chinese Collection, Harvard Yenching Library Rare Book Collection

The talismans potentially released powerful, protective forces; however, the talismanic images themselves recorded within the pages were merely templates. In order for the talisman to be effective, the nightmare sufferer needed to follow the written instructions given in the encyclopaedia and actually write the talisman by hand. What was arguably most important was acknowledging or naming the source of the nightmare. Once the source of the problem was clear, it was possible to regain control of the situation and alleviate physical and mental suffering. Correctly naming the problem allowed the nightmare sufferer to choose the correct talisman, which would then drive away whatever had caused the nightmare in the first place.

These dream treatments were all forms of social therapy, of first acknowledging a problem that manifested in dreams and then treating the problem based on information presented within the pages of 'Dream Exorcism'. This implies that bad dreams or nightmares were perhaps not private; rather, it may have been the case that sharing this information with family members might have helped alleviate dream-related suffering.

Before detailing the talismanic techniques presented in *Forest of Dreams*, it is important to briefly introduce the function of talismans in China. Scholars have noted that in ancient China, talismans were formed of two pieces, each held by one party of a given contract. Connecting the two pieces together served to identify the authority of the two parties, thus legitimating the contract.[17] Modelled after official imperial injunctions, talismans refer to mandates, orders, or injunctions issued under seal, designed to invoke the intervention of spirits or gods. Talismans were and are commonly used in conjunction with incantations and serve as a manifestation of cosmic energies, representations of a particular deity or deities, and edicts for the spirit world. Written in abstract or diagrammatic form in rectangular and simple composition (or so-called celestial writing *tian shu* 天書), talismans use stylized characters, figurative elements, geometrical patterns and symbolic signs, drawn in combination. Commonly used symbolic elements are small circles representing stars or constellations; curves representing water, fire and the flow of energy; spirals and curls representing clouds and cosmic movement.

Talismans vary greatly in their composition and can represent all the forces in the universe, as well as the words and symbols that grant power or control over said forces. According to some scholars, talismans revealed the workings of the universe in a raw and undiluted state, showing adepts the interior structure, the true shape and quality of things.[18] The timing of the application of talismans was important; incantations were to be activated at precise times in order to support, promote or change the flow of cosmic energies.[19] In order to operate with effect, the talisman often denoted thunder, lightning, the sun and the moon. Stellar deities and the constellations were, and are, depicted by black spots or dots linked in clusters. Generally, the evil to be combated or destroyed was, and is, written at the end. Talismans belonged to a tradition of occult, symbolic art over 2,000 years old and represented the visual remnants of the belief in the spiritual powers of calligraphy and the written word.[20]

Taken alone and without reference to the accompanying text, the talismanic images in 'Dream Exorcism' provided little clue as to their purpose or latent power. These talismanic images were accompanied by the texts of incantations, which acted to impart power to the talisman. The implied reader was one who likely suffered from chronic or debilitating bad dreams or nightmares and was literate enough to seek out self-help or treatment. The compilers explained that Laozi taught methods for avoiding nightmares (*bi e meng fa* 避惡夢法) and included them in the work.[21] In the explication of Laozi's method, the compilers stressed the importance of beginning treatment the moment a person is aware of having had a nightmare. The method required the nightmare sufferer to use the left hand to twist the philtrum fourteen times, gnash the teeth together fourteen times, and repeat an incantation aloud. The incantation consisted of a chain of commands, which ordered a protective army to guard specific meridian points and prevent evil spirits or influences from penetrating the body.[22]

After saying the incantation, 'Dream Exorcism' recommended that the person who had the bad dream or nightmare write the accompanying talisman, which would then suppress the evil causing the nightmare, blocking it outside the 'three passes' (*san guan* 三關) meridian point, and consequently help the person attain auspiciousness, which would then presumably alleviate the problem.[23]

Just before writing the talisman, the nightmare sufferer was to click together his or her teeth, face east, focus internally and recite the provided incantations. 'Dream Exorcism' then offered a brief step-by-step instruction in talisman writing, first visually depicting the proper brush-holding technique. Next, it explained how to draw the three dots representing the three Pure Ones (*san qing* 三清). Although the instructions did not specify, it would seem that the nightmare sufferer would draw the talisman with the right hand while using the left hand to move through the gestures. The compilers suggested using a clean writing table, ink stone, paper and brush, which implies the reader must have had access to such items. The text does not specify a size for the talismans; perhaps this was left to the discretion of the reader and paper availability.

The next section of 'Dream Exorcism' included ten talismanic samples or templates from which to choose, based on dream content (see Figure 1.1). This particular set of ten talismans is grouped under the category 'to suppress' (*yan* 厭), which derives from 'suppress' or 'dominate' (*yansheng* 厭勝), a Daoist technique of gaining control over people or things.[24] The goal of this technique of suppression was aimed at benefitting oneself and avoiding or deflecting disaster. The forms of the ten talismans are similar, with three black dots representing the three Pure Ones at the top; empty circles connected with single black lines representing a particular constellation (such as the Big Dipper *beidou* 北斗 or the Southern Dipper *nandou* 南斗); and stylized, blocky characters at the bottom which represent either the creation of a sacred, protected space or the names of the evil influences which the talisman promised to exorcize. These ten talismans specifically acted against the after-effects of inauspicious dreams (*bu xiang zhi meng* 不祥之夢) about specific subjects.

Each of these talismans purportedly suppressed a particular kind of inauspicious dream. Based on the content of the inauspicious dream, the reader was presumably expected to choose the most appropriate talismanic model. The ten talismans were listed in the following order:

yan tian ri feng yu bu xiang zhi meng 厭天日風雨不祥之夢 [Suppress Inauspicious Dreams about the Sky, Sun, Wind or Rain]

yan shan chuan qiao lu bu xiang zhi meng 厭山川橋路不祥之夢 [Suppress Inauspicious Dreams about Mountains, Rivers, Bridges or Roads]

yan ren gui xian bu xiang zhi meng 厭人鬼仙不祥之夢 [Suppress Inauspicious Dreams about People, Ghosts or Immortals]

yan fushi shenmao bu xiang zhi meng 厭服飾身貌不祥之夢 [Suppress Inauspicious Dreams about Clothing, Adornments, the Body or Outer Appearances]

yan shi zhai qi min bu xiang zhi meng 厭屋宅器皿不祥之夢 [Suppress Inauspicious Dreams about Rooms, Dwellings, Household Utensils or Tools]

yan sha dou xing yu bu xiang zhi meng 厭殺鬬刑獄不祥之夢 [Suppress Inauspicious Dreams about Killing, Fighting, Punishments or Jail]

yan yan yue si zang bu xiang zhi meng 厭宴樂死喪不祥之夢 [Suppress Inauspicious Dreams about Banquets, Music, Death or Burials]

yan hua guo gu cai bu xiang zhi meng 厭花果穀菜不祥之夢 [Suppress Inauspicious Dreams about Flowers, Fruits, Grains or Vegetables]

yan chan yun cai bo bu xiang zhi meng 厭產孕財帛不祥之夢 [Suppress Inauspicious Dreams about Giving Birth, Conceiving, Wealth or Money]

yan shui huo dao zei bu xiang zhi meng 厭水火盜賊不祥之夢 [Suppress Inauspicious Dreams about Floods, Fires, Robbers or Bandits]

The next set of twelve images of talismans related specifically to nightmares (*e meng* 惡夢) and listed the nightmare exorcism methods of the Supreme Lord Laozi (*taishang laojun rang e meng fuzhou shuo* 太上老君禳惡夢符呪說) (see Figure 1.2). The introduction to the set of twelve talismanic templates stressed the time the nightmare occurred, rather than its specific content or subject matter. Categorical differentiation distinguished this set of twelve talismans from the previous set of ten talismans.

Interestingly, part of the process would have required at least a semi-public visual acknowledgment of nightmare suffering. Those talismans to be hung on the walls of the residence compound would have been visible to other family members and co-residents. Although it may not have been obvious that the talisman was specifically directed toward nightmares, it would have been clear that the talisman was directed at healing. It may have been the case that sharing this information with family members helped prevent disaster. An entire family might have suffered from the predicted ill effects of an individual family member's nightmare; therefore, family members had a collective, vested interest in the nightmares of individuals. Talismanic production visually implied the need of a cure or purge, indicating the presence of a problem, albeit a solvable problem. In that sense, talismanic cures were a form of dream-related discipline or, at an extreme, perhaps of stigmatization. In the general advice section we have a sense of the shared social space of dreams and nightmares; readers of 'Dream Exorcism' were exhorted to avoid startling somebody who was having a nightmare or who was snoring. Sleeping, and, by extension, dreaming were not private affairs.

If a person had a nightmare, upon awakening in the morning, they were to write the talisman that corresponded to the date. Next, the nightmare sufferer was to visualize Laozi wearing a crown and dark robes and then say the following incantation seven times: 'Brilliant and vast, the sun rises in the east. I command this talisman to break up and drive away nightmares and inauspicious dreams, as quickly as [imperial] statutes and orders do! Ha!'[25]

The text then explained that the nightmare sufferer should first say the incantation and then write the corresponding talisman. If these steps were followed, the nightmare sufferer's heart's red *qi* would grow as large as a chicken's egg (*xin you chi qi ru jiluan da* 心有赤氣如雞卵大).[26] The text then recommended raising the *qi* upwards until it permeated outwards. At this point, the reader was instructed to knock the teeth together and spit out the *qi* in one breath into the centre of the talisman. Afterwards, the reader was instructed to drink water flowing in an eastward direction and spit to the east. This series of actions would dispel any inauspiciousness associated with the dream.

The nightmare-avoidance talismans in this section are divided according to the twelve earthly branches (*shi'er dizhi* 十二地支): rat, ox, tiger, rabbit, dragon, snake, horse, sheep, monkey, rooster, dog and pig. The visual structure of this set of talismans is quite similar to the talismans included in the previous portion of this *juan*, with three black dots representing the three Pure Ones at the top and stylized, rectangular characters at the bottom. The talismans divided according to the twelve earthly branches, however, do not contain shorthand versions of constellations. Another difference between this set and the previous one is that this set of talismans gives brief, yet specific, handling instructions based on the date of the nightmare.

According to the days (such as rat, ox, tiger, rabbit and so on) mentioned with images, nightmare sufferers were instructed to write the talismans. For example, if a nightmare had occurred on a rat day, the nightmare sufferer was to write the rat day talisman according to its provided template. When writing out the talismans as instructed, nightmare sufferers were told to repeat the given incantation once and breathe life into the talisman.[27]

The third and final set of talismans consisted of three talismans designed to break (*zhan* 斬) the Three-Corpse Gods (*san shi* 三尸) (see Figure 1.3). Unlike the talismans in the previous two sections, the Three-Corpse Gods talismans were intended for consumption, to be physically taken into the body. In this way, they closely resemble herbal prescriptions contained in medical casebooks. These were anti-nightmare prescriptions that were first visually depicted and then physically imbibed.

The Three-Corpse Gods are located in three places in the body: the Upper of the Three-Corpse Gods resides in the Clay Pellet (*ni wan* 泥丸); the Middle of the Three-Corpse Gods resides in the Heart and Abdomen (*xin fu* 心腹); and the Lower of the Three-Corpse Gods resides in the Stomach and Feet (*wei zu* 胃足). On *gengshen* day (庚申), the Three-Corpse Gods are believed to ascend to Heaven to report on individual transgressions and good deeds.

According to the explanation preceding the three talismans in this section, illness was explained as caused by the Three-Corpse Gods and nine worms. Thus, when sick people dreamed of struggles and fighting at night, it was because the worms and the Three-Corpse Gods resided within the physical body. Here, the focus was not on inauspicious dreams or even on nightmares, but rather on the nightmares of those already suffering from physical illness. Based on the language used, it seems that, at least for the compilers, dreams lay on a spectrum, with inauspicious dreams viewed as relatively more innocuous than nightmares, which were in turn construed as being less problematic than illnesses caused by the Three-Corpse Gods.

In order to stop the Three-Corpse Gods, 'Dream Exorcism' recommended using the wood of a peach tree as the talismanic writing surface. Because of its purported exorcist properties, peach wood was, and is, used in many Daoist rituals. After writing the talisman on the bark of the peach wood according to the instructions, nightmare sufferers were to bury the talisman under the doorsill. On a *gengshen* day, which occurred every sixty days, or six times a year, the nightmare sufferer was to wear the talisman. *Gengshen* day was no doubt chosen because this was the day that the Three-Corpse Gods ascended to Heaven to report on individual transgressions. If an individual was found wanting, his or her life span was shortened. On *gengzi* 庚子 days, if the nightmare sufferer swallowed the talisman (it is likely that the talisman itself was ingested only symbolically), the Three-Corpse Gods would be eliminated.[28] Also, nightmare sufferers were told to write the names of the Three-Corpse Gods on each sixth *geng* 庚 day and the Three-Corpse Gods would cease wreaking havoc on the dreamer's health. Each talisman included in 'Dream Exorcism' promised to sever a particular one of the Three-Corpse Gods.

Preface to 'Dream Exorcism'

Based on the division between the talismanic sections, it seems that dreams, inauspicious dreams and nightmares were conceived of as existing along a spectrum, with an implied perception that nightmares caused by the Three-Corpse Gods were the most problematic health-wise among the three. The introductory preface to 'Dream Exorcism' provided more nuance. As is evident from the preface to 'Dream Exorcism', the presence of dreams and nightmares indicated individual moral corruption. It was apparently up to the individual in question to re-shape his or her moral fibre based on the messages from dreams. Indeed, as the preface claimed, it was the case that 'those people who have not yet turned to goodness and who cannot attain fortune, or for those who have become evil and are not able to turn to prayer, or even for people who have good intent, heaven must create the circumstances of trivial nightmares, which cannot be explicated or exorcized'.[29]

The preface claimed that all phenomena (disasters, pestilences, disease, and, by extension, all dreams and nightmares) could be exorcized, however, dreams and nightmares alike could only be truly and completely exorcized by a change in personal deportment or by cultivating virtue. Talismanic cures, herbal prescriptions and prayers might be efficacious, but the implication was that long-term cures required more than a quick fix:

> If, upon awakening from a dream, demons come, and [you] immediately speak to the demons of morality and justice and then pray against wrongdoings or transgressions, but [you] are actually not repentant, then how can simply taking herbal prescriptions and saying a few incantations to dispel demons help [you] toward the path to true auspiciousness and healthy rest? Early *Ru* scholars said: 'In order to exorcise the inauspicious, doesn't one need to cultivate virtue?' As for rubbing together auspicious mulberry [wood] in order to cause bewilderment and confusion to retreat, Heaven will banish and end evil. The evil in your spirit and *hun* will escape. It is not enough to sweep away and clean. I, however, have examined myself critically and have cultivated virtue. This can be called the path to great virtue and knowledge ... Isn't it the case that nothing is better than adopting an intent of self-reflection and cultivation? Those who are in the midst of using the talisman of Hei-yu to suppress and escape [dreams] say that it is easy to follow. However, they do not know if they have already reached the shore of awakening or not.[30]

From the passage above, it is clear that nightmares were perceived of as indicators of personal failings, of exhortations from the gods or spirits to improve or suffer the consequences. Sole reliance on the toolkit of dream-related lore in 'Dream Exorcism' would not put readers on the 'shore of awakening', although it did promise to provide relief. Rather than simply taking herbal prescriptions or following incantations, the preface exhorted nightmare sufferers to undertake a path of critical self-reflection and examination.

The preface continued, claiming that although people are inherently ignorant and therefore suffer from envy and fear, the Buddha proved that holiness and virtue triumph over evil. The compilers conceded that nightmares were indeed a reality, but they maintained that heaven was able to exorcize nightmares from virtuous people. Exorcist methods relied on yang principles. The compilers asserted that this was the reason sages used the doctrine of yang virtue to encourage people to follow paths of goodness and cultivation:

> therefore, these magical talismans and methods of exorcism and other such techniques – which were handed down for hundreds and thousands of years – are still able to quell evil in people and are still able to cure those people who suffer from fevers and illnesses. All this is only possible because what the *qi* of pure yang absorbs is numinous, auspicious, and eternal.[31]

Conclusion

In conclusion, this chapter argues that the compilers of *Forest of Dreams* domesticated dreams by creating a visible system of meaning surrounding invisible desires, anxieties, and fears. Compilers also placed dreams firmly within the social sphere, suggesting that dreams must be regulated on a communal and not just individual level. By situating dreams firmly in the realm of accessible knowledge, the compilers returned to apprehensive readers the power they might have previously found in a more stable social structure. Moreover, the compilers also enacted a new social order in written form, in which the discussion and treatment of dreams served as a means of both individual and communal regulation.

In the roughly 5,000 dream examples quoted in *Forest of Dreams*, emperors worried over their physical health or the uncertainty of ascending the throne. Examination candidates hoping to embark on a civil service career worried over whether or not they would pass or fail the upcoming examinations. The compilers of *Forest of Dreams* worried over the future of their country and the worsening political situation. These anxieties first manifested in dreams were subsequently alleviated, but only after the dream had been properly understood and shared with others in the community. Untreated dreams and nightmares had repercussions at both the individual and social level.

Forest of Dreams also illuminates the relationship between dreams, nightmares, and healing practices in late Ming China. Indeed, it can arguably be read as a medical how-to text. The compilers rendered public esoteric knowledge on talismans and incantations. Highlighting dream and nightmare treatments (such as general sleeping and dreaming advice as well as specific talismans) contained in 'Dream Exorcism' illuminates the relationship between dreams and health in late Ming China. 'Dream Exorcism' delineated what could and should be done with dreams, inauspicious dreams, and nightmares and provided the vocabulary and tools to educate readers on how to view and treat dreams and nightmares. Thus, the work offered readers the ability to discipline themselves, offering not only a concrete means to comprehend the world of dreams, but also the methods necessary to alleviate anxiety through the exorcism of inauspicious dreams and nightmares.

2 EMOTIONAL THERAPY AND TALKING CURES IN LATE IMPERIAL CHINA

Hsiu-fen Chen

The Chinese have recognized the importance of emotions in health and sickness since antiquity; in late Imperial China, assessments of emotional states remained significant in both medical theories and clinical encounters.[1] In addition to aetiology and diagnostics, physicians also developed unique therapeutics for treating illnesses caused by emotional imbalance. These treatments were widely recorded in both medical texts and literary jottings. They lay the foundation of the discussions in this chapter.

An early medical treatise on emotions can be found in the first received medical classic, *Huangdi neijing* 黃帝內經 [Inner Canon of the Yellow Emperor] (*c.* first century BC – first century AD; hereafter the *Inner Canon*). This work sets out the theory of the five major human emotions, known as the 'Five Intents' (*wuzhi* 五志), which was broadly followed by later physicians. The medical views of emotions seemed largely unchanged before mediaeval China. In the late imperial period, however, both medical theories and practices of emotional disorders underwent drastic changes. Firstly, physicians not only extended the 'Five Intents' into the 'Seven Emotions' (*qiqing* 七情), but also expanded the category of 'emotions' (*qingzhi* 情志) and 'mental states' (*shenzhi* 神志) by including some other emotional disorders into their nosology. Secondly, some physicians even went further to reinterpret an old therapeutic principle, 'announcing causes' (*zhuyou* 祝由) in terms of a psychotherapy-like perspective. No less important was the application of a healing art involving emotional manipulation and talking cures. Therefore, when one sixteenth-century physician stated that 'when emotions go extreme, no drug can cure [the resulting disorders]; [they] must be overcome by emotions' (*qingzhi guoji fei yao ke yu xu yi qing sheng* 情志過極　非藥可愈　須以情勝), it signifies not only a quotation of an old saying from the *Inner Canon*, but rather a new perspective of emotional therapy.[2] In late Imperial China, this treatment, with its appeal to emotional manipulation, was referred to both as the 'Principle of Mutual Conquest of the Five Phases/Intents' (*wuxing/wuzhi xiangsheng zhi li* 五行/五志相勝之理), and 'overcoming one emotional state by another' (*yi qing sheng qing* 以情勝情).[3] Two recent studies identify it as 'emotional counter-therapy' or 'therapy by counter-affect'.[4]

Due to the scope of this chapter, discussion will focus on, though not be restricted to, emotional disorders treated by emotional therapy and talking cures in late Imperial China. To begin with, the medical views of emotions and sickness will be traced since antiquity, showing how they were transmitted in later ages. Secondly, emphasis will be placed on late imperial medical cases, in which therapeutic techniques of emotional manipulation and talking cures were applied. An overall review, finally, will estimate the extent to which this way of emotional therapy worked. As will be argued in this chapter, a successful emotional therapy always depends on close interaction between doctors, patients and their families. Without scrutinizing the specific circumstances in which a Chinese healer-patient relationship was situated, it is unlikely to explain fully why emotional therapy, despite its success in quite a few clinical encounters, remained less prevalent than drug remedies in pre-modern China.

Emotions and Sickness in Classical Medical Thought

The relationship between emotions and sickness is frequently discussed in Chinese medical works. In early China, the *Inner Canon* depicts anger (*nu* 怒), joy (*xi* 喜), pensiveness (*si* 思), sorrow (*you* 憂) and fear (*kong* 恐) as the five major human emotions. From the perspective of the correspondence system, these five emotions, or the 'Five Intents' in later physicians' terms, correspond to the 'Five Viscera' – the Liver, the Heart, the Spleen, the Lung and the Kidney.[5] If any of the five emotions reaches an extreme state, its corresponding visceral organ will be injured too: anger injures the Liver; joy injures the Heart; pensiveness injures the Spleen; sorrow injures the Lung; and fear injures the Kidney.

As the theory of the 'Five Intents' and the 'Five Viscera' derives from the concept of the 'Five Phases', consequently, the constructed relations of 'mutual conquest' amongst the 'Five Phases' also apply to that of the 'Five Intents'. The authors of the *Inner Canon* suggested that Wood/anger 'overcomes' (*ke* 克) Earth/pensiveness; Earth/pensiveness overcomes Water/fear; Water/fear overcomes Fire/joy; Fire/joy overcomes Metal/sorrow; Metal/sorrow overcomes Wood/anger. However, the identification of specific emotions is not always consistent, as recorded in the *Inner Canon*. One example is 'sorrow', which is sometimes replaced with 'worry' in certain texts of this work.[6] What follows is a table to show the corresponding relations between the 'Five Phases', 'Five Viscera', and 'Five Intents':

The Five Phases	**The Five Viscera**	**The Five Intents**	**The Intent that it overcomes**	**The Intent that overcomes it**
Wood	Liver	Anger	Pensiveness	Sorrow/Worry
Fire	Heart	Joy	Sorrow/Worry	Fear
Earth	Spleen	Pensiveness	Fear	Anger
Metal	Lung	Sorrow/Worry	Anger	Joy
Water	Kidney	Fear	Joy	Pensiveness

Table 2.1: The 'Principle of Mutual Conquest of the Five Phases'

In a *qi*-dominated cosmology, the *Inner Canon* also suggests the key role of *qi* in human health. In this view, all medical disorders arise from abnormal states of *qi*. Any change in the emotions also affects the movements of *qi*. As it is stated in the *Inner Canon*, 'anger makes *qi* ascend; joy relaxes it; grief (*bei* 悲) dissipates it; fear makes it descend; cold contracts it; heat makes it leak out; fright (*jing* 驚) makes it chaotic; exhaustion consumes it; and pensiveness congeals it'.[7] When a person indulges in any of the Five Intents, such indulgence injures his *qi* and hence his visceral organs.[8] In short, not the emotions themselves, but the *qi* is affected by the imbalanced emotions, which results in various illnesses. This medical opinion echoes the mind-and-body holism of classical Chinese medicine. As Kuriyama put it, '[w]hen doctors in the *Neijing* subsequently spoke of *qi* rising in anger, sinking in fear, seeping away in sorrow, they weren't so much trying to *explain* [sic] emotions, objectively, as relating what they knew from their own bodies, describing what they felt, subjectively, within themselves'.[9]

Numerous medical works follow the medical theories of emotions in the *Inner Canon* with minor modifications. One of them is the aetiological canon *Zhu bing yuan hou lun* 諸病源候論 [The Treatise on Causes and Symptoms of Medical Disorders]. According to it, the accumulation of the 'Seven *qi*' (*qiqi* 七氣) caused by different factors – including anger, wrath, worry, joy and distress – may result in illnesses beneath the Heart or in the abdomen. When they occur, it is so painful that one is unable to eat and even feels like dying.[10] This medical view of the mutual influence between *qi*, emotion, and illness was further elaborated in the twelfth and thirteenth centuries. Certain physicians expanded the category of the 'Five Intents' into the 'Seven Emotions' by inclusion of the emotions of grief and fright. They were seen as the 'inner causes' (*neiyin* 內因) of illnesses, in contrast to the environmental factors, namely, the 'external causes' (*waiyin* 外因).[11] Since then the term 'Seven Emotions' has become more widely used than the 'Five Intents'. The category remained important in aetiology even in the nineteenth century, though medical discussions were not restricted to only the seven emotions.[12]

Apart from aetiology, the nosology of emotions also underwent development between the sixteenth and the eighteenth centuries. Wu Kun 吳昆 (*b.* 1551) was probably the first doctor to create a new category for the classification of illnesses originating in emotional disturbance. In his *Yifang kao* 醫方考 [Research on Medical Formulas], Wu illustrated eleven cases to show how physicians and laymen alike had applied emotional therapy in earlier times.[13] Wu was not the only one who had noted the classical medical doctrine about the 'Mutual Conquest of the Five Emotions' from the *Inner Canon*. Zhang Jiebin 張介賓 (1563–1640), one of Wu's contemporaries, also proposed a category of 'emotional disorders' (*qingzhi bing* 情志病) in his annotation on the *Inner Canon*.[14] One century later, the great imperial encyclopaedia, *Gujin tushu jicheng yibu quanlu* 古今圖書集成 [Past and Present Synthesis of Books and Illustrations], again demonstrates a wide range of medical treatises on 'emotions' throughout the ages.[15] All these works featuring a new category of emotions/emotional disorders suggest that physicians and medical writers in late Imperial China appeared to have new perceptions of emotions/emotional disorders.

To be sure, the identification of 'emotional disorders' as a new category was not limited to nosology only; discussion now turns to the therapeutics of emotions, showing how late imperial physicians elaborated upon the old notion of the 'Principle of Mutual Conquest of the Five Phases' by the development of a healing art with recourse to 'talking cures'.

'Talking Cures': Old Doctrine and New Practice

In modern psychology and psychoanalysis, 'talking cure' is an important therapeutic technique that aims to cure mental illnesses by verbal communication and emotional catharsis. Despite the lack of psychotherapy equivalent to that in modern medicine, pre-modern Chinese physicians did cultivate unique healing arts involving oral skills and emotional manipulation for certain emotional disorders, as the evidence of certain medical case records and the jottings of literati suggests.

As for verbal communication, the *Inner Canon* provides a therapeutic outline for doctors: 'loathing for death and desire for life are common human feelings (*ren zhi qing* 人之情). If a doctor informs his patient what is malevolent, tells him what is benevolent, instructs him in what is appropriate and relieves him from what he is suffering from, then how can one, even if he is an unjust man, not listen to him?[16] This principle emphasizes the importance of communication between doctors and patients. It also stresses that a good doctor should come to know how his patients feel, and then speak to them appropriately to suit their individual need. No specific illness is noted, however.

In late Imperial China, Zhang Congzheng 張從正 (1156–1228) was one of the most skilful physicians in the healing arts of emotional catharsis. Based on the doctrines of the *Inner Canon*, he firstly explained the 'Principle of Mutual

Conquest of the Five Phases' in detail, followed by his elaboration of 'talking cures' as follows:

> sorrow can cure anger, i.e., by affecting one by misery and distressed talks; joy can cure sorrow, i.e., by pleasing one by mocking and teasing talks; fear can cure joy, i.e., by frightening one by forcing and threatening talks; anger can cure pensiveness, i.e., by offending one by insulting and cheating talks; pensiveness can cure fear, i.e., by drawing one's attention from here to there by talking.[17]

For disorders caused by fright, Zhang had different advice. He argued that

> only familiarity (*xi* 習) can cure fright. The *Inner Canon* states that 'the frightened one should be calmed'. 'Calmness' means 'ordinariness'. Fright is caused simply by a sudden occurrence. Nothing can frighten a person once he is familiar with what he sees and hears.[18]

Zhang suggested that a doctor should play tricks on his patients by cheating them and using deceitful language where applicable. These remedies should be so cunning and unpredictable that they are capable of distracting the patients' attention and changing their way of looking at things. However, he also cautioned that the 'Principle of Mutual Conquest of the Five Phases' is not suitable for everyone. That is, physicians should have a certain kind of 'competence' (*caiqi* 材器), so that their verbal interactions can produce a positive result in combination with treatments. Physicians who are unable to identify patients' emotions accurately cannot make this psychotherapy successful.[19] The manipulation of emotions by talking cures and affective language plays a key role in Zhang's emotional therapy. Zhang claimed that he had successfully cured several patients by emotional therapy: 'I have treated these cases [so easily] as if 'delving into a pocket to fish out [something]' (*ru tan nang ran* 如探囊然).[20] His medical views and clinical experiences of emotional therapy became so renowned that they were widely recorded in Ming-Qing medical works.[21]

Zhang Congzheng's 'talking cure' was echoed by the modified therapeutic practice of 'announcing causes'. In early China, the method of 'announcing causes' was rather a diagnostic means that aimed at tracing the origins of illnesses through prayer. By contrast, the late Ming physician Zhang Jiebin interpreted this old ritual healing from an emotion-oriented perspective. As he explained,

> [announcing causes] is the so called [technique] to know where the illness comes from (*suo cong sheng* 所從生). Only when [a doctor] traces the origin, then [he knows] the way to treat it. None of the treatments will fail if [he] detects what [the patients] loathes (*e* 惡), adores (*mu* 慕), competes (*sheng* 勝), and [where his illness] comes from.[22]

His view was followed by another doctor, Wu Jutong 吳鞠通 (*c.* 1758–1836). Wu believed that it was necessary to announce causes whenever a doctor treats 'inner injury' (*neishang* 內傷). He should firstly detail where the illness comes from and make this known to the patient, so that the latter can avoid having another fit. The doctor should also examine how the illness develops in meticulous detail, as well as scrutinize the hidden feelings of 'exhausted men' (*laoren* 勞人) and 'pensive women' (*sifu* 思婦). He must exhort his patients with amiable words, caution them with solemn words, and inspire fear in them with words of danger. This is the way to make them delightful at heart, after which effective results of treatment can be obtained.[23] Lin Peiqin 林佩琴 (1772–1839), one of Wu's contemporaries, held a similar opinion. He argued that one should detect the roots of illness before treating them, regardless of whether they stem from unfulfilled wishes, frustrated encounters, accumulated thoughts or unhappiness at heart. If these symptoms cannot be relieved until they result in 'fatigue by accumulated repression' (*ji yu chenglao* 積鬱成勞), there will be nothing one can do to help.[24] Again, 'announcing causes' was viewed as an important approach to the therapy of emotional disorders.

In short, the practice of 'announcing causes' evolved from its original usage of ritual healing into a means for physicians to observe the mental states of patients in late Imperial China.[25] The reinterpreted medical views above remind us that examining patients' emotional disorders and knowing their origins became crucial in arriving at medical judgments in this period. Emotional manipulation, 'talking cures' and 'announcing causes' are therapeutic techniques of particular importance to emotional therapy. But how would these ideas be applied in clinical encounters? The following medical cases provide some hints.

Emotional Therapies in Clinical Encounters

As mentioned earlier, Zhang Congzheng was arguably the most talented doctor specializing in the 'Principle of Mutual Conquest of the Five Phases'. When treating various disorders generally categorized as 'inner injury', Zhang demonstrated unique insights in the application of emotional therapies. One of his most successful medical cases was about a governor of the City Xi 息; hearing his father being murdered by thieves, the man cried out with grief and soon after he stopped crying, he began to feel pain in his heart. A lump gradually formed within the course of a month, swollen like a cup beneath his heart, causing him great pain against which no prescribed medicine worked. Acupuncture and moxibustion were suggested as treatments but the patient was loath to undergo them due to his pain. Then Zhang Congzheng was requested to come and neither medicine nor acu-moxa did he recommend. When he arrived, a shaman happened to be there, probably at the governor's invitation; Zhang simply imitated the shaman's performance, accompanied by mad ravings, in order to entertain the patient. The latter could not help but laugh out loudly, until he felt embarrassed and turned his face to the wall. In one or two days, his lump disappeared completely. Just as Zhang explained,

> the *Inner Canon* states that 'worry causes *qi* stagnation and joy leads to the relaxation of a hundred vessels'. It also states that 'joy overcomes sorrow'. As the *Inner Canon* already stipulated this method, why did people continue to use acupuncture and moxibustion? They just increased the patient's pain.[26]

He thus applied such a therapy since all other treatments had failed. This success enabled Zhang to claim his superiority over that of other healers by his excellent therapeutic techniques. It is particularly significant in the circumstances in which Zhang had to compete with shamans. As he once complained, 'ancient people viewed doctors as teachers, so the Medical Way worked; people nowadays despise healers as servants, therefore the Medical Way has been abolished'. If most of the 'ambitious gentlemen' (*youzhi zhi shi* 有志之士), as he claimed, regarded learning medicine as something shameful in his era, it is no wonder patients never knew how to distinguish between good and bad doctors.[27]

Zhang Congzheng's distinctive psychological techniques were also demonstrated in the case of Lady Xiang 項. A wife of a chief-official at the City Gate, she had been afflicted by outbursts of anger and loss of appetite, often shouting and scolding with fury as if she would kill her servants. Her loathsome words never ceased. Various doctors prescribed medicine for her, but her condition remained unchanged for nearly half a year. Then Zhang was sent in. In his diagnosis he said to her family that 'this [illness] was hard to cure'. Surprisingly, Zhang seemed to have prescribed a treatment of 'performing arts': he instructed two singing-and-dancing girls to put red powder on their faces and behave like actresses. The lady watched their performance and laughed loudly. The next day Zhang changed his tricks and asked these girls to engage in wrestling (*jiaodi* 角觝) in front of the lady. Again, she laughed loudly. Zhang arranged for two other women with great appetites to appear beside her and exaggerate how delicious their food was. Because of their antics, the lady asked to have a taste. In a couple of days, the fury of her anger diminished and her appetite increased. Her illness was eventually cured without medicine. Later, she became pregnant and finally gave birth to a son.[28] Rather than showing that 'sorrow overcomes anger' based on the Principle of 'Mutual Conquest of the Five Phases', this medical case exemplifies that 'joy overcomes anger'. It suggests that emotional manipulation may be practiced in a flexible way. Similar to the former case, emotional manipulation became a 'magic bullet' in a difficult case when no other medicine worked. No less interesting is the lady's childbirth. Obviously, not only the lady's bad temper but her relationship with her husband improved. The couple were able to produce a son, thanks to the doctor's 'dramatic' treatment.

A similar case yet with a different treatment is described in Zhang's medical case book. A wealthy woman was unable to fall asleep for two years. Again, no medicine prescribed could cure her. Her husband then turned to Zhang for help. When reading her pulses, the doctor found them relaxed. He regarded this as a sign of a Spleen disorder arising from pensiveness. Based on the principle that 'pensiveness can be restrained by anger', he secretly instructed the woman's husband to make her angry. Later, the man indeed made off with her money and indulged himself in drink for several days. These actions indeed drove the lady into a state of rage. On that night, she sweated much and began to feel sleepy. She went to bed and continued to sleep for more than eight days. When she woke up, she felt hungry and started eating. Later, Zhang examined her again and found her pulses normal, showing that she was completely cured.[29] Obviously, this is a case which demonstrates that 'anger overcomes pensiveness'. It also shows the importance of a patient's family members in cooperating in such an emotional therapy.

Zhang Congzheng also cured an emotional disorder of Wei Dexin's 衛德新 wife. Once she stayed in a lodge when travelling. That night, the house was robbed and set afire. She was frightened and fell from her bed to the floor. Since then, she became so scared that she would lose consciousness when she heard any sound. Her family had to walk on tiptoe to avoid making any noise. Her symptoms persisted for over a year. Various doctors treated her symptoms as heart disease, but none of the remedies of ginseng, pearl powder or the 'Pill of Pacifying the Emotions' (*dingzhi wan* 定志丸) was effective. Zhang diagnosed her and explained her condition to the family: 'fright refers to *yang* and rises externally; fear refers to *yin* and rises internally. One is frightened because one is not aware of the situation; one is fearful because one is aware of it'. Zhang then asked two maids to grasp the patient's hands and place her in a high chair. He put a small table in front of her and said: 'Your lady, please watch this!' When he hit the table with a stick, the woman became greatly frightened. Zhang asked her: 'why were you so shocked when I hit the table with a stick?' He hit it again and this time she looked slightly pacified, and her fright appeared to diminish. After a moment, he repeated the same action several times. Besides the table, he also struck the door with a staff, and stealthily asked someone to make noise by tapping on the windows. When her fright was gradually pacified, she asked the doctor with a smile: 'what kind of treatment is it?' The doctor replied, 'the *Inner Canon* states that 'the one who is frightened should be calmed'. Calmness means ordinariness. One should not be frightened by what one regards as ordinary'. On that night, he asked someone to keep striking the doors and windows until dawn. After one or two days, the lady was no longer frightened even at the roar of thunder.[30] This example shows the principle that 'familiarity overcomes fear'. As Zhang Congzheng's emotional therapy was so extraordinary, certain later physicians paid tribute to him by quoting from his treatise and citing his treatments on emotional disorders in their own works.[31]

In addition to his own medical case records, Zhang Congzheng also recorded two other cases before his time. In the first case, a certain Mr. Zhuang 莊 once treated a man who had suffered from 'extreme joy and happiness' (*xi le zhi ji* 喜樂至極). In his diagnosis, he read the patient's pulse and pretended to exclaim in surprise. Then he told the patient that he would get the appropriate medicine. But, he just disappeared and never returned. The sick man began to worry that his illness might be so critical that the doctor had simply given up on the medication. He even cried out to his relatives and friends, saying he would die soon. Mr. Zhuang knew the patient was going to recover soon, so he appeared again. The patient asked him why he had gone away. Mr. Zhuang explained it was because he had intended to treat the patient's joy by inducing fear, based on the theory of emotional therapy in the *Inner Canon*.[32]

In the second case, an unknown governor had been afflicted by 'persistent diarrhoea' (*dongxie bu yi* 洞泄不已). A Mr. Yang from Shandong was called to examine him. As Yang was already aware of the governor's symptom, he did not talk to the patient directly upon entering the house. Rather, he chatted for several hours about astronomy and the weather with others present; the patient was so attentive to these subjects that he nearly forgot to go to the toilet. Mr. Yang later explained to the patient why he had administered such a treatment. He said that it is better to know a patient's hobby before treating his illness; he simply talked about what the latter loved in order to distract his attention from the illness itself.[33] At first glance, these two medical cases do not follow the 'Principle of Mutual Conquest among the Five Phases' closely. However, they both involved a therapy based on 'talking cures' and emotional manipulation. Just as the *Inner Canon* states, none of the treatments will fail if a doctor detects what his patients loathe and adore.

One of Zhang Congzheng's followers, the Yuan physician Zhu Zhenheng 朱震亨 (1282–1358), was also renowned for the emotional therapy by 'counteraffect'.[34] Clinically, Zhu's most remarkable medical case was his treatment of a woman's love sickness. In this case, a lady's illness had been marked by a loss of appetite, lying in bed and facing north all day for half a year. None of the physicians called upon could cure her. In his diagnosis of her Zhu Zhenheng found that her liver pulse was string-like and over the top of the left wrist. It was a sign indicative of a congealed *qi* in the Spleen. Zhu was told that the woman had been promised in marriage, yet her husband-to-be had travelled away to Guangdong and had been absent for five years. Zhu thus judged that all her symptoms were caused by her 'wanting a man but not being able to get one' (*si nanzi bu de* 思男子不得). To cure her pensive disorder, Zhu told her father: 'this illness can only be cured by anger because the blow of anger *qi* can rush the stagnation of earth. Now you should drive her into a rage'. But the father did not agree with the doctor's judgment. Zhu then entered the chamber and gave three slaps on her face, falsely accusing her of being involved with someone. The woman became so angry that she cried aloud. When her anger and sense of shame eased up, she asked for food. Again, Zhu stealthily told her father: 'although her *qi* of pensiveness is relieved, she should be treated by joy. Then her symptoms will never occur'. They deceitfully told her that her husband would return soon as mentioned in his letter. Three months later, her husband finally came back. She completely recovered.[35] As Zhu explained, the lady's various symptoms were owing to her lovesickness and unrequited yearning: when pensiveness injures the Spleen and causes various illnesses, it can only be 'restrained' (*sheng* 勝) by anger and 'relieved' (*jie* 解) by joy.[36] This case became so famous that it was widely transcribed in several Ming medical works, their slightly different contents notwithstanding.[37] One reason that makes it so remarkable is the unusual healer-patient relationship it depicts. Without gaining the patient's family's approval, surprisingly, Zhu applied a treatment that might be regarded as aggressive or offensive and might have caused him considerable trouble in the event that his treatment had proved unsuccessful. Another aspect of this case is that Zhu seemed to believe that being deceptive was necessary for the sake of her cure. This goes against normal medical ethics, yet he found support in his predecessor Zhang Congzheng.

Zhu Zhenheng took on another medical case of emotional disorder. Mr. Chen, a top degree holder of the National Civil Service Examination, once requested Zhu to treat his younger brother, who had been suffering from coughing up and vomiting blood. His face also had a dark complexion due to excessive worry. He had taken medicine for ten days but his condition remained the same. After his diagnosis Zhu told Chen: 'this ailment is caused by damage to the Kidneys due to frustration. It can be relieved by joy and is therefore curable'. Hence they moved the patient to a secluded place where he could easily have access to whatever he wanted, particularly food and clothing. He became so happy that his dark face regained its normal colour. Not long afterward, all his symptoms disappeared without any medication.[38] According to Zhu's judgment, this patient had been suffering from both worry and frustration. Although it is not clear whether his frustration came about from the pressure of his elder brother's achievement, we do know that the therapeutic method that 'joy overcomes worry' suggested by Zhu was effective.

In the Ming dynasty (1368–1644), some doctors showed no less interest in emotional therapy than their predecessors had. For example, Wan Quan 萬全 (1499–1582) believed that emotional disorders could only be cured by emotional manipulation and catharsis. In his view, it was easy to cure diseases caused by physical desires or daily exhaustion. By contrast, illnesses developed from the 'Five Intents' and the 'Seven Emotions' were more difficult to treat. These 'illnesses of spirit and thought' (*shensi zhi bing* 神思之病) cannot be restored, unless one is 'contented with one's lot' (*letian zhiming* 樂天知命) and 'irrespective of success or failure, good or bad' (*chengbai lidun zhi zhi duwai* 成敗利鈍 置之度外).[39] Zhang Jiebin held a similar opinion. As he put it, women's emotional illnesses can be relieved only when their wishes are fulfilled; they can also temporarily be freed when their pensiveness is restrained by anger. Men, on the other hand, cannot ultimately be cured unless they know 'when to yield and when not to' (*nengqu nengshen* 能屈能伸), or unless they have 'a detached mind and supreme wisdom' (*daguan shangzhi* 達觀上智)'.[40] In short, not only healers' therapeutic experiences but also patients' characters play a decisive role in the success of emotional therapies. Zhang Jiebin's viewpoint also highlights the gender difference in cases of emotional imbalance.

In medical practice, the emotional therapy applied by certain Ming doctors did not always follow the 'Principle of Mutual Conquest of the Five Phases'. *Shishan yian* 石山醫案 [Stone Mountain Medical Case Histories], 1519, records several cases of emotional therapy attributed to Wang Ji 汪機 (1463–1539) and other physicians. One of them involved a governor of nobility who had suffered from ailments when a drought and subsequent famine afflicted the land he governed. He called in more than ten doctors and none of them could cure him. Then one final doctor arrived. After reading the patient's pulse, he counted on his fingers, saying that 'in one day's evening it will rain'. Then he left without another word. The sick man thus wondered: 'does it mean that my illness is untreatable? Why did the doctor only mention the rain and not any medicine for me?' In the evening of the designated day, it actually did rain. The governor, overjoyed, got up and walked about his courtyard. By dawn his illness seemed to have gone away. Later, the doctor came again. He gladly asked the doctor the reason why he felt fully recovered when the rain began to drop. The doctor replied: 'Your Highness caught the illness due to excessive worry. I surmise that a faithful and compassionate high governor like you must worry about your people. If your illness was caused by worry about the drought [which had afflicted the people], it is also sensible that your illness would be cured by falling rain'.[41] The doctor in this case did not use any method of emotional manipulation. He simply accurately predicted the result of the treatment based on his superb medical reasoning and his ability to forecast the weather.

The *Stone Mountain* provides another case to demonstrate the principle that 'joy overcomes sorrow'. It is said that a district government runner once arrested a criminal, chained the criminal's neck with an iron cord and dragged him back to his office. When they were halfway there, the criminal suddenly jumped into the river and drowned. His family made false accusations against the runner, suing him for having tried to get money out of the criminal and forcing him to jump to his death. The lawsuit was later dismissed, but the runner was sentenced to pay an indemnity to the victim's family. As he had little money, he became 'ill from worry and anger, looking drunk and idiotic, speaking in a chaotic and absurd manner, and even losing consciousness'. When a doctor was sent in, he realized what had caused the patient's illness. As it could not be cured by medicine, he suggested that the patient's family have tin cast in the shape of silver ingots. When he put them beside the patient's bed, the latter regarded them as real silver. He grapsed them in his hands immediately and was filled with joy. Not long afterwards, he recovered.[42] This case is remarkable since the doctor applied a deceitful strategy to cure the patient's emotional disorder. We cannot tell whether the patient's illness would have recurred once he discovered the truth. In fact, not all doctors are willing to deceive patients for the sake of curing them. Yu Zhen 俞震 (1709–?), for example, argued that deception can only be a tentative means for treatment. A doctor should enlighten his patients' with 'proper principles' (*zhengli* 正理) when treating their 'mental illnesses' (*xin bing* 心病).[43]

Another recorded case involves a young woman's illness due to pensiveness. She and her mother deeply loved each other. Unfortunately, her mother died when she was just about to marry. Since then she could not stop thinking of her mother and lost her vitality, appeared tired and desired rest. Her chest and diaphragm were 'vexed and oppressed' (*fanmen* 煩悶), and she often felt feeble. No prescribed medicine worked. When one final doctor was called in, he judged that 'this illness was caused by pensiveness and no medicine can cure it'. The doctor knew that people preferred engaging 'witches' (*wu* 巫) for fortune-telling in the region where the patient live and thus asked the lady's husband to find a female spirit medium. They paid her stealthily and instructed her in what to say in her meeting with the patient. When the spirit medium visited the patient, firstly, she pretended to be possessed by the lady's deceased mother. Then she told the afflicted daughter: 'You and I feuded in our former lives. So you were born to harm me in this life. As your destiny got the better of mine, I died earlier than you. Now I am in Hell, thinking about revenge. Your sickness is critical simply because I brought it to you'. The patient was so angry at these words that she began to scold her false mother: 'I have been ill because of you. If you intend to harm me, why should I think of you?' Afterwards, she ceased suffering from pensive disorder and eventually recovered.[44] Again, this case provides evidence to show that anger overcomes pensiveness. It also reveals the doctor's deceptive tactic despite his good intention. Without the cooperation of the patient's family, however, this tactic could not have succeeded. Besides, the paradox of this case lies in the different conceptual frameworks of physician and patient. As Joanna Grant put it, the physician, while not necessarily believing in the power of the spirit medium, felt obliged to employ a medium in whom his patient deeply believed in order to achieve the effect based on his prognosis and medical rationale.[45] Indeed, this strategy worked.

In late Imperial China, owing to the rapidly growing population, an increasing number of men competed with each other in taking the Civil Service Examination. Very few of them were lucky enough to pass the Examination while most of them failed. The results of the examination produced very different degrees of emotional impact on the candidates. An unknown scholar suffered from a laughing disorder after passing the county exam sometime at the turn of the sixteenth century. Yuan Tian 袁體庵, a physician of Gaoyou 高郵 (in present Jiangsu Province), was called upon to treat him. During his diagnosis the doctor pretended to be surprised, stating: 'this illness is incurable and you have not long to live. You had better hurry back home or it will be too late'. He also asked the patient to bring his letter to a Mr. He 何 when passing by Zhenjiang 鎮江 (in present Jiangsu Province). When the scholar arrived in Zhenjiang, his laughing disorder was almost cured. He brought Yuan's letter to Mr. He, who read the letter and showed it to him. In it Yuan wrote that the scholar had become mad because of his excessive joy. To cure him the doctor decided to manipulate his emotions, causing worry and depression by the threat of death. The scholar realized why the doctor had done so and was so grateful to Yuan that he bowed to the North (where Yuan lived) several times before he departed.[46] This case demonstrates the principle that 'fear cures joy'. Yuan simply echoed Zhang Congzheng's therapeutic view: 'to frighten one by using force and threatening words'.

Not all of the practitioners of emotional therapy were physicians. In the renowned novel, *Rulin waishi* 儒林外史 [The Scholars], Fan Jin 范進, a middle-aged man, had failed several times in taking the Civil Service Examination. One year, he finally succeeded and attained the rank of Juren 舉人, but was so overjoyed that he unfortunately went mad. His family and neighbours were helpless. Later, they sent someone to find Fan's father-in-law, Butcher Hu 胡, the person of whom Fan was most fearful. When Hu arrived on the scene, he gave his son-in-law a slap on the face. Fan lost consciousness because of this blow and, when he had woken up, had regained his sanity.[47] Although Hu was not a physician, he cured Fan of his madness in a way that corresponds with the principle that 'fear overcomes joy'.

Likewise, another case caused by excessive joy was also cured by a non-physician. According to the record, a respected official, Li Qixing 李其性, was a native of Luyi 鹿邑, Guidefu 歸德府 (in present Henan Province). His ancestors had worked as farmers for several generations. In a year, Li passed the county examination. His father was very happy and he often laughed loudly. In the next spring, Li passed a higher examination and obtained the Jinshi 進士 degree. His father's laughing disorder became worse. Ten years later Li was promoted to the higher rank of censor, upon which his father's laughing disorder had become critical, with the laughing occurring all day and never ceasing. Li worried a great deal about his father and discussed his condition with a distinguished doctor at the Royal Academy of Medicine. Based on the doctor's advice, he asked his family to write a letter to his father, telling him that the son had just passed away. His father was so grieved that he nearly died of it, but over the course of ten days, he gradually recovered from his laughing disorder. Li then fabricated a post again to notify his father that 'the official was saved from death by a Doctor Zhao'. Li's father was no longer grieved and his laughing disorder never appeared again.[48] Once again, Li Qixing treated his father's illness caused by extreme joy simply by employing 'force and threatening words'.

Similar to the three cases described above, an eighteenth-century man was also afflicted by an illness due to extreme happiness. However, his illness was treated in a different way. Based on the record of a jotting, a 'district governor' (*fanxian* 藩憲) suddenly became blind one thousand days since his inauguration. He sent a runner to summon the physician Ye Tianshi 葉天士 (1667–1746). Doctor Ye asked the runner: 'Has the governor ever ruled elsewhere?' The runner replied: 'The Capital'. Ye asked again: 'Has he ever ruled anywhere else (besides the Capital)?' The man answered 'no'. Then Ye said: 'Please return and tell the governor immediately that I will not appear, unless the governor greets me with insignias of rank carried in procession'. Upon hearing this from the runner, the governor felt angry. His attendants tried to comfort him and said that Ye was a superb physician, almost a god, and that he should request the doctor to come. The governor thus said: 'Fine, let's heed what he said. If his treatment does not work, I will definitely punish him'. A procession was sent to greet Ye, but when they arrived at Ye's house, Ye told them that 'You should return and tell the governor immediately that I will not respond to such an invitation, unless the governor's wife comes to greet me in person'. In particular, Ye emphasized to them that 'you should tell the governor exactly what I had said. In case he blames someone, I shall be the one to be held responsible'. The runners could not help but return. When they told the governor Ye's words, he went mad and shouted loudly, causing all of his servants to tremble. In his rage, suddenly, his lost eyesight was recovered. At that very moment, Ye arrived at the door to ask for forgiveness. As he explained:

> I would not dare to be so aggressive, if not for the sake of therapy. The human spirit (*shen* 神) is lodged (*cang* 藏) in the Heart, and its intent (*zhi* 志) is joy. If a man's happiness is boundless, his spirit is dispersed and cannot lodge in the Heart. The eyes are the messengers (*shi* 使) of the Heart; the Heart is the lodge of the spirit. (Due to your recent promotion) you were so happy that your spirit was dispersed and you lost your eyesight. The *Inner Canon* states that sudden joy injures *yang* and sudden anger injures *yin*. When *yang* is injured, *yin* becomes flourishing. Only anger can make *yang*

> *qi* ascend; only great anger can repress *yin* and stretch *yang*. If I were not so bold, you would not have been so angry. I was obliged to do so. There was no other strategy.

The governor listened to Ye's words and decided to reward him.[49] This dramatic case reminds us that a doctor might make a medical judgment by oral queries without seeing the patient in person, although this is not always the case in reality. Moreover, it shows that practicing emotional therapy of this kind may risk the doctor's life. If fact, this case precisely exemplifies how risky it is to drive a patient – in particular one with a higher social status and official rank – mad. As Ye finally succeeded in his treatment and escaped the sentence threatened by the governor, these dramatic narratives certainly help to make the legend of his healing arts appear as cunning as a god. To some extent it satisfies what readers expect to read from a jotting that records 'the strange'.

Conclusion

In this study, it is argued that emotional therapy was interpreted and practiced in a rather 'psychologized' perspective in late Imperial China. On the one hand, the category of 'emotions' is created in nosology, and the 'Seven Emotions' were often viewed as sources of various illnesses. On the other hand, 'emotional counter-therapy' based on the theory of the 'Five Phases' became more popular in therapies of medical disorders originating in the emotions. No less important is a reinvented interpretation of the old therapeutic techniques of 'announcing causes' in terms of proto-psychotherapy. All these features help to characterize the realm of the mind in the late imperial period.

In general, emotional therapy with an appeal to emotional manipulation and communicational techniques seemed to have received positive effects. Nevertheless, given the fact that the genre of medical case histories only records successful cases, we should not underestimate the prevalence of drug therapy in the late imperial medical landscape. Although some physicians paid more attention to talking cures, this does not necessarily mean that they applied herbal remedies less than they did previously, regardless of whether the illnesses were related to emotions or not. None of the physicians discussed in this study went beyond this medical scope.

Returning to Zhang Congzheng, his *The Scholar Serving His Kin* illustrates several excellent and successful medical cases of 'counter-affects' therapy. Yet, it is also true that he treated patients' madness and emotional disorders more frequently in non-psychological ways. One instance is that he used a method of catharsis with salt water to treat one woman's laughing disorder. In another case he prescribed a herbal recipe to cure a woman who was unable to stop crying. In Zhang's medical work, the number of drug therapies is obviously much higher than that of talking cures.[50] The reasons why most Chinese physicians, despite their acknowledgement of emotional therapy, preferred drug remedies, require explanation.

The first factor to be explained should be the physicians themselves. In his research of the eleven cases in Wu Kun's *Research on Medical Formulas*, Nathan Sivin characterizes the medical practice of 'emotional counter-therapy' as follows: Doctors need a great deal of clinical resourcefulness in order to respond to dynamic pathological and physiological processes. The therapy of first resort was usually material, i.e. the use of drugs. When some dysfunctions of emotional origin are so serious that conventional means will fail, then this residuum can yield only to powerful counterbalancing emotions. In other words, emotional manipulation was just one – and usually the last one – of the doctors' options. Hence Sivin concludes that the 'emotional counter-therapy' in Wu's work is not represented as a 'theoretical innovation', but as a 'practical expedient'.[51]

Sivin's general observation is quite true, since it can also be applied to the cases in this study. Nonetheless, there is more to say about the complicated circumstance of the physician-patient encounter. Emotional therapy and talking cures can apply to patients of both lower and higher status. Yet, some earlier cases show that the doctors who had employed the method of emotional therapy had to pay a high price for their treatment; sometimes it even cost them their lives. A good example is Wen Zhi 文摯 (the Warring States), who was finally killed when his emotional therapy had enraged King Qi 齊王. Another instance is Hua Yuanhua 華元化 (Hua Tuo 華佗), who had luckily survived an official's attempt to kill him owing to a similar therapy. These two doctors' talents were rare and precious such that patients could hardly expect to find from among a hundred thousand people; nevertheless such doctors encountered unexpected disasters because of their emotional therapy. Ye Tianshi, who was almost punished after he had driven a high official into a rage, is also such a case. Zhang Congzheng thus laments: 'If a doctor cannot protect himself by his most subtle medical skills, does it not mean that medicine is no more than 'undignified techniques' (*jian ji* 賤技)?'[52] It is somewhat true that medical practitioners were despised by the majority of societies since the days of antiquity. In Zhang's times, the status of doctors remained no higher than that of other kinds of 'healers', given the fact that both doctors and shamans might be summoned together. Emotional therapy did not become the preferred choice of doctors, probably because their life could be endangered, if their treatment proved unfavourable.

However, the factor of unequal social status between physicians and patients seems insufficient to explain why the therapy by 'counter-affects' was not popular among patients of low rank as well. As Zhang Congzheng claimed, the therapeutic methods based on the 'Principle of Mutual Conquest of the Five Phases' must be tricky and unpredictable: if one has no 'competence', one cannot use these five methods. Zhu Zhenheng and Wu Kun held similar attitudes. The success of talking cures thus depends on a doctor's talent and the power of his language. Sometimes he is even obliged to apply deception or use threatening language to change a patient's abnormal behaviour. In short, physicians' accurate diagnostic and sophisticated psychological techniques were certainly the key to emotional therapy. A qualified doctor always knows how to detect and distinguish his patient's emotional states, and then he applies appropriate emotional manipulation by subtle language skills. In such circumstances, the practice of emotional therapy is obviously more complicated and even more difficult than drug therapy.

Not only a doctor but a patient needs to be competent. Whether a patient's emotional states are suitable to talking cures is also crucial to the effectiveness of emotional therapy. Emotional manipulation will not work if a patient' mind is too dull to receive his doctor's messages. Other factors of the physician-patient relationship should also be taken into account. Gender is an important facet. In late Imperial China, some male doctors complained that women's emotional disorders were particularly hard to cure. The sense of shame that distanced the female patients from their male physicians added to the difficulty of communication between both sides.[53] In an age when patients often change their healers again and again, the extent to which a physician can obtain full information about his patient becomes questionable. As it was not always easy for a doctor to fully grasp his patient's history and make a medical judgment promptly, he would have to acquire necessary information from other sources, e.g. his patient's family members and attendants. In this study, several cases show that the patients' family members and attendants chose to trust and follow the doctors' therapeutic suggestions. Without their mutual consent and cooperation, the doctors' therapeutic tactics would not have possibly worked. The father of Zhu Zhenheng's female patient, Li Qixing's family and the attendants of Ye Tianshi's patient are all such cases. Li's case also indicates there is no sharp line between therapy performed by doctors and emotional manipulation carried out by laymen.

The last, but by no means least, factor to be taken into account is the aetiology of illness. As stated earlier, ancient Chinese doctors tended to believe that imbalanced emotions caused different motions of *qi* and therefore resulted in corresponding symptoms. That is, emotional disorders were necessarily involved in the disturbance of *qi*. Apart from emotional manipulation based on the 'Principle of Mutual Conquest of the Five Phases', drug therapy aimed at the regulation of *qi* can certainly be applied to these illnesses as well. As a fourteenth-century medical work comments, officially compiled books of pharmaceutics since the Song dynasty (960–1279) always suggest a drug therapy aimed at regulation of imbalanced *qi* in the treatment of the 'Seven Emotions'. As a result, doctors could neither distinguish the symptoms of heat, phlegm, depletion or repletion along with the Seven Emotions; nor did they acknowledge the different states of patients' emotions.[54] Yang Jizhou 楊繼洲 (1552–1620) expressed a similar complaint. He said that the *Inner Canon* states clearly the therapeutic methods for the healing of emotional disorders, but most doctors just abandoned them, which appeared to him to be really odd.[55] These observations remind us of pre-modern doctors' general ignorance of emotional manipulation despite a few exceptions. In the late imperial period, most doctors – including Wang Kentang 王肯堂 (1549–1613) who provided a systematic nosology of 'mental states' (*shenzhi* 神志) in his medical work – tended to regard various emotional disorders as *qi* disorders and therefore generated drug recipes as their prescription.[56] From an overall view, the devising of an 'emotions' category in Wu Kun and some other works does not result in a split between mind and body or between what moderns would call somatic and psychological symptoms.[57]

In conclusion, body-and-mind holism remained influential in doctors' aetiology, diagnostics and therapeutics in late Imperial China. Many doctors emphasized that the illnesses caused by extreme emotions could not be cured by normal drug therapy. Some of them even went further in applying subtle skills of talking cures for the manipulation of patients' emotions. Yet, due to the restrictions of aetiology and various factors of the healer-patient relationship, these doctors' 'psychologized' approaches to emotional disorders could not go beyond the frame of *qi* cosmology. They never prevailed in pre-modern Chinese medicine, while their counterpart – drug therapy – did.

3 MEDICAMENTS AND PERSUASION: MEDICAL THERAPIES FOR MADNESS IN NINETEENTH-CENTURY CHINA

Fabien Simonis

> 'Emotionless herbs and plants cannot treat emotional illnesses'.
> (無情之草木　不能治有情之病)
>
> Wu Tang 吴瑭, 1836

The first time physician Wu Tang (1758–1836) went to examine him, Mr. Bao was chained to a large grindstone in an empty room, hands and feet shackled, dirty and dishevelled, his lower parts exposed and the rest of his emaciated body barely covered by garments he had tried to shred.[1] If his wife refused to see him daily as he demanded, Bao would yell himself hoarse and wail so unbearably that a family member would have to attend to his needs, after which he would be slightly appeased, but he would later resume his uproar, without one day of lull. Dozens of doctors had failed to cure him of his mania, which had lasted for seven years.

How did pre-twentieth-century Chinese physicians understand this kind of insane behaviour and how did they attempt to treat it? On what conceptions of the body and its pathologies were these approaches based? Were some therapies more common than others, and if so, why? This chapter starts with a historiographic and conceptual survey, and then draws from Mr. Bao's case several themes that will help to answer these questions. These themes include the nature of the medical object 'madness' in pre-psychiatry China (and how it differs from 'mental illness'), the complex ties between emotions and insanity in Chinese medical representations, the relative importance of medication and exhortation in the treatment of psycho-behavioural pathologies, and the construction and enactment of efficacy in therapeutic relations. By the end, readers will be able to discern what was typical from what was unique in Wu Tang's approach, and will therefore have grasped the main medical ways of handling insanity in late Imperial China.

Partly because madness was considered similar to other illnesses in both patho-mechanisms and treatment, it was the object of no specialized medical literature, and no debate concerning it had any major impact on broad doctrinal developments. As shown in my previous work, changes in the understanding and therapy of insanity can be explained only if we are aware of broader transformations in medical thinking.[2] The study of a single disorder can thus help to elucidate broader issues in Chinese medical history. By the same token but in reverse, a single case file by Wu Tang will serve here as a hub of issues that will allow us to explore Chinese medical approaches to insanity at large.

When they discussed acts, words and people that they considered mad, Chinese physicians, officials and ritual specialists alike used an array of intelligibly related concepts at the centre of which were *kuang* 狂, *dian* 瘨/顛/癲 and *feng* 風/瘋.[3] In various pre-imperial texts, *kuang* had meant anything from extravagant or impetuous to crazy or furious. The *Shuowen jiezi* 說文解字, a lexicon that was compiled around AD 100, glosses it as 'a rabid dog' (*zhi quan* 狾犬). Yet starting around the first century BC when the *Huangdi neijing* 黃帝內經 [Yellow Emperor's Inner Canon] was first compiled, *kuang* in medical texts stabilized to mean something like 'mania'. One of the earliest instances of *dian* I have found is from the Mawangdui medical manuscripts (copied around 200 BC), where it is written 瘨 and refers to an epileptiform disorder that Donald Harper translates as 'seizure sickness'.[4] The character *dian* 癲, which is now the orthodox graphy for the illness associated with *kuang*, does not appear in the *Shuowen jiezi* and probably did not exist at the time. It only became common in the Song dynasty (960–1279), probably as a result of the merging of *dian* 瘨 with *dian* 顛 ('upside down'), a term that writers from the Six Dynasties used, sometimes in conjunction with *kuang*, to refer to eccentricity. *Feng*, for its part, originally meant 'wind' in expressions like *fengkuang* 風狂 (Wind mania) and *xinfeng* 心風 (Heart Wind), both of which refer to something like madness. By the fourteenth century, mainstream medicine had stopped attributing insanity to Wind, but the sound *feng* had become so associated with madness that it was lexicalized in expressions like 'crazy monk' (*feng seng* 風僧) or 'to have a fit of Wind/madness' (*fa feng* 發風). In the seventeenth century, a doctor from the Huizhou region in Anhui identified *fengzi* 風子 (which is now written 瘋子 and means 'madman') as a popular term for *kuang*.[5] By the nineteenth century, *feng* in all expressions referring to madness was usually written 瘋 (composed of 風, 'wind', and the disease radical 疒), but this was a graphic novelty, not a semantic one.

Despite their different origins, these words were often used interchangeably. Their specific referents, connotations and performative force depended on the practices within which they were deployed. What Qing law referred to as 'madness illness' (*fengbing* 瘋病), for instance, differed from medical 'insanity' (*diankuang* 癲狂), but their differences derived from the functioning of judicial and legislative operations rather than from the terms themselves.[6]

My wider study of mad acts, mad speech and mad persons in late Imperial China highlights the disunity of 'madness' in various Chinese fields of practice and refashions the resulting dispersion into an intelligible research object. Here, the focus is on explaining how late Imperial Chinese doctors understood and treated psycho-behavioural disorders. For lack of space, this chapter will discuss neither the legal handling of crimes committed in a state of insanity, nor the abundance of ritual treatments for mad behaviour that pervaded China in the nineteenth century, such as 'trials of the insane' (*shen fengzi* 審瘋子), the chanting of Buddhist sutras, Daoist exorcisms and other apotropaic methods.[7]

Like psychiatrists, Chinese physicians faced and handled deeds, words and people that they labelled mad. Yet this article is not a history (or even a prehistory) of 'Chinese psychiatry'. The material presented can nonetheless serve as ground for comparison with the psychiatric concepts and practices that translators, specialists and a few institutions imported into China starting in the late nineteenth century, in order to appreciate how Chinese doctors themselves understood insane behaviour.

Psycho-Behavioural Pathologies in Chinese Medicine

Until recently, there had been no serious historical work on that which may be called madness in Chinese medicine. The many studies that tried to identify precursors to modern psychiatry did not take original Chinese categories seriously.[8] Because symptomatic descriptions are more likely to give China a place in a 'grand titration' of medical discoveries than obsolete explanations and treatments, this scholarly literature focused primarily on the way ancient treatises described insanity.[9] Even Chinese historians have mostly concentrated on new discoveries, on categories that have survived into the modern field of 'traditional Chinese medicine', and on views that they consider compatible with those of current science. Such research often praises ancient physicians' 'achievements' and 'contributions' to Chinese understanding of 'mental illness' or to the development of 'Chinese psychiatry'.[10]

Yet 'traditional Chinese psychiatry' never spoke of itself, was not represented by any institution and was not manifested in any specialized text. If we collect observations and techniques from various texts and treat them as precursors of something to come, we risk reducing the activities of Chinese medical writers to having hovered around – and ultimately failed to find – something they were not even looking for, for instance a full-fledged concept of 'mental illness'. Besides the difficulty of claiming that people contributed to solving problems they never posed, that approach only identifies superficial resemblances with psychiatry and interprets them, as if by default, through the frames of either modern psychiatry or 'traditional Chinese medicine', neither of which existed before the twentieth century.

In recent Western scholarship, *dian-kuang-xian* 癲狂癎 has replaced mental illness as a centre of attention, a typology that echoes recent Chinese compilations in which these illnesses also form an inseparable trio.[11] This approach suitably avoids the dead end of 'traditional Chinese psychiatry', but it rests on two fragile assumptions: 1) that *dian-kuang-xian* was a natural unit valid for all of Chinese history, and 2) that *dian*, *kuang*, and *xian* were 'types of madness'. Instead of saying that *xian*, which medical sources consistently described as a convulsive disorder, was a form of madness, why not claim (perhaps even more plausibly) that madness was a form of seizure? But even this would be missing the point, which is that *dian*, *kuang*, and *xian* were not sub-types of any higher-order category like 'madness'.[12]

Whereas modern psychiatrists give different names to distinct clusters of behavioural and psychological symptoms, for most of Chinese history there were no 'types of madness', but only one or two insanity disorders – *kuang* and *dian*, or simply *kuang* or *diankuang* on its own – characterized by a variety of pathological acts and affects. Although medical historians usually interpret *dian* as a form of madness distinct from *kuang*, a clear symptomatic distinction between *dian* and *kuang* only crystallized in the nineteenth century, when *dian* came to refer to an extreme apathy contrasting with manic *kuang*.[13] Even then, not all physicians accepted this demarcation. The colloquial term *feng* 瘋 (crazy, mad), which is widely used in modern Chinese, rarely appeared in late imperial medical texts, not because it referred to a different kind of insanity, but because it was a vernacular term rather than a classical illness category.

Despite the simplicity of the nosology of madness in Chinese medicine, and marked differences in how psychiatrists and Chinese physicians produced knowledge, *dian*, *kuang* and *feng* refer to the same kinds of overt behavioural pathologies on which psychiatry has focused most of its attention, from the era of 'mad-doctoring' to the latest editions of the DSM. Regardless of whether it was called *kuang*, *dian*, *diankuang* or *feng*, insanity was an obvious disorder, a blatant loss of social competence. Physicians focused on such overt 'behavioural dislocations' probably because they were mostly called to treat openly insane men and women – a spinster who escaped to the market naked, a failed examination candidate who sang all day, or an innkeeper who believed a white monkey was fanning his wife's feet with a large fan.[14] Vaguer feelings of mental discomfort are seldom discussed in medical documents, probably because they were rarely reported to doctors.

To avoid the notion of 'mental illness', these pathologies shall here be called 'psycho-behavioural'. 'Psycho' is used as a prefix because most treatise writers and physicians attributed insanity to dysfunctions of the Heart (*xin* 心), the command centre of mental activities. The term 'psycho-behavioural' may remind some readers of 'psycho-behavioural therapies' in contemporary behavioural science and psychology, but here it is used only to characterize the most typical *symptoms* of madness in Chinese medical texts, not to allude to an unrelated modern field.

Supervenience and its Consequences

To help make sense of Chinese understandings of psycho-behavioural disorders, and to dispel the impression that they stood alone as a category of illness, let me borrow the concept of 'supervenience' from modern philosophy of mind. For our purposes, it can be simplified as follows: process A is said to 'supervene' upon process B when changes in process A (a delusion or an emotion, for instance) are always accompanied by changes in process B (say, brain chemistry or the dynamics of bodily fluids).[15]

In Chinese medicine, both the regular functioning of the Heart and its dysfunctions (manic behaviour, delirium, anxiety, forgetfulness, etc.) supervened upon a somatic process. Put in the broadest terms, Chinese physicians attributed mad symptoms either to invasion by external forces ('deviant Qi', Wind, ghosts) or to internal imbalances strong enough to generate pathological effects. They claimed to cure patients by expelling these external invaders or redressing these imbalances, sometimes both. Because of this emphasis on dynamic situations, the medical tradition considered permanent disorders anomalous. Chinese physicians thus rarely medicalized personality and almost never called patients 'mad people' or 'madmen' (*kuangren* 狂人, *fengzi* 瘋子) and the like.

An important difference between Chinese medicine and modern psychiatry is that whereas the latter identifies imbalances – in neurotransmitters, for example – that almost exclusively produce psychiatric disorders, Chinese doctors claimed that the imbalanced fluids that triggered insanity or underlay excessive emotions could also generate symptoms that psychiatrists would consider purely physical. Excessive inner Fire could produce not only anger and hallucinations but also nosebleeds, ticklishness and constipation.

For complex reasons that shall not be explained here, *kuang*, which was classified as a Wind disorder in all important pre-Song treatises and discussed under anti-Wind remedies in most Song formularies, was by the fourteenth century almost always attributed to the action of Fire and mucus.[16] Although demonic etiologies remained prominent even in mainstream medicine, many physicians attributed possession-like symptoms to the sudden blocking of the 'Heart's openings' (*xinqiao* 心竅) by mucus.[17] Doctors who attributed madness to the action of Fire and mucus used purgatives and emetics to wash out Fire and expel mucus. These aggressive therapies could go hand in hand with replenishing when Fire was diagnosed to be rooted in depletion.

To a crucial extent, the supervenience between mental and physiological processes in Chinese medical thinking was inscribed in medical terminology. Most physicians thought that madness occurred when the Heart (*xin* 心) or its residing Spirit (*shen* 神) could not fulfil their functions. The common translation of *xin* as 'heart-mind' highlights the uneasiness of rendering into English what was self-evident in Chinese: the junction of mind and structure in a single word. As a hinge between the 'mental' and the 'physical', *xin* allowed Chinese physicians to trace insanity to a somatic imbalance, to mental processes or to both at the same time without cognitive dissonance. We find the same double denotation in *shen*, which could refer to spiritual or vital functions but also to the numinous fluid that underlay them. Common medical expressions could accentuate either meaning of Heart or Spirit. *Shi xin* 失心, for instance, is better rendered as 'loss of mind' than 'loss of heart', not only because 'loss of heart' implies dejection rather than mindlessness in English, but also because what was 'lost' according to the Chinese expression was not the heart as an organ but the functions it was thought to assure. When, on the other hand, a medical text claimed that 'failed Blood flushed the Heart' (*bai xie chong xin* 敗血沖心), the physical organ was unambiguously involved.

The two notions of Heart and Spirit provided an established semantic path and a ready-made conceptual schema for tracing psycho-behavioural pathology to physiological processes. They allowed seamless shifts between the mental and the somatic, two domains that English speakers usually describe with different sets of terms even when they do not adhere to the dualism of mind and body.

This being said, both ancient Chinese texts and late imperial physicians could discriminate between the body and mental activities when needed. Chapter Twenty-Five of the influential *Suwen* 素問 [Basic Questions] version of the *Yellow Emperor's Inner Canon* (first century BC), for instance, explains the difference between 'Spirit' and 'somatic form' (*xing* 形). In a roughly contemporaneous text, we read that 'in madness, the somatic form is not damaged' (*kuang zhe xing bu kui* 狂者形不虧), whereas the preface to an eighteenth-century treatise states that 'in past and present there have been two great [kinds of] illnesses: those of the Heart [mind?] and those of the body' (*gu jin you da bing er, qi yi zai xin, qi yi zai shen* 古今有大病二 其一在心 其一在身).[18]

Yet the distinctions that some medical writers sometimes made between 'Heart' and 'Spirit' on the one hand and 'embodied person' (*shen* 身) or 'somatic form' on the other – or even between mental and somatic illnesses – did not shape the social organization of therapy. Indeed, late imperial physicians were expected to treat all disorders.[19]

Because of the common grounding of all illnesses, including those of the Heart, in physiological imbalances, there was no independent notion of mental or behavioural illness in Chinese medicine. *Kuang* was discussed next to illnesses that were neither mental nor behavioural, and was considered treatable by similar means, chiefly medicinal decoctions. In *Yitong* 醫通 [Comprehensive Medicine] for instance, Zhang Lu 張璐 (1617–99) recommended three recipes for curing madness that could also respectively treat 'tremors' (*zhanzhen* 顫震), 'blood accumulations' (*xuxue* 蓄血) and headaches.[20]

Though all Chinese physicians would have agreed that madness always had a somatic substrate – excessive inner Fire, depletion of Cardiac Qi, etc. – that could be detected by pulse taking, they differed in the degree of supervenience they accepted. Most doctrinal explanations and clinical accounts reduced madness to the non-mental processes that underlay it and gave the impression that all that was needed to cure it was drugs that acted directly on these processes. But not all physicians were reductionists. For most doctors, emotions were just one kind of internal imbalance among others. Emotions could supervene upon (or co-vary with) their underlying fluids without being reducible to them. The fact that medical writers rarely attempted to specify how, in organic terms, people reacted emotionally to the outside world suggests that they found it difficult to explain affects purely as products of somatic flows.

Because the main focus of psychodynamics in Chinese medicine was the realm of emotions, it is tempting to take them as the core of a comparison with psychiatry, but I prefer to view Chinese understanding of emotions as a peninsula of mental and behavioural content attached to a continent of somatic medicine. I shall explore this continent in more detail when I discuss the case of Mr. Bao, to which we are now ready to turn.

Wu Tang and His Case Files

Though his family was registered in the Huai'an 懷安 area in northern Jiangsu, Wu Tang – also known as Wu Jutong – lived mostly in Beijing from 1783 until his death in 1836, and practiced medicine there for at least forty years starting in 1793.[21] An avid admirer of Suzhou physician Ye Gui 葉桂 (1667–1746), Wu was particularly struck by Ye's work on Warm-factor illnesses (*wenbing* 溫病).[22] Following a friend's advice, in 1798 he started to collate his own treatise on these pathologies and named it *Wenbing tiaobian* 溫病條辨 [Systematic Distinctions on Warm-Factor Illnesses] upon completing it in 1813. Late in his life, Wu also compiled a short doctrinal work titled *Yi yi bing shu* 醫醫病書 [Curing the Ills of Medicine] and a collection of case histories that includes Mr. Bao's case.

Case files rose in popularity in late imperial times following the spread of the notion that illness was an ever-changing phenomenon whose facets could never be exhaustively described. In this view, each morbid event potentially required a unique therapy. The disciples and admirers of Zhejiang physician Zhu Zhenheng 朱震亨 (1282–1358) were the leading transmitters of this flexible art of prescription in the fourteenth, fifteenth and sixteenth centuries.[23] By the early nineteenth century when Wu Tang was practicing, a large number of doctors were keeping records of their clinical encounters, both for their own reference and for their patients. Once assembled into books, these records could be brought to bear on the doctrinal issues of the day.[24]

Wu Tang's *Wu Jutong yi'an* 吳鞠通 [Medical Case Files] were not a simple clinical companion to his treatise on Warm illnesses. Like most Chinese case collections, it aimed to demonstrate the doctor's ability to treat all illnesses, from furor to furuncles. Because Wu and his contemporaries believed that most disorders arose from similar bodily imbalances, the way they handled any disorder depended on their general understanding of human vitality, pathogenesis and therapeutic principles.

Case files were also more than illustrations of general doctrines. Records of clinical encounters describe specific symptoms rather than the formulaic ones found in doctrinal compilations. When discussing insanity, medical treatises usually borrowed formulations from the venerable *Yellow Emperor's Inner Canon*, a disparate textual corpus which, for most of the two millennia that followed its compilation in the first century BC, served as a repository of authoritative doctrinal statements. In excerpting this text, physicians probably assumed that educated readers would immediately recognize these turns of phrase and what they referred to. Case records, on the other hand, were designed to demonstrate a practitioner's diagnostic perspicacity and accurate prescriptions. The case form therefore encouraged physicians to write about unique cases rather than prototypes. Case files also provide information on the social and moral significance of madness and on gender differences in the treatment of an illness that treatises typically portrayed as un-gendered and morally neutral.

In Wu Tang's case collection, a section called 'Insanity' (*diankuang*) appears in Fascicle 2 between sections on 'Liver-related swellings' (*ganyong* 肝癰) and 'Depletion and wasting' (*xulao* 虛勞). As we saw above, the placing of such symptomatically diverse illnesses side by side is by no means surprising as all of these disorders were attributed to similar patho-mechanisms. Every case in the insanity section of Wu's collection provides the name and age of the patient (with one exception) and continues with a description of the symptoms, multi-levelled discussions of etiology (food, emotions, cosmic configurations), and details on diagnostic and therapeutic strategies.[25] All cases contain follow-up treatments and all but one end with a successful cure. The case of Mr. Bao appears between cases dated 1809 and 1827.

Madness, Emotions and Social Disappointments

At the beginning of his narrative, Wu Tang notes in formulaic language that Mr. Bao 'had first become ill because his achievements did not follow his ambitions' (*xian yin gong ming bu sui er bing* 先因功名不遂而病). Most late imperial medical writers interpreted this kind of distress as an emotion. Insanity had not always been discussed alongside emotions, or emotions considered as possible causes of madness. One of the earliest explicit connections of *dian* or *kuang* with emotions in a Chinese medical text appears in Wang Bing's 王冰 eighth-century annotated edition of the *Suwen* 素問 [Basic Questions], one version of the *Yellow Emperor's Inner Canon*.[26] On a textually corrupted passage (or one Wang incorrectly emended) that read 'mineral drugs: fits of *dian*; herbal drugs: fits of *kuang*' (*shi yao fa dian, fang cao fa kuang* 石藥發瘨 芳草發狂), he glossed: 'Excessive joy is [makes?] *dian*, excessive anger is [makes?] *kuang*' (*duo xi wei dian, duo nu wei kuang* 多喜為瘨 多怒為狂).[27] Wang Bing's association of *dian* with emotions diverged from contemporary medical texts, which described *dian* as an epileptiform illness, but found support in non-medical usage, where *dian* and *kuang* had become close equivalents or were used together in the compound *diankuang*, which referred broadly to 'insanity'.[28] Perhaps Wang's description of *dian* as excessive joy derived from the *Inner Canon*'s frequent tying of *kuang* with anger and the perceived need to describe *dian* as the converse of *kuang*.

Wang Bing's interpretation of *dian* and *kuang* remained obscure until the twelfth century. A physician and medical writer called Liu Wansu 劉完素 (*c.* 1120–1200), who lived in northern China under the Jin dynasty (1115–1234), brought it back into visibility by reinterpreting it. In his *Suwen xuanji yuanbing shi* 素問玄機原病式 [Method for Tracing Illnesses to their Origins with the Mysterious Mechanism of the Basic Questions], completed before 1186, Liu approved of Wang's association of *dian* with joy and *kuang* with anger, but because he understood all emotions as rooted in excessive inner Heat, he concluded that, 'because all five emotions can generate Heat, *kuang* can be triggered by any of the five emotions. It is simply that anger is [a] more common [cause]' (*kuang wu zhi suo fa jie wei re, gu kuang zhe wu zhi jian fa, dan nu duo er* 況五志所發皆為熱 故狂者五志間發 但怒多爾).[29] Liu's view of both madness and affects diverged from the *Inner Canon*, which had explained emotions as processes of Qi (not effects of inner Heat) and had only associated *kuang* with anger (not with excessive emotions in general). The pathological scenario Liu proposed created a hinge between insanity and emotions – as cognate products of inner Heat – that made it natural for them to be discussed together.

To Liu's teachings on the pathological power of Fire and inner Heat, Zhu Zhenheng – the fourteenth-century physician who put so much value on case records – added ethical and cosmological precepts from the Neo-Confucian school known as the 'Learning of the Way' (*Daoxue* 道學), whose main upholders also viewed emotions as rooted in inner Fire. Zhu's purposely syncretic teachings became the most prestigious set of medical doctrines from 1350 to at least 1550.[30] Though most of the texts attributed to him and his disciples did not articulate the connections between madness and emotions any further than Liu had, they spread the Fire-mucus etiology of insanity through China's medical circles.

Despite Zhu's authority, until the sixteenth century few cases of madness in the Chinese medical literature were given an emotional content. One could become crazy from excessive heat, sudden fright or mucus encroaching upon the Heart, and there were routine ways of explaining how emotions supervened upon these processes, as when despondency left the Heart depleted and vulnerable to a mucus attack. Most emotionally grounded cases of madness were treated with medicinal decoctions that acted on these imbalances rather than on the emotions that had triggered them. Even the manipulation of emotions in 'therapy by counter-affect' was rooted in a particular understanding of how the viscera interacted inside the body.[31]

Wu Tang's formulaic tracing of Mr. Bao's insanity to social disappointments ('his achievements did not follow his ambitions') emerged in the writings of sixteenth-century physicians from the Jiangnan region, where low examination quotas were failing to accommodate the rising number of candidates, creating a large number of men frustrated by their thwarted careers. Those medical writers tended to call this form of insanity *dian* rather than *kuang*.[32] To distinguish these two illnesses, Sun Yikui 孫一奎 (1522–1619), from Huizhou in Anhui, proposed to understand *dian* as rooted in depletion – itself interpreted as a result of emotional setbacks – and *kuang* as triggered by pathological over-repletion. Although Sun's distinctions were often retained in later medical treatises, even physicians who called emotional madness '*dian*' 顛/癲 rarely abided by this definition in their case files.[33] By the nineteenth century, it had become routine knowledge that emotions could lead to madness, but the taxonomic travails surrounding *dian* and *kuang* still had not been settled. This is why Wu Tang could refer to Mr. Bao's madness as *kuang* and still attribute it to frustration, though, as we shall now see, he saw Bao's emotion as rooted in somatic excess rather than the more usual depletion.

Diagnosis, Etiology and Drug Therapy

In the next segment of the case file, Wu Tang claimed that more than a hundred doctors had come to see Mr. Bao, including the best in the capital as well as illustrious physicians from several regions in the Lower Yangzi delta, but that they had all failed to cure the patient.[34] He was the latest doctor to visit, and would presumably be sent away like the others if he fell short.

Wu remarked that most healers had used replenishing drugs. Although manic symptoms like Bao's usually called for aggressive therapies, other physicians had probably decided to replenish because – following medical treatises – they had diagnosed his madness caused by failed ambitions as being rooted in depletion. By stating that most doctors had chosen a replenishing therapy, Wu of course implied that they were wrong and prepared to emphasize the extent of his own success where so many of the best had failed.

In interpreting Bao's symptoms, Wu Tang did not make use of what Jan Goldstein calls 'the power to classify', that is, the ability to choose accurately between different illness entities in a context in which identification of the illness by name has great explanatory power.[35] Indeed, as we saw above, there were effectively no types of madness in Chinese medicine, just one multifaceted psycho-behavioural disorder – *kuang* or *diankuang* – that could manifest itself in a variety of ways and for a variety of reasons. Simply naming *kuang* therefore ensured no more than superficial intelligibility and had no therapeutic consequence.

Physicians like Wu Tang decided on a therapy only after they had identified the imbalance that was generating the illness at hand. They usually grasped the root of a disorder by feeling the patient's pulses. Because the doctors palpated the pulse looking for signs of 'mucus and Fire', 'stasis' or 'Liver Wind', problems that had arisen from interpersonal even were often reduced to imbalances in the organism.

Characteristically, Wu Tang interpreted Bao's insane behaviour through categories that drew diagnosis away from the patient's daily context: 'I examined his pulses: the Six Sections were strung, extended and sturdy. I said: 'This is a manifestation of over-repletion, not depletion'' (*zhen qi mai, liu bu xian chang er jing, yu yue ci shi zheng, fei xu zheng ye* 診其脈 六部弦長而勁 余曰此實症 非虛症也). Wu recognized that social or emotional frustrations could cause serious madness, but he still viewed this process as somatically grounded: Bao's disappointments had turned into an excess of inner Fire that Wu would now try to eliminate with 'extremely bitter' cooling drugs decocted into a potent purgative.[36] This was not a revolutionary diagnosis. Indeed, an excess of inner Fire and mucus had by Wu's time become the most commonly identified medical root of insanity. Also typically, the target of Wu's therapeutic intervention was the same body that suffered from headaches or urinary discomfort.

Two doses of the cooling prescription proved successful: Bao's 'rash talking diminished and he carried himself more calmly' (*wang yu shao er ju dong an jing* 妄語少而舉動安靜). Perhaps the purgatives made Bao excrete until he became weak and subdued, but this weakness was part of the expectations created by the etiological conceptions on the basis of which Wu had prescribed the purgatives, which was that psycho-behavioural symptoms could be treated by acting on the somatic processes they supervened upon. The widespread Chinese use of purgatives and emetics to treat insanity must have stemmed in part from their perceived efficacy. These drugs 'worked' insofar as they produced a visible effect on the patient. Bao's calmer state must have been seen not as the temporary result of a debilitating purge, but as the quick and successful reduction of the Fire that had been feeding his insanity.

The day after he calmed Mr. Bao with purgatives, Wu Tang prescribed Yin-replenishing drugs, a strategy he frequently adopted in his treatment of Warm illnesses.[37] Although Wu did not give the detail of his new prescription, we know that he was trying to keep the purgatives from 'breaking' (*zhe* 折) the patient, whose vitality had been drained by a long illness. Wu's altered recipe illustrates the therapeutic dynamism of Chinese medicine, by which remedies are adapted to the changes in illness configuration that result from the ingestion of drugs.

Persuasion and Efficacy

The effects of the adjusted prescription were probably more unexpected than Wu cared to admit in his well-woven narrative. As Bao's relatives came to report the next day, the patient's

> 'wailing and chaotic talk are many times worse than before, and there is not a moment of calm. We think these symptoms are impossible to treat and we are afraid he will almost certainly die. You need not examine him again'. (*jiao qian zhi jiao xiao wang yu jia shu bei zhi duo, wi yi ke zhi jing, ci zheng xiang by neng zhi, liang qi bi si, xian sheng ke bu bi zai zhen yi* 較前之叫哮妄語加數倍之多　無一刻之靜　此症想不能治　諒其必死　先生可不必再診矣)

On the verge of being dismissed like his predecessors, Wu affirmed his grasp on the therapeutic process by convincing Bao's family that the imbalance that was causing the illness was being invisibly modified even as the patient appeared more vehement. We can also hypothesize that Bao's madness resumed simply because he was no longer weakened by the purgatives. In any case Wu prudently renounced replenishing Yin for the moment and went back to prescribing Fire-draining drugs in heavier amounts and for a more sustained stretch than the first time. A few days later, the patient had become 'largely lucid' (*da wei ming bai* 大為明白).

In treating madness the goal of most Chinese physicians was to put an end to disabling symptoms rather than to foster their patients' well-being or to reinstate them into meaningful social relations. They may have judged the latter to be the task of the patient's family. Indeed, most medical case records end when the patient has stopped acting madly.

In the case we are discussing, however, Bao's return to lucidity marks a sudden turn in the narrative. As both the clinical encounter and the case record draw to a close, for the first time Wu reports talking to his patient.

> He contracted his illness because his ideas fell short and because he could not reach the highest degree in the knowledge of texts. [But] since being able to reach the apex is not something one can forcibly achieve, what is there to be angry about? In life, filial piety means to be concerned for the heart of one's parents. I severely reprimanded

> him: he lowered his head, without reply. After that, I progressively decreased the bitter drugs and added Yin replenishers. Half a day later we removed his penal implements, he put on his clothes and cap, and we kneeled and bowed together. His spirits were no different from those of a healthy person. He became much stronger after he took one course of the 'Special harmonizing and vitalizing paste'. He even succeeded in the following session of the examinations! (於是將其得病之由　因伊念頭之差　因未識文章至高之境　即能至高　非人力所能強為　何怒之有　人生以體親心為孝　痛乎責之　俯首無辭　以後漸減苦藥　加補陰　半日以後　去刑具　著衣冠　同跪拜　神識與好人無異　服專翕大生膏一料而大壯　下科竟中矣)

The 'Special harmonizing and vitalizing paste', which was prescribed in the form of pellets, was of Wu's own invention. It contained dozens of ingredients, some quite expensive. Wu typically used it at the end of his treatments of Warm-factor disorders to replenish Yin and balance Yang.[38] The entire treatment lasted two weeks at most. As the crucial last sentence stressed, Bao's fits did not resume as they had after the other physicians left. The cure lasted.

Clearly no bedside jotting, Wu Tang's case file was carefully emplotted to lead to final success.[39] It is a typical example of the therapeutic optimism we find in Chinese medical records: the physician designs the appropriate therapy from a correct diagnosis and expertly modulates drugs to rectify the physiological imbalances that had been causing illness. Wu may have been lying or embellishing, but let us assume for now that he really cured Mr. Bao of his seven years of manic behaviour. How are we to explain this recovery?

Whereas other Chinese doctors usually thought it sufficient to intervene on physiological processes, Wu Tang's treatment attended to the personal roots of his patient's suffering. After Bao had become 'largely lucid' as a result of repeated purges, Wu both rebuked and exhorted him. Proper filial behaviour, Wu proclaimed, was both easier to achieve and of greater consequence than examination success. By reacting angrily to his failure in the pursuit of something he could not control, Bao had failed his family.

Wu's moralizing was more than *ex post facto* embellishment for his elite audience. The re-assertion of proper social roles was part of the cure. The donning of clothes and cap, for instance, was the first thing that Zhu Xi 朱熹 (1130–1200) – whose texts and commentaries Mr. Bao had read since childhood like all other Chinese men who prepared for the civil examinations – had declared should be taught to children.[40] And when Wu and Bao kneeled together, they were probably facing Bao's ancestral tablets. Wu's emphasis on the culturally powerful notion of filial piety afforded Bao a new social position that did not depend on examination success.

Wu Tang's treatment of Mr. Bao resembles ritual therapies 'in which the values of traditional roles and responsibilities are reaffirmed as more important than the individual grudges, griefs, and fears cathartically released in the rite', except that Wu relied on exhortations and enactment rather than catharsis for effect.[41] Ritual and symbolic cures are crucial ways in which the elusive afflictions some of us call 'mental disorders' are treated in all societies, including our own.[42] As Thomas Csordas has observed, ritual healing often consists not in removing an illness, but in transforming the suffering person.[43] Wu gave Mr. Bao a chance to re-symbolize his experience so that it was no longer defined purely by failure. Bao's case reminds us of 'the potential of symbols to affect and reorganize experience', and that we are 'interactive', not 'indifferent' kinds.[44]

Wu Tang's 'Chatty Three-inch Tongue'

As has already been hinted, the use of exhortation to treat insanity was extremely rare in China's clinical literature. In cases of madness, *behaviour*, not emotional or cognitive dispositions, was the primary target of treatment, and it was modified mainly with drugs. Many late imperial physicians accepted that all kinds of disorders could be triggered by emotional imbalances, but few worked on their patients' emotions during therapy, and even fewer found this issue worth discussing.

Wu Tang's attempt to reinstate Bao into a meaningful social role is also exceptional in Chinese medical records. Remarkably, Wu did not view these efforts as an isolated therapeutic success. In a section of his book *Curing the Ills of Medicine* titled 'On the necessity of invoking the cause when treating inner harm' (*zhi nei shang xu zhu you lun* 治內傷須祝由論), he emphasized the importance to the healing process of making patients change their point of view on themselves.[45] 'Inner harm' (*neishang* 內傷), a notion that Li Gao 李杲 (*c.* 1181–1251) had defined as pathological depletion triggered by hunger or exhaustion, had by Wu's time been broadened to include emotionally induced disorders.[46] 'Invoking the cause' (*zhuyou* 祝由) usually referred to the ritual removal of ghosts, but Wu gave it a peculiar meaning better suited to his medical orientation.

Wu's text is a rare articulation (at least in Chinese medical records) of the therapeutic importance of transforming emotions through spoken guidance.

> I say that in treating inner harm, it is necessary to 'invoke the cause', to announce in detail where the illness came from and to make this known to the sick person so that [he or she] will dare not have another fit. In addition, one must meticulously examine and understand departures from the correct and scrutinize the hidden emotions of exhausted men and pensive women. [One must] guide them with amiable words, caution them with solemn words, and inspire reverential fear in them with words of danger. You need to make them happy at heart and sincerely compliant, after which marvellous results can be obtained. (吾謂凡治內傷者　必先祝由　詳告以病之所由來　使病人知之　而不敢再犯　又必細體變風變雅　曲察勞人思婦之隱情　婉言以開導之　莊言以驚覺之　危言以悚懼之　必使之心悅誠服　而後可以奏效如神)

This description is consistent with what Wu Tang reported doing with Mr. Bao. He scrutinized and understood Bao's 'hidden emotions' – detecting anger – and found a way to make him 'sincerely compliant' with both amiable and solemn words. He thus helped Bao to recognize and eliminate the root of his illness. Wu's next words about 'invoking the cause' display the confidence of hindsight:

> In my life, I have been served by this [approach] in innumerable instances of illnesses that could not be treated, such as lone abdominal swelling [abdominal distension not accompanied by the swelling of the limbs], Wood-riding-on-Earth,[47] dry-Blood phthisis [consumptive symptoms attributed to 'dry Blood'], dysphagia [suffocation resulting from the inability to swallow food], upturned stomach, *and insanity*. This is what is meant in Mr. Ye [Gui]'s case files when it is said that herbs and plants without emotions cannot treat emotional illnesses. (余一生得力於此 有必不可治之病 如單腹脹 木乘土 乾血癆 噎食 反胃 癲狂之類 不可枚舉 葉氏案中謂無情之草木 不能治有情之病 亦此義也)

After a disquisition on four fractious types of patients and four challenging types of illnesses, Wu concluded: 'To treat people and illnesses that are difficult to treat, you must rely on that chatty three-inch tongue!' (*nan zhi zhi ren, nan zhi zhi bing, xu ping san cun bu lan zhi she yi zhi zhi* 難治之人 難治之病 須憑三寸不爛之舌以治之).[48]

Several collections of case files attributed to Ye Gui – the physician whose work on Warm-factor disorders had compelled Wu to compile his own – circulated in Wu Tang's time, but it has been impossible to locate the one in which Wu Tang found the statement on 'herbs and plants without emotions'. Wu presented a similar idea as his own in his case collection:

> 'I think that emotionless herbs and plants cannot treat emotional illnesses. To be efficacious in all cases, one must first dispel perplexity and make the emotions flourish unimpeded' (*yu si wu qing zhi cao mu, bu neng zhi you qing zhi bing, bi de kai qi yu meng, shi qing zhi chang sui, fang ke ji jian xiao yu wan yi* 余思无情之草木 不能治有情之病 必得开其愚蒙 使情志畅遂 方可冀见效于万一).[49]

Wu worked on his patients' emotions to ensure that even illnesses that had no emotional manifestations – nausea, abdominal swelling – would not recur after they had been suppressed by drugs.[50] Madness was only one among several illnesses that could be rooted in emotional excesses.

Conclusion

Sick persons who meet a physician engage in an interaction that may transform how they understand their own condition. Participants may carry the result of these transient encounters into their later lives. Unfortunately we have no access to the 'identity-making processes' by which Bao refashioned himself in response to Wu's inculcations.[51] We shall never know if he overcame his past disappointments by convincing himself that success in the examinations was outside his control, whether he made a strong personal commitment to the core ethic of filial piety, or whether Wu Tang was simply boasting.

Wu Tang's treatment of Mr. Bao was in any case highly atypical. Like most Chinese physicians, Wu understood madness as the destruction of social roles, placed the burden of diagnosis on pulse taking, and relied on drugs to treat behavioural symptoms, but his belief that exhortations played a crucial role in treating illnesses that had been triggered by excessive emotions stands out among his contemporaries. Indeed Mr. Bao's case is among the few that explicitly discuss the dynamics of identity that unfolded between late Imperial Chinese doctors and their mad patients.

Even though Wu Tang spoke to his patient, his therapy was no 'talking cure'. For there to be a talking cure, as in psychoanalysis or some forms of psychotherapy, the patient needs to verbalize something. Yet both in Mr. Bao's case and in the way Wu explained how he treated other instances of emotionally induced illness, the patient remains completely voiceless. As a therapeutic weapon, speech was wielded solely by the doctor, whose words were just another way of acting on his patient's condition.

Few pre-twentieth-century Chinese physicians explained mad acts and mad words in reference to the dynamic self. They tried to cure insanity chiefly with medicinal decoctions, giving the impression that they were treating imbalanced bodies rather than distressed persons. Reductionism was more common than we might assume in this 'holistic' tradition that supposedly treated patients as integrated mind-body entities. As argued above, medical doctrines that interpreted mental activities as supervening upon somatic processes did not encourage physicians to focus on the psychology of patients.

Chinese approaches to madness should not be compared too hastily with psychiatric understandings of 'mental illnesses'. Chinese physicians shared 'psychiatry's time-honoured concern with alterations of social behaviour', but they did not consider mental and behavioural illnesses as a separate kind of disorder.[52] All disorders happened to the same body. Even Wu Tang, who paid special attention to the emotional roots of illness, did not single out madness as more mental than abdominal swellings, headaches and nausea. His therapeutic use of exhortation could have challenged the reductionist approach that typically traced mad behaviour to organic imbalances, but Wu never thought of persuasion as a rival to medicaments. As therapeutic tools, words were simply complementary to drugs.

4 PSYCHIATRIC SPACE AND DESIGN ANTECEDENTS: THE JOHN G. KERR REFUGE FOR THE INSANE

Peter Szto

> Of all the 12 buildings which have been erected during these two years, nine are dwellings for patients, two are attendants' quarters and one is the bathrooms and cooks' quarters. Two are built of boards, but ten of them are built of the very best of brick with concrete floors and tiled roofs and are in every way most substantial. They should last for fifty or one hundred years, at least, and with little outlay for repairs as they are of very simple design.[1]

The last sentence in the above quotation proved prophetic regarding China's accommodation of psychiatric space. In this chapter psychiatric space refers to the intentional use of architecture to shape therapeutic outcome. More than 100 years have passed since China first built a separate space to house the insane. Also known as madhouses, insane asylums or psychiatric hospitals, knowledge of these built environments have been based on scholarship focused on European and American architecture than China.[2] Unfortunately, China's insane asylums have been overlooked in the literature despite their significant role in the history of psychiatry.[3]

This chapter responds to the paucity of research on insane asylums beyond the Western context. The aim is to examine linkages between Western and Eastern ideas on psychiatric space vis-à-vis China's first insane asylum – The John G. Kerr Refuge for the Insane.[4] Special attention is given to three American social welfare institutions because of their influence on the design of the Kerr Refuge: The Pennsylvania Hospital (1755), the Friends Hospital (1817; originally Friends Asylum, hereafter Friends Hospital) and the Pennsylvania Hospital for the Insane (1841). All three were established in Philadelphia to provide Kerr design options for China. The focus here is on the Kerr Refuge's formative years, 1872 to 1901, when unique cultural dynamics shaped China's accommodation of psychiatric space. The contours of this accommodation are examined to shed light on the continuities and discontinuities of asylum design.

China's first insane asylum did not emerge out of a cultural vacuum. The founder of the Kerr Refuge, Dr. John Glasgow Kerr, overcame great odds to build China's first psychiatric hospital. In the course of time he did succeed, as indicated below:

> The trees which stand in the grounds afford shade, which is very grateful to the patients during the summer months ... The grounds are surrounded by a wall. This is indispensable here and, as the grounds of the Chinese are usually thus surrounded, it probably does not offend the feelings of the patients as it would at home.[5]

The reference to American patients taking offense to a wall is an interesting comparison, suggesting the role of culture in the design of psychiatric space. Culture is important to understand how design shaped the Kerr Refuge. The following questions are addressed to explore the design links between east and west: 1) What specific architectural designs influenced China's first insane asylum? 2) What design ideas did Kerr embrace and reject? 3) Who were the developers of these asylum designs? 4) Why did the creation of psychiatric space in China happen in the late Qing period and not prior? Two key concepts are used to examine these design links: social technology transfer and cultural context. Both recognize that psychiatric space involved the transfer of knowledge across societies and cultures and how historical and comparative analysis is useful to describe the transfer process.

Social Technology Transfer

The concept of social technology transfer is used to examine the accommodation of the insane asylum in the southern port city of Canton.[6] The insane asylum is unique among social welfare institution and emerged in nascent form in Europe, notably, as the St. Mary of Bethlehem in 1247 – a priory at Bishopgate, in London.[7] Religious clerics, motivated by Christian teachings on compassion and care towards the insane, promoted the idea that a separate space was needed to restore an insane mind to sanity. They believed the best place was in a safe and structured environment. Without a separate space to handle one's insane kin, families were hard pressed to deal with difficult and dangerous cases at home.[8] Historically, the Chinese preferred kinship-based care as the best social location for the insane. 'Social technology' expresses the need for society to solve social problems such as insanity within an institutional or extra-familial setting. Szto defines social technology as 'the development of human resources to enhance societal wellbeing'.[9] Institutions like the insane asylum were 'the locus of intervention...where human resources are organized to enhance societal wellbeing'.[10] This definition assumes social welfare institutions are more efficient for solving social problems than individuals. An institution provides regulated and routine care for a large number of individuals not related by birth better than individuals acting alone. Social technology transfer explains how the Western approach to insanity replaced China's longstanding kinship-based approach to insanity.

The Sociocultural Context of Late Qing China

A major factor for successful social technology transfer is cultural context: how the local environment supports and sustains transfer. In late Qing China (1644–1911), Canton provided an accommodating cultural context for the Kerr Refuge. During the later years of the Qing dynasty, imperial power was waning due to widespread corruption and the encroachment of foreign exploitation. China's Confucian culture largely tolerated the insane based on the social virtues of filial piety, social harmony, and mutual aid.[11] Filial piety is an attitude of deep veneration for one's elders. It views social relationships embedded within a hierarchy of respect and deference. The goal is to create balance among competing roles and responsibilities to create social harmony. One important dynamic of filial piety is mutual aid, or the practice of assisting someone that sets in motion a reciprocal process of helping in return. When one helps someone based on genuine regard it creates a moral obligation for that person to return the favor in the future.

Confucian social philosophy taught that the preferred social location for the insane was a kinship-clan obligation. Moral suasion and ritual codes obligated care of the insane within the sphere of family rather than an institutional setting.[12] Evidence for this practice is that for 4,000 years the Chinese never created an insane asylum on its own but instead relied on Confucian social mores. Neglect of filial piety would result in 'loss of face', an intense feeling of social embarrassment, shame or status.[13] To avoid the perception that others had a diminished view of one's moral character, it was important to project the impression that everything was fine, even though this was not actually the case. The strategy of 'saving face', according to social psychologists Bond and Hwang, 'represents the confidence of society in the integrity of ego's moral character, the loss of which makes it impossible for him to function properly within the community'.[14] Thus, to avoid 'loss of face', Chinese families cared for their insane kin rather than face humiliation and ridicule. In everyday life this meant allowing insane relatives to freely roam the village under the watchful eyes of family members. Fortunately, the slow rhythm of agrarian life help to tolerate often bizarre and erratic behavior of insane kin. Only in extreme and rare circumstances did family members beat, chain, tether, or physically confine their relatives. The Chinese approach to insanity held sway until the eighteenth century when the social order weakened family ties.[15]

The Emergence of Psychiatric Space

Psychiatric space did not emerge in Europe independent of context and culture. Italian architect Vittorio Gregotti observed 'the worse enemy of modern architecture is the idea of space considered solely in terms of its economic and technical exigencies indifferent to the ideas of its site'.[16] An examination of psychiatric space indifferent to site and context will misread insane asylums as disconnected from their design antecedents.[17] For example, thirteenth–century priories, madhouses and charity asylums in Europe were a response to diminishing familial and community supports. It wasn't until the 1890s that psychiatric space was accommodated in China, occurring in Canton as a result of the city's southern location, openness to things foreign and an earlier exposure to overseas communication and influence rather than China's hinterland and northern urban centers. Urbanization, housing shortages, and political corruption also affected Canton's rapid social change, while undermining Chinese families' capacity to care for their insane kin at home. The Western approach of isolating the insane into spaces built especially for them offered Canton's families an attractive alternative to China's Confucian kinship-based approach.

When Protestant missionaries began arriving in China at Canton in 1804 they brought with them distinct social welfare ideas regarding salvation and sanity.[18] They also assumed their ideas were epistemologically superior and thus culturally necessary for the Chinese to adapt, particularly regarding the need for psychiatric space. This presumption of superiority raises two concerns. First, the shift in care from an informal to formal approach presumed that the Western insane asylum was an appropriate alternative to traditional Chinese practices. Whether therapeutic outcome always necessitates an architectural solution is debatable and requires closer scrutiny before concluding that 'safe confinement and imprisonment of lunatics' is universally efficacious.[19] Second, care of the insane outside the sphere of family questions the balance among government, economy and religion to support psychiatric space. Is it always the primary function of family to care for insane kin, or can other social structures also be involved? These are important questions as detractors of the Kerr insane asylum argued that missionary work should never commingle with government services or secular charitable obligations.[20] They believed that evangelism should only be about saving 'lost souls' and not involve social services, especially for the insane.

Expectations for outward expressions of faith were different in the homeland than for China. In America, asylum building was an acceptable manifestation of faith and charitable relief, as championed by Dorothea Dix (1802–87) and Quaker asylum-designer Thomas Story Kirkbride (1809–83). In fact, justification for asylum care was very much a religious argument.[21] Creating space for the insane was considered strategic for a young nation aspiring to create a society grounded in reason and religion. The idea of the mad aimlessly roaming America's streets did not bode well with an eschatological self-image of a 'city on a hill'.[22] Psychiatric space was important for America to create a rational social order. From where though did America view institutionalization as the preferred approach to handling the insane?

Embryonic forms of psychiatric space appeared in medieval Europe where hospitals hosted the sick and housed the destitute. When medieval families could no longer care for insane kin, space outside the home was sought. Hospitals, at first, offered alternative physical space for families to practice hospitality towards the sick and the stranger. Architectural historian Nikolaus Pevsner explains that the words 'Hospitals, hospice, hostel, hotel are all derived from the Latin hospes, the guest or the host'.[23] Hospitality signified both a physical and spiritual act of kindness. In Latin, the idea was expressed as *omnes superveni-entes hospites tamquam Christus suscipiantur*, meaning that every arriving guest must be welcomed as if he or she were Christ.[24] People believed that God himself directly blessed the poor and protected the vulnerable through individual acts of hospitality. Hospitality, in effect, exemplified a 'Christ-like' attitude, by making strangers guests and the alien an integral member of the community. In medieval European society, hosting outcasts and embracing strangers created an informal social safety net without having to build a separate location for the insane. Cathedrals and monasteries hosted the poor as physical manifestations of the Church's social teachings:

> In monasteries the custom was, as at St. Gall, to have the guest-house west of the claustral precinct and the infirmary east. Kirkstall, the Cistercian abbey outside Leeds, can serve as an example. The infirmary was aisled and had at its east end the chapel so that the sick could see the altar and the services. It must never be forgotten that medical treatment was inadequate and communication with God more urgent than with a doctor or a medically active monk.[25]

Furthermore, religious beliefs informed the design and operation of hospitals in medieval Europe. For example, the Cruciform Plan followed the shape of a cross and was easy to build yet rich in religious symbolism.[26] Each section of the cross contained a separate ward to create a total of four patient wards. In the center of the cross an altar was placed to remind the sick of God's presence in the midst of their suffering. By the late seventeenth century, spokes were attached transforming the simple cruciform pattern into the Radial Plan (see Figure 1.0). The additional spokes also provided economic benefit by creating more hallways and bed space within the same space. Early nineteenth century American insane asylums adhered to the Cruciform Plan.[27]

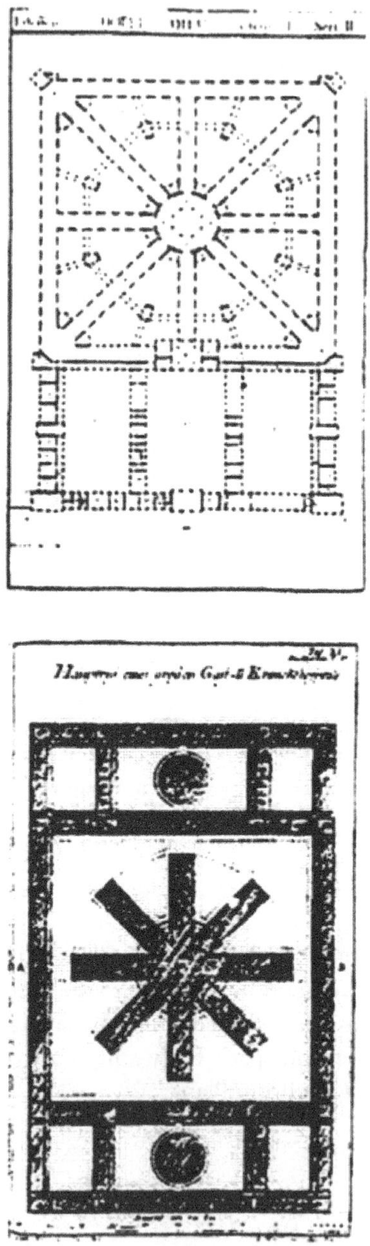

Figure 4.1: From Cruciform Plan to Radial Plan. J. D. Thompson and G. Goldin, *The Hospital: A Social and Architectural History* (New Haven: Yale University Press, 1975), p. 46. © Grace Goldin

Hospice Differentiation

Medieval social philosophy began to lose its influence with the rise of Renaissance and Reformation thought. New ideas challenged conventional hospital architecture by replacing the influence of theology with science.[28] As Europe moved further away from its religious moorings towards a secular understanding of insanity, the rationale for confinement would also change. For example, space came to be understood in terms of utility rather than sacral value. Space was something to be manipulated and maximized for functionality and performance. French scientist Jean-Baptiste Le Roy describes this new attitude in his 1773 comment on hospital architecture: 'A ward is, as it were, a machine for treating the sick'.[29] Science asserted that society was like a machine that could be measured, calibrated, and designed for total efficiency. This reductionist perspective saw the design of hospitals in terms of body parts and the workings of a machine:

> Foundling hospitals, asylums for the insane, lying-in hospitals had already existed before 1800; now – to take London as an example – we get the Eye Hospital in 1805, the Chest Hospital in 1814, the Ear Hospital in 1816, the Cancer Hospital in 1835, the Orthopaedic Hospital in 1838 and so on.[30]

Although the size and shape of psychiatric space varied between European and American insane asylums and the Kerr Refuge in China, their histories are linked by design.

Transfer of Psychiatric Space

Psychiatric space was an exclusive model of Western practice until American medical missionaries transferred it to China.[31] Throughout China's history, the Chinese had never developed its own psychiatric space but instead cared for the insane within the purview of family. A separate space for the insane was anathema to Chinese practice. In traditional Chinese society the insane were not a neglected or under-served group but rather beneficiaries of Confucian morality and virtue. Why then did the Chinese accommodate Western psychiatric space in the late Qing? The American city of Philadelphia offers answers.

Philadelphia was the hub of American Enlightenment activism where prominent social welfare institutions originated. America's first medical hospital and private insane asylum were established in Philadelphia.[32] These institutions were not just local products but modeled after European designs.[33] The colonialists wanted America to be an enlightened society just like Europe, that is, free from lunatics cluttering its streets. Social reformers Dorothea Dix (1801–87) and Horace Mann (1796–1859), among others, advocated for 'architecture to embody and advance their respective collective ideals' of treating the insane in confined space.[34] Their advocacy produced scores of insane asylums that championed architecture as a symbol of progressive social ideals. The Kerr Refuge was an extension of three Philadelphia insane asylums: the Pennsylvania Hospital (1755), the Friends Hospital (1817), and the Pennsylvania Hospital for the Insane (1841). Each influenced the Kerr Refuge in some way regarding design and function.

Kerr studied medicine at Thomas Jefferson Medical School in Philadelphia, where he graduated in 1847 at the age of twenty-three. Medical education at the time followed a preceptorship model that emphasized apprenticeship and experience over academic studies. When Kerr was in Philadelphia it was small enough that he was aware of the city's only three insane asylums. It is reasonable to infer that the three insane asylums influenced the design of the Kerr Refuge.

The Pennsylvania Hospital – 1755

Benjamin Franklin founded America's first private medical facility in 1755 – the Pennsylvania Hospital. One of its founding goals was to treat the insane in a rational and civilized environment. Adhering to Enlightenment-inspired institutions of eighteenth–century Paris and London, Franklin imagined similar voluntary institutions in Philadelphia. He believed only a private and non-sectarian approach to social welfare institutions would create an enlightened society.

Dr. Benjamin Rush (1783–1813) was the first head physician at the Pennsylvania Hospital. Rush believed responding to the insane with compassion and kindness was necessary as opposed to inhumane cruelty and bitter indifference, as apparently was the case at the Pennsylvania Hospital. Nancy Tomes describes the 'zoo-like atmosphere' at the Pennsylvania Hospital where conditions were akin to harsh incarceration than therapeutic milieu. For Rush, however, moral treatment was 'a medical regimen employing psychological techniques that emphasize the human, rather than beastlike, nature of the insane'.[35] Rush argued that the insane had different needs and required special attention they could not receive if mixed in with other hospital patients – as was the practice at the Pennsylvania Hospital.[36] In 1792 he successfully lobbied the government to finally build a public insane asylum.

The major lesson for the Kerr Refuge from the Pennsylvania Hospital was that comingling medical and mental cases in the same building was fraught with risks. Staff found it difficult to give equal time and attention since symptoms and behaviors were so different. For example, the view that the insane were similar to wild beasts and should be treated as such was how the insane were handled before Rush taught otherwise. When the Pennsylvania Hospital opened, it had only two classifications of patients – sane and insane. Mixing and confusing the two types easily led to 'techniques to subdue lunatics that effectively cast the physician as an animal tamer'.[37] By 1832, the hospital finally realized that each classification needed its own space and treatment protocols. When Kerr began his medical studies in the mid-1840s, the idea of a separate space to treat the insane had already become established architectural precedent and standard asylum design. Gerald Grob explains how 'educated and upper-class laypersons, physicians, intellectuals, and others had become aware of the newer views associated with the advocates of a hospital-based system of care'.[38] It is presumed here that Kerr was among these enlightened and educated individuals.

The Friends Hospital – 1817

In 1817, Thomas Scattergood, a devout Quaker layman, founded America's first private, non-profit, and faith-based insane asylum – the Friends Hospital. Built in a remote rural area north of Philadelphia, the city's second insane asylum was 'for such of our members as may be deprived of their reason'.[39] For a city of 100,000 to have two insane asylums was unique.[40] The Quakers felt only an insulated moral community run by and for Quakers could treat their insane and thus warranted an exclusive faith-based institution.

Design sensitivity was markedly different from the Pennsylvania Hospital. The first building of the Friends Hospital followed the Cruciform Plan. Later buildings re-created the intimacy of a small farming village: 'An important aspect of moral treatment was the realization that different types of patients could be better cared for if housed in different areas'.[41] The goal was to create a separate space to retreat from the exigencies and harshness of a fallen world. To achieve this, Scattergood paid special attention to architectural detail to insure quality comfort and care, whereby ventilation, lighting and social space were designed to maximize healing.

Kerr also shared a similar moral framework and religious worldview with the Quakers. They both believed in social change inspired by religious conviction and the best social location for the insane was in an institutional setting. In addition, they endorsed asylum design of small structures rather than a central large structure on a secluded campus far removed from the city. Perhaps the most significant similarity was the belief in a separate sectarian space for moral treatment in a cottage-like setting.

Pennsylvania Hospital for the Insane – 1841

Asylum care had become well established in America by the 1840s. Asylum doctors saw in this an opportunity to elevate their low social status as 'mad-doctors' to one of professional respectability. The pubic perceived them more in terms of quackery and superstition than science. The 'medicalization of madness' sought to use disease concepts instead of spiritual or moral categories. This scientific perspective enhanced psychiatry's public image justifying the need for psychiatric space. Grob explains the scientific worldview and institutionalization:

> Since the disorder was in large part precipitated by improper behavioral patterns or a deficient social environment, it followed that treatment had to begin with the creation of a new and presumably appropriate environment. Home treatment was ineffective, for the physician had no means of controlling or eliminating the causal elements that produced the disorder. Institutionalization, therefore, was a sine qua non. Once in a hospital, the patient could be exposed to a judicious mix of medical and moral treatment.[42]

Asylum care paved the way for 'asylum medicine' to develop. This new approach synthesized architectural design with medical science and developed at the Pennsylvania Hospital for the Insane (hereafter PHI).[43] The leading practitioner of asylum medicine was Quaker physician Thomas Story Kirkbride (1809–83). Kirkbride graduated from the University of Pennsylvania Medical School (1828–32) and then completed his one-year residency at nearby Friends Hospital. His residency exposed him to Scattergood's model of moral treatment and the design sensitivity and cottage-like atmosphere of Friends. The year instilled a lasting impression, before leaving to accept a position at PHI as superintendent between 1840 and1883. As superintendent he placed great value on plumbing fixtures, ventilation systems, window size and wall color as active treatment ingredients. Kirkbride practiced what Rothman labeled 'moral architecture', the idea that the buildings themselves were curative. Noted Kirkbride historian, Tomes, observed:

> He well understood the importance of first impressions in securing a patient's confidence and willingness to submit to the hospital regimen, and continually worked to give the buildings a 'pleasant and cheerful' character ... Each Report invariably included some pleasant description of the building or the pleasure grounds surrounding it, which Kirkbride repeatedly characterized as 'highly cultivated and improved'.[44]

Kirkbride was unrelenting about asylum design. His design came to be known as the 'Kirkbride Plan' and defined insane asylums as 'a therapeutic community modeled on the outside world, yet operating according to hygienic principles'.[45] The Plan advocated a single elongated building, linear in form, and designed to house all patients under one roof. If additional buildings needed to be constructed, they were then attached to the main structure to make the linear design even more elongated. The design took hold in America but not in Europe. The Europeans instead preferred small individual cottage structures that promoted individual attention in a communal setting. Kirkbride published his linear plan as an architectural guide in 1854 and became the industry standard for asylum design in the United States. Carla Yanni points out, 'For most of the nineteenth century, from about 1840 to about 1900, he was the single most important nineteenth-century psychiatrist when it came to matters of architecture'.[46]

Kirkbride's influence on asylum design was widespread, yet had less sway on Kerr than the Friend's emphasis on personal attention and community. Kerr was highly motivated to build an asylum in China informed by impressions shaped while a medical student in Philadelphia:

> To complete the sphere of medical work as a mission agency there is needed the establishment of asylums for the helpless classes. As yet nothing has been done in heathen lands (except in India by the British government) in this department of medical work considered so important in Christian lands.[47]

Design Continuity and Discontinuity

After Kerr graduated from Jefferson Medical College in 1847, he returned to his native Ohio. He wanted to practice medicine in an area of high need and rural Ohio met this desire. One day, a Chinese national passed through to lecture on China. The gentleman spoke passionately on the need for foreign medical missionaries in China. The talk was compelling enough to inspire Kerr to give up Ohio for China. Soon afterwards Kerr signed with the American Presbyterian Board of Foreign Missions (hereafter APBFM) to become their first medical missionary to China. He sailed for Canton in 1853, but would return often to visit his alma mater in Philadelphia. On his furlough visits back to Jefferson, Kerr would impress his colleagues and former professors with exotic cases from China. His compassion and curiosity for medical education never waned while in China, as he wanted to share and stay abreast of the latest in medical research. The school's Alumni Bulletin remembered him well:

> one of the most robust characters ever to receive a diploma from Jefferson. He and his wife left for China in 1853 on a sailing vessel of six hundred fifty tons, and arrived in Hong Kong after a voyage of six months ....In 1897, Dr. Kerr was called to Peking to perform a serious operation on the United States Minister, His Excellency, Charles Denby. The diplomat had already gone to Europe for treatment which had not been successful. Dr. Kerr was seventy years old then and probably the world's foremost surgeon in vesical calculus.[48]

Given the frequency of his furloughs that included visits to Jefferson, his own interest in creating psychiatric space in China, and Kerr's known curiosity about best practices, only if he were extremely disinterested in asylum design would he not be aware of Philadelphia's two premier insane asylums. When he graduated from Jefferson, the Friends Hospital had been already treating patients for thirty years, and the Pennsylvania Hospital for seven.

Whatever expectations Kerr had about practicing medicine before leaving for China, after he arrived he was alarmed by the high number of Chinese insane coming to the Canton Medical Hospital for treatment. Deeply concerned about the lack of an appropriate space to treat them, he became resolute about finding a viable solution. One wonders if he remembered the risks of mixing sane with insane patients and the miserable consequences that resulted in patient abuses at the Pennsylvania Hospital decades earlier. Kerr fortunately understood the pitfalls of mixing medical and mental health cases in the same building, which is partly why he was such a staunch advocate for psychiatric space.

Kerr first broached the idea of developing psychiatric space in 1872 in the *Canton Medical Hospital Annual Report to the American Presbyterian Board of Foreign Missions*.[49] The Board flatly rejected his idea, as well as Kerr's repeated overtures, arguing that lunatic care was not the responsibility of missionary benevolence and should instead be shouldered by the Chinese. The Board assumed a narrow definition of missionary activity, that is, only evangelism proper and absolutely no social services. Despite the Board's rejections, Kerr was undeterred and instead set out on his own to procure support. For the next twenty-six years Kerr developed support, studied asylum design and methods to treat the insane in China. The long wait certainly allowed Kerr to carefully mull over different designs for China, i.e., Kirkbride's linear design versus Scattergood's cottage system.

Finally, in 1891, Kerr took his life savings, plus a small amount of privately donated dollars, and purchased three Chinese acres (equivalent to 4.5 English acres) in the Fong Tsuen suburb of Canton.[50] He planned to purchase more acreage in the near future expecting the need for psychiatric space to grow. In 1892 he would purchase more land just before taking his final furlough. After all these years Kerr's vision for psychiatric space was becoming real. This vision was made clear in the Refuge's 1898 inaugural report:

> The design is to begin with a small number, until attendants can be trained to take care of them. With kind and careful attention, comfortable surroundings, good food and out-door exercise, the change from the treatment and influences of heathen relatives will have a beneficial effect, and will be sufficient in some cases to result in cure.[51]

The above report is evidence of Kerr's preference for a small-scale (Scattergood's Friends Hospital) rather than a large-scale (Kirkbride's Pennsylvania Hospital for the Insane) approach to psychiatric space. Critics of the Kirkbride Plan and, indirectly, Dorothea Dix's campaign to establish a public insane asylum in every state, warned that large-scale insane asylums would unintentionally become custodial and impersonal. They were simply too big, inhospitable and machine-like. Kerr disliked the idea of warehousing insane patients, preferring instead the moral vision treatment of the Friends Hospital. He also liked the Quaker approach because it valued work-as-therapy and viewed community as a means of moral reform. Kerr embraced moral treatment, seeing it as relevant for the Chinese context and consistent with his missionary convictions.

Location

For thousands of years Canton's coastal location made it an attractive place for farming, commerce and maritime trade. When, in the eighteenth century, European traders also discovered Canton's resourceful location, they came in droves. The Europeans liked the business acumen of the Cantonese and the shorter travel route Canton afforded versus the arduous route of the Silk Road (see Figure 4.2, below). In addition, Canton's long distance from Peking provided political advantages for traders weary of government control stifling their pursuit of wealth.

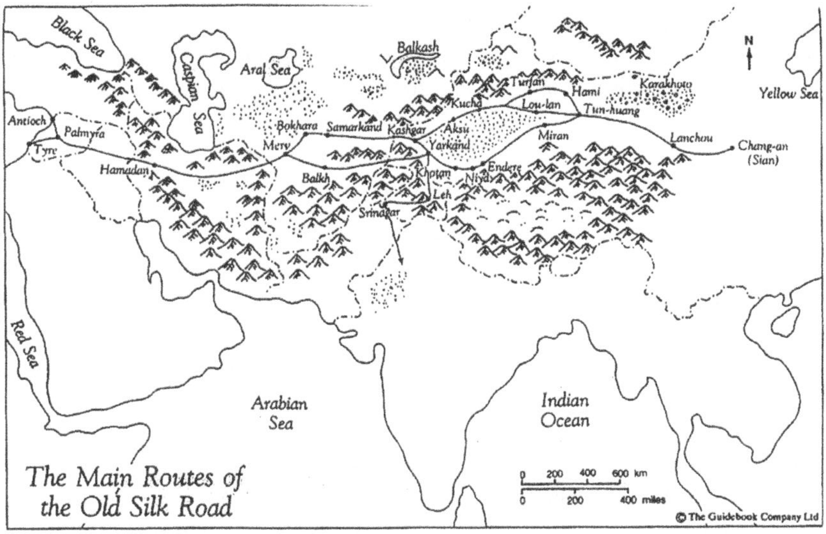

Figure 4.2: The Main Routes of the Old Silk Road. C. Chan, *China* (Lincolnwood, IL: Passport Books, 1995), p. 171.

The APBFM stationed Kerr at Canton because of its geographic advantages and established foreign presence. The Canton System of Trade (1757–1842) and two Opium Wars (1839–42 and 1856–60) placed legal restrictions on where foreigners could reside that essentially limited them to Canton. The Treaty of Tianjin (1858) also stipulated that foreigners could not purchase property within city limits, making the Fong Tsuen locale ideal (see Figure 4.3, below). Fong Tsuen offered plush farmland endowed with large shady trees, placid rolling hills and was a short boat ride from Canton's central district, the Bund. It was also lush with decorative flowers, rice paddy fields, lychee trees and bananas as cash crops for a thriving local economy. Kerr liked Fong Tsuen because of its easy access for both patients and staff; it was only a ten-metre boat ride from Shamian Island, 'the chief residence of Europeans'.[52] Building the Refuge close to Shamian Island was a pragmatic decision. The small narrow island was the main foreign commercial district that housed consulates and foreign support services. Due east of Shamian Island was the Bund, the central waterfront where the Canton Medical Hospital stood. Kerr was superintendent at this hospital for some forty years and was very familiar with the area. Easy access to the hospital was critical in cases of emergency medical relief and to get additional staff support when needed. Fong Tsuen also allowed families and patients to arrive by boat or foot from the western outskirts. This was important for the occasional obstreperous patient when families needed to strap insane kin to ladders, haul them in pig baskets, or bring them in chicken coops for care.[53] In more ways than one, Fong Tsuen reflected the Anglo-American bias for a rural location. Rural areas provided a pastoral atmosphere that supported sequestration and recovery: 'As regards our own treatment we depend upon the regular, quiet life of the asylum'.[54]

The Design

Landscaping and construction of the Kerr Refuge began in 1894. Four years later the building was completed and, on 20 February 1898, the Kerr Refuge admitted its first two patients: one male and one female. The opening was historic and, because of Kerr's persistence, strong personality and financial resources, psychiatric space became a reality. Kerr overcame a myriad of obstacles to turn the concept of psychiatric space into brick and mortar: he had to buy the right materials, hire skilled laborers, garner local support and, most importantly, have a design in mind that was suitable to Canton's social and cultural environment. He miraculously accomplished all this without any support from his mission board and without a vernacular asylum model to follow. Fortunately, Kerr was superintendent at the Canton Medical Hospital where he gained invaluable experience and knowledge about local construction management. While there he helped build hospitals, chapels, dispensaries, schools and private homes.[55] Each building project provided Kerr with cultural insights into Canton's arcane government procedures that enabled him to get things done. It did not hurt that Kerr was a senior member of the missionary and foreign business community, a prominent role that gave him access to local contractors and political connections. Yet despite his connections and knowledge of local ways, unless he had the right asylum design, all things would not have come together.

Despite differences of opinion on missionary polity, Kerr remained loyal to the foreign missionary community. He therefore upheld his Mission Board's policy of building structures so they complimented local tastes and mores. Canton's architectural vernacular involved unadorned low-lying buildings placed close together:

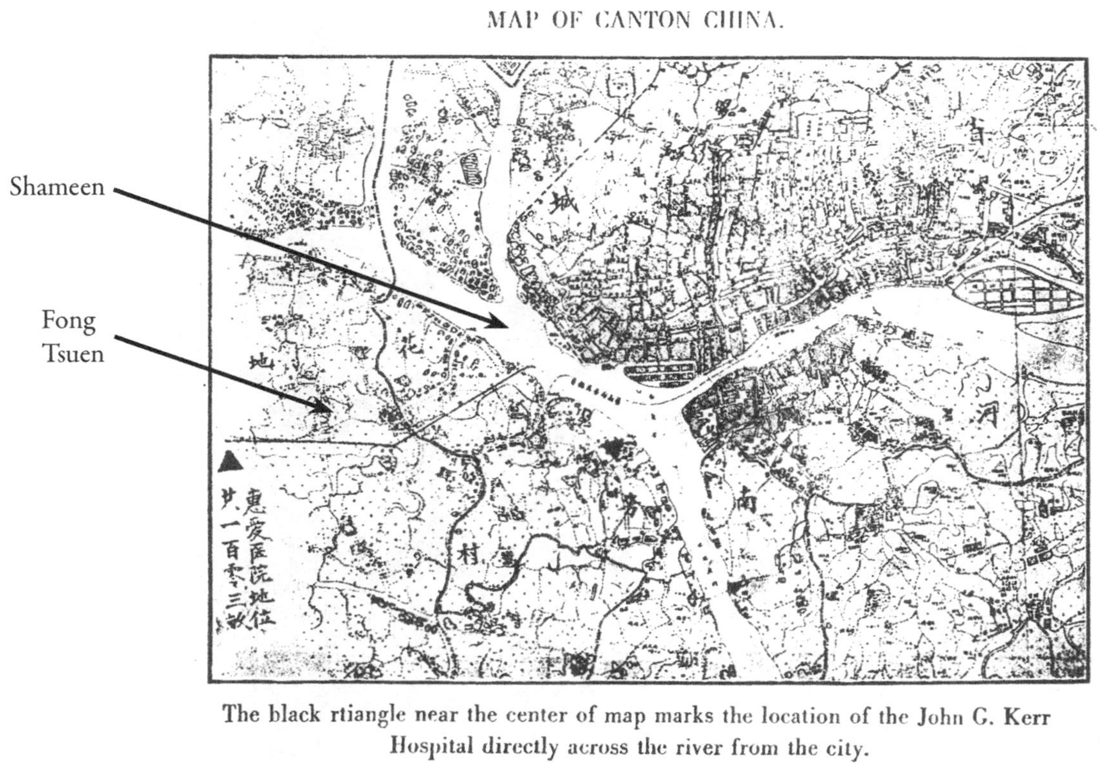

Figure 4.3: The John G. Kerr Hospital in Canton, China. 'Report for 1924 – The John G. Kerr Hospital for the Insane, Canton China,' Guangzhou Psychiatric Hospital archives, Guangzhou, China.

> The houses in which the people live are all after one general plan, the only difference between rich and poor being in the size, material, and ornamentation. There are usually no windows in the front, only a door set in the middle, opening on a short hall-way, with small rooms on either side that leads into a court open to the sky.[56]

For a foreigner to build a large, ornate structure in Canton for the insane would have been not only culturally offensive but totally out of place. This was especially the case considering Canton's high population density and Fong Tsuen's rural environment. For Kerr the goal of psychiatric space was to create a feeling of safety, comfort and intimacy – not a symbol of foreign imposition or oppression. Thompson & Goldin characterize the attitude Kerr held towards design in terms of *designed* and *derived* space. The former uses space to perform particular functions, such as nursing care for psychiatric patients.[57] The latter refers to the inheritance of built forms and then adapting them for alternative purposes. Kerr creatively integrated both, by inheriting the legacy of American insane asylum design and adapting them to Canton.

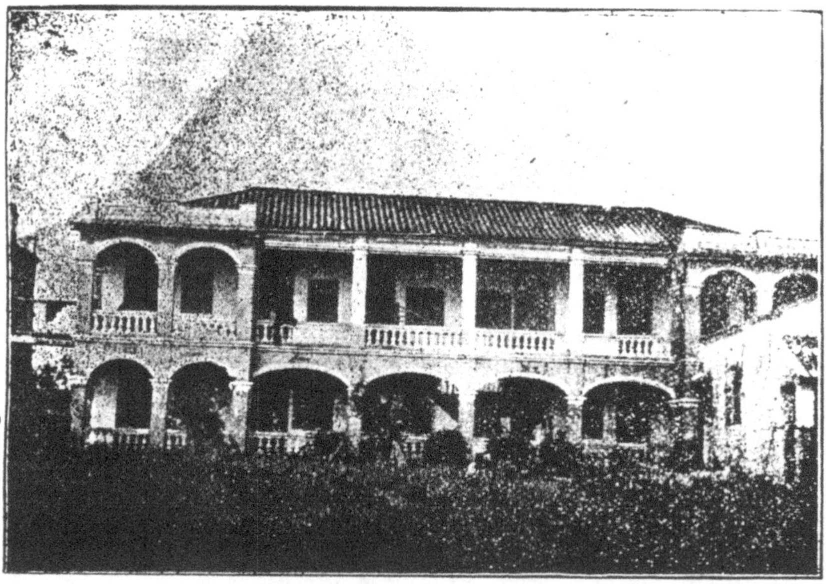

One of the two first buildings, with portion of chapel on the right

Figure 4.4: One of the First Two Buildings of the Kerr Asylum. *Report for the years 1907 and 1908* (Canton, China: China Baptist Publication Society, 1909), inside cover.

Kerr's asylum design involved three elements: a box-shaped exterior, broad-arched verandas and upturned tiled roofs (see Figure 4.5). Stylistically, the design was consistent with other colonial architecture in south China. Many of these colonial structures still stand in Macao, Hong Kong and Guangzhou, such as schools, colonial administrative offices, hospitals or orphanages. The box-shaped design Kerr preferred was modest and functional. Its simple square design encouraged freedom of movement within a confined space. The cost-benefit was also not lost on Kerr, who had a limited budget. From a therapeutic perspective the design promoted a feeling of safety and comfort for patients and families. The boxy design achieved this with high ceilings and ample windows to insure healthy ventilation and plenty of ambient light. The rooms were also large and could comfortably hold four to six patients each. Depending on ability to pay and whether interpersonal space was an issue, private rooms were available. The accommodations at the Kerr Refuge were definitely more amenable for healing insanity than staying confined at home.

The exterior of the buildings were designed for therapeutic effect as well (see Figure 4.5). Kerr believed the physical appearance of each building should look and feel inviting. To achieve this he wrapped the building with verandas, trimmed with a baluster-ornamented handrail and arched openings. The veranda space was functional in how it created an open hallway for patients to stroll or sit. Freedom of movement was important because Canton's intense weather involved unrelenting heat, humidity, sun and rain. The extra veranda space allowed patients to safely mill about yet sheltered from the elements.

The building roofs were covered with green up-turned shingles. The shingles shielded the patients from the summer's drenching heat, as well as protection from any evil spirits. The Chinese long held that spirits float above and it was important to be protected from evil attacks. Kerr had a dual purpose in mind with the roof design. Sensitive to Chinese cultural beliefs, the curvature of the roof could recycle evil spirits back into the atmosphere and could also drain off heavy rains.[58] Proper building materials were important to weather Canton's intense sub-tropical climate. Summer and autumn brought withering heat and heavy humidity; winter and spring involved life-threatening monsoons and typhoons. Timber frames were not used because of their susceptibility to fire and decay. Instead, red brick and mortar were used to fortify the walls against high winds and occasional abuse from violent patients. On the ground level, the floor walls were laid three bricks deep and the second floor walls two bricks deep. The floors were tiled and wooden frames trimmed all doors and windows. The exterior of the windows originally had wooden shutters attached for extra protection, but these and the floor tiles were removed after violent patients used them as weapons.[59]

Kerr made every effort to integrate Cantonese habits to operate the Refuge. He hired indigenous staff and promoted local cultural practices surrounding food, bathing and toilet rituals. To build trust and maintain local support, he practiced the proven strategy of first building a dispensary. The idea was that by offering familiar healing agents to the Cantonese, they would later accept strange and unfamiliar practices, that is, Western medicine. The strategy worked. The first building housed a dispensary on the ground floor with patient rooms on the upper floor. Kerr also promoted local leadership and hired Dr. Wan Tun-mo, a Kerr-trained physician as manager of the dispensary Dr. Wan's role was to 'conciliate the goodwill of the neighboring shopmen'.[60] When the second building opened, it was designated for patients only.

Kerr's commitment to cultural competency was well known, but to leave no doubt of his belief in psychiatric space, he moved his entire family into the first building. A bold move to convincingly demonstrate that asylum care was absolutely safe and secure. Kerr's asylum design worked, '... for the buildings were both filled to comfortable fullness. We now have something over sixty inmates'.[61]

Building Expansion

Three years after the Refuge opened, Dr. Kerr turned from his bed to fellow medical missionary, Charles Selden, and said, 'I give this institution into your hands'.[62] Selden willingly accepted Kerr's offer and immediately set out to fulfill Kerr's vision of developing comprehensive psychiatric space:

> The amount of space at our command affords room for several more buildings, together with a lawn and shaded walks for recreation and exercise. As the benefits of the institution become appreciated by the Chinese, and the necessity for it is understood by benevolent men and women in Christian lands, we have faith to believe that funds will be forthcoming to build up a model institution, and that others of its kind will multiply until this form of Christian benevolence will permeate this vast empire. At the lowest percentage of insane to the population in Western lands, 300 asylums with capacity for 1,000 patients each are required for China.[63]

Like Kerr, Selden was adamant about asylum care as a legitimate field of medical missions:

> The history of the institution cannot be concluded without recording the fact that it was planned, opened, and has been carried on in prayer to the Wise Master Builder and Chief Physician. He has shown His approval and has given His presence; has always in His own time – not always in ours – provided men and means.[64]

Selden remained superintendent until the hospital temporarily closed in 1934 because of widespread social unrest. War with Japan and Communist-inspired labor disputes made it dangerous for missionaries to continue their work at the Kerr Refuge.[65] Before permanently returning to the United States, Selden had transformed the two-building Kerr institution into a European-style cottage system with bungalows, gardens, 'modern' amenities, a chapel and ample space to exercise.

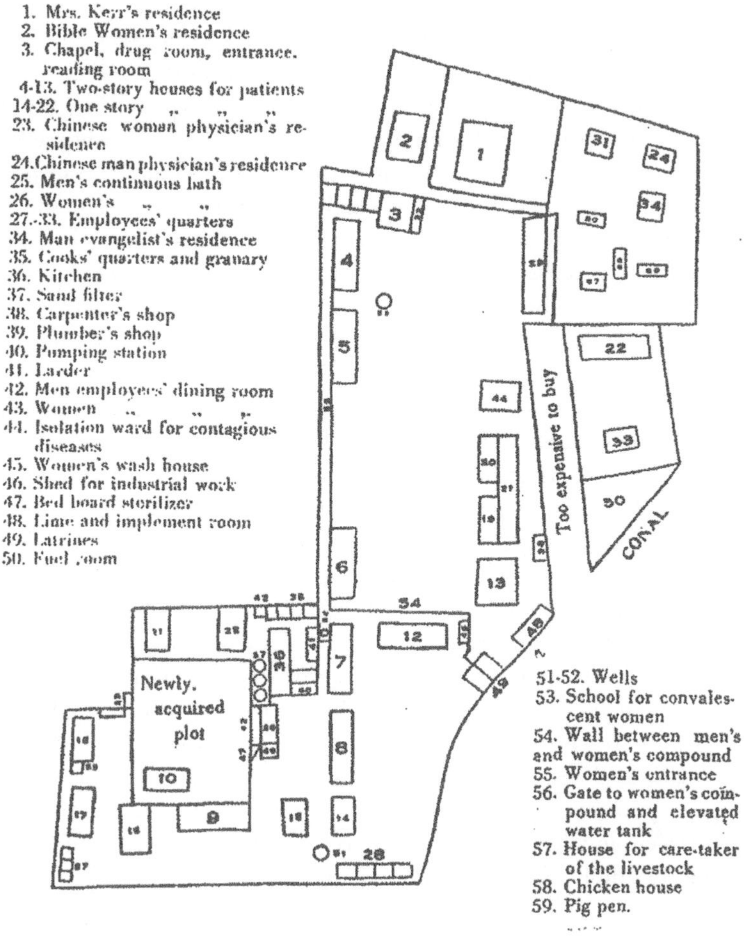

Figure 4.5: A Schematic Rendering of the Kerr Asylum. 'The John G. Kerr Hospital for the Insane - Report for the Years 1922 and 1923', Guangzhou Psychiatric Hospital archives, Guangzhou, China.

Figure 4.5, above, is a schematic rendering of the insane asylum in 1922. The sketch shows the efficient use of space for psychiatric ends and how the missionary designers sought to redeem every square inch.

Conclusion

This study examined the design links between Eastern and Western expressions of psychiatric space. The links unveiled design continuities and discontinuities between nineteenth–century insane asylums in Philadelphia, USA and the Kerr Refuge in Canton, China. The links make clear the historic role of the Kerr Refuge in insane asylum architecture and how social technology transfer shaped China' spatial location of the insane. Further study is warranted on the development of psychiatric space in China after the foreign missionaries left and native personnel replaced them. The absence of foreigners introduced a period when very little is known about the Kerr Refuge. In the first half of the twentieth century, China's political economy and social environment sparked radical change that directly affected care of the insane. It would be fascinating to know how China's shifting cultural identity, power relationships among elites and changing social welfare ideology unfolded during China's brief Republican era, the post 1949 Liberation years and Cultural Revolution to effect psychiatric space.

What is known is that Kerr and Selden believed good design was integral to sustaining psychiatric space. They built the Kerr Refuge to withstand decay, dereliction and disaster. Selden predicted, 'They should last for fifty or one hundred years, at least, and with little outlay for repairs as they are of very simple design'.[66] Long-term spatial performance and permanency for psychiatric space is what Kerr and Selden strived. If the Kerr Refuge was to be an instrument of care and evangelism, then its transfer as social technology was worth every effort. Finally, investigation into how visual discourse of the Kerr Refuge advanced evangelism and ameliorated insanity deserves attention. Without visual evidence of the Refuge, supporters were hard pressed to 'see' for themselves the fruits of their support. Kerr and Selden worked hard to avoid the image that their buildings in China were simply a 'container for outcasts'.[67]

5 AN IRON CAGE OF CIVILIZATION? MISSIONARY PSYCHIATRY, THE CHINESE FAMILY AND A COLONIAL DIALECTIC OF ENLIGHTENMENT

Zhiying Ma

In November 2011, the *New York Times* published two articles on the inadequacies of mental health treatment in China. In the first article, the authors discussed the 'dearth of care' in the dark Chinese household:

> Left to their own devices, some relatives resort to heartbreaking solutions. In 2007, He Jiyue, a government psychiatrist, discovered a 46-year-old man locked behind a metal door in a stinking room in a rural Hebei Province home. The man was mentally ill, his aged parents told Dr. He. They had locked him up after he attacked his uncle.
>
> That was 28 years earlier. The man, a high school graduate, could no longer speak. 'I said to the parents: 'How could you do this to somebody?'' Dr. He recalled. They replied, 'We had no choice'.
>
> In the past three years, Chinese mental health workers have rescued 339 other people whose relatives were too poor, ignorant or ashamed to seek treatment. Some, shackled in outdoor sheds, were 'treated just like animals', said Dr. Liu Jin, of the Peking University Mental Health Institute.[1]

In a nutshell, the article portrayed mentally ill Chinese as treated like animals, locked up by his ignorant and heartless families, awaiting a liberating and humanitarian rescue by the psychiatric science. The authors of the article used this image to lament the shortage of professional mental health care in China, to establish psychiatry's authority against other practices of care, and to legitimize the profession's expansion. This international discourse of psychiatric liberation vis-à-vis familial constraint has been circulated and utilized within China as well. For example, Dr. He quoted in the *New York Times* article was very likely a participant in the 'Unchaining Movement' (*Jiesuo Xingdong*), a national mental health campaign that began in 2006, and that is aimed at replacing domestic confinement with free or low-cost treatment for rural patients.[2]

This nationally and globally circulated discourse of the dehumanized patient, the constraining family, and a liberating psychiatry echoes the discourse of the missionaries who were the first to practice psychiatry to China. On 28 February 1898, John G. Kerr, an American Presbyterian missionary doctor, opened the first refuge for the insane in China. In an often-cited documentation describing the Kerr Refuge's opening, Charles Selden, who directed the Refuge after John Kerr, vividly portrayed the family induced suffering of the first two patients:

> In his home this man [the first patient] had been chained for three years to a stone in such a way that he could not take a single step, and had lost his power of walking. The second patient, a woman, was found sitting on the floor of a hut with a chain around her neck, the end of which was fastened to a staple in the floor behind her... she was sitting on the floor of a little hut built over water, with a chain around her neck and with a dejected expression of countenance.

Staff at the Kerr Refuge immediately unchained the two patients upon admission and, in his writing, Selden celebrated that 'for the first time in the history of China a mind-diseased patient was to receive special care'.[3] If the birth of psychiatry in the West is often symbolized by the image of Philippe Pinel ordering the chains to be removed from patients at the Paris Asylum for insane women, chains that represent the barbaric practices of the public institution, then the arrival of psychiatry in China is marked by John Kerr removing the chains that symbolized neglect and abuse that was going on in the private household.[4] After the Kerr Refuge was shut down in 1926 because of a labor strike, missionary psychiatrists in other parts of China continued to talk about the insane being restrained with ropes, with chains, or in 'an iron cage'.[5] Today, Chinese-trained psychiatrists still celebrate Kerr's symbolic unchaining of the patient from the familial 'iron cage' as the beginning of '*modern Chinese* psychiatry', and reproduce this emancipatory discourse in their own work.[6]

This chapter will examine medical missionaries' establishment of psychiatry in China from the 1890s to the late 1920s. In particular, it will show, first, how missionary representations of 'the Chinese family' were formed by the colonial encounter and by elisions of historical dynamics, and, second, how these psychiatric epistemologies, trapped in logics of rationality and governance, tended to become 'iron cages' of control themselves. To these ends, the chapter will examine missionary correspondences regarding the need for mental hospitals in China, the Kerr Refuge's annual reports and its staff's memoirs and publications on insanity in China in major globally-circulated medical journals (such as *The China Medical Journal*) from the 1890s to the late 1920s. While this paper cannot analyze epistemologies of and social arrangements for insanity beyond this designated period in great detail, it nevertheless will briefly illustrate some more extensive continuities and shifts brought in train by the dominant category of the Chinese family.

Previous studies have examined the birth of modern Chinese psychiatry in the Kerr Refuge. For example, Kao and Szto have both looked at this process through the lens of 'technology transfer', i.e. 'the dissemination of Western concepts of institutional psychiatry in China',[7] and Yang has analyzed the spatial politics involved in the establishment of the Refuge.[8] Their work has influenced my conceptualization of Chinese psychiatry. However, this study departs from the impact-response framework implicit in these previous studies, a model presuming that a pure and unchanged essence of psychiatry from the West is imposed on an inert and similarly essentialized Chinese culture.[9] In this rather ahistorical framework, there are some timeless characteristics to Chinese society's management of insanity. These lie especially in the character of the Chinese family, and they await reform by modern, scientific psychiatry. In contrast to the impact–response framework, a more dialectical analysis of psychiatry's establishment in China, particularly its knowledge making and the ensuing power effects, will reveal that medical missionary knowledge and local care practices dynamically configured and reciprocally determined each other in the colonial encounter.[10] Note that to avoid reifying 'the Chinese family' yet again, the term 'local care practices' will be used to refer not only to various ways in which relatives handled the insane, but also a constellation of other closely related factors such as religious practices, government policing, and legal provisions. In what follows, I will lay out the theoretical tools that will be employed to conduct such a dialectical analysis of missionary psychiatry, including critiques of rationality, conceptualizations of colonialism, and the knowledge/power complex of biopolitics.

The Family: Rationality, Colonialism, and Biopolitics

Medical missionaries' charge upon the Chinese family at the turn of the twentieth century ironically resonates with Max Weber's contemporaneous criticism of modern Western civilization as an 'iron cage'. For Weber, the Enlightenment project that marked the beginning of modern Western civilization took as its ultimate value the establishment of free and rational humanity unfettered by customs, blind faith, and cruelty; in other words, individual freedom and dignity constituted modernity's value rationality, that is, pursuits 'determined by a conscious belief in the value for its own sake ... independently of its prospects of success'.[11] Gradually, the metamorphosis of value rationality into instrumental rationality – that is, procedures held to be rational to the extent that they are effective in serving calculated ends[12] – and the domination of the latter over the former have trapped people in systems of bureaucracy, technical management, and institutional control.[13] In this paper, Weber's analysis is apposite for the history of Chinese psychiatry, in that, as will be shown, missionary psychiatry's value rationality of liberation and humanitarianism also became entangled with an instrumental rationality of social control and bodily discipline.

Diverging from Weber's argument about the *self*-alienation of rationality, however, it can be contended that the 'iron cage' of psychiatric rationality in China was closely tied to its identically named other, i.e. the 'iron cage' of the Chinese family. This is because in many colonial situations, the family was targeted a pivot for Enlightenment projects, a key site to fashion modernity/ies against tradition(s).[14] For example, at the turn of the century both liberal and socialist reformers endeavored to bring about a 'Chinese Enlightenment' by destroying the traditions of an oppressive patriarchy, such as concubinage, familial authority, ritual propriety, that symbolized the local bondage of ignorance and custom.[15] They would emancipate the individual with universal reason, companionate love and the nuclear family. However, as many feminist historians have pointed out, because this emphasis on the individual and the nuclear family was ultimately aimed at strengthening and modernizing the nation-state, rather than promoting individual freedom for its own sake, both liberal and socialist discourses ended up reproducing the family-state homology characteristic of 'traditional' China, constructing a new patriarchy, and failing to fully live up to their promises of Enlightenment and emancipation.[16] Missionary psychiatry worked similarly as a modernizing project, beginning by positing the Chinese family as a cultural indicator of backward tradition from which the suffering individual should be saved, and ending up educating and working with the family as a primary site to control the insane.

Yet the familial 'iron cage' is not just a steady departure point that psychiatric rationality resembled and, unfortunately, returned to. While some previous feminist historians have assumed a pre-existing Chinese patriarchy, here it is argued that the Chinese family as an object and psychiatry as a knowing subject co-constituted each other over time in what can be called 'a colonial dialectic of Enlightenment'. In their work *Dialectic of Enlightenment,* Horkheimer and Adorno further developed of Weber's initial notion of the paradoxical relationship between value rationality and instrumental rationality. They point out that in order to ensure the knowing subject's victory over the world, Enlightenment reduces the multiplicities and specificities of objects so that they can be seen as manifestations of a pre-existing, self-standing law, a law that is accessible to rationality and in a 'happy match' with it.[17] In this reduction and unification, everything is measured by its degree of conformity to rational constructs, figured as a mere repetition of the law that we already know. This form of repetition 'amputates the incommensurable'.[18] The 'other' of Enlightenment is thus *created* in a process of measurement, amputation, and domination. In this case, the 'other' is 'the patriarchal Chinese family', an indicator of local backwardness against the universal, progressive Enlightenment reason, an object of psychiatric intervention.[19] The modern configuration of the other, this failure to recognize alterity beyond rationality and identity, in turn comes to define the knowing subject – psychiatry in our case – and conditions the paradoxical metamorphoses of reason into a coercive law.

Some readers might find it strange that the word 'colonial(ism)' has been chosen to discuss how medical missionaries dealt with Chinese patients and families, as China was never fully ruled by a single colonial government, and as many medical missionaries were engaged in promoting humanitarianism or advanced technologies rather than imperial invasion or colonial government. However, in this article, the word 'colonial(ism)'is used in three interrelated senses: first, colonialism involves establishing a hegemony of the West over the rest, promoting a supposedly universal Law over particular (non-Western) cultures. Culture here is posited as an ahistorical and essential whole, of which every part is a metonym of the whole. Figured as 'the region of conjuncture where society necessarily meets biology',[20] the family is a key metonymic that anchors the whole culture (at the lower end) along an evolutionary scale.[21] Second, the historical dichotomy and hierarchy between the West and the rest, in East Asia as elsewhere, simultaneously facilitates and conceals an intricate game of power, domination, and regulation between different social forces in a colonial society. In Barlow's words, rather than a simple pressure of the West over the rest, '[t]he so-called particular (colonial or not-Western nation) and the so-called universal (colonizer) turn out not to be opposites after all, but rather a married pair that endorse each other's defects in order to conceal their own'.[22] In this case, 'the patriarchal Chinese family' as an object of colonial intervention was formed in, and in turn fueled, the interactions and interlocking of social powers. Third, colonialism elides its epistemological hegemony and power dynamics of colonialism, causing the colonized to reiterate cultural essentialism and the West's failed promise of emancipation.[23] In other words, ignoring the first two senses of colonialism and focusing only on the 'absence of an intrusive colonial regime', people in a so-called semi-colonized society may be 'intensely addicted to the idea of science [or any other universal Law] because science promised to offer a new kind of epistemological certainty to replace the crumbling cosmological order'.[24] As we will see later, contemporary Chinese psychiatry's constant invocation of the unchaining discourse may at times signal such an addiction.

Psychiatry's attention to the family also contributes to the growing literature on biopolitics in China, which examines how medicine and other technologies of life constitute subjects for institutional discipline and regulation through discursive practices about the body. So far most studies have only focused on the biologized individual and the statistically enumerated population as the subjects of biopolitics, and few have looked at the medical and hygienic construction of the family.[25] This is a regrettable lacuna, because as 'a hinge between the biological and the social', the family is a key site for political regimes to simultaneously govern the individual and the population, and thereby to reproduce and regulate their political economy.[26] A Foucaultian genealogy can, however, be done, indicating how the Chinese family emerged as a purported cultural essence that 'was fabricated in a piecemeal fashion'[27] from diverse discursive and material techniques: including, vitally, those related to the making of a modern medical science.[28] Although the main sources for this genealogy of the family are hospital reports and academic journals written by missionary doctors, these accounts have been scoured for vestiges and fragments of domestic practices, legal provisions, and cosmological forces which missionary psychiatry attempted to silence.[29] These traces in turn might suggest networks of local power that were part and parcel of the dynamic configurations not just of the Chinese family, but also of modern psychiatry.

To anticipate the conclusion, it will finally be argued that missionary psychiatric reason, with its essentializing tendencies and tendentious alignment with networks of local power, framed the Chinese family not only as an oppressive and maddening space, but also as a calculative agent of biological survival and sexual reproduction, as a site for enacting eugenic projects. This configuration of the Chinese family then facilitated psychiatric reason's own transformation into an institution of risk containment, and motivated the intermeshing of medical and legal apparatuses. As such, the familial 'iron cage' and the psychiatric 'iron cage' shaped each other throughout the twentieth century in a colonial dialectic of Enlightenment.

Domestic Confinement, Psychiatric Liberation?

In the late nineteenth century, when most missionaries supported medical evangelism, some nevertheless expressed anxieties regarding the benefit of scientific reason and the mandate of Western civilization, troubling missionary discussions on whether to establish refuges for the insane in China. From 1872 onwards, John Kerr, a well-respected medical missionary in Canton, repeatedly proposed the establishment of such a refuge to the Presbyterian Board, curiously provoking much opposition from his colleagues. Besides doubts about the feasibility of converting insane people who lack basic faculties of understanding, some missionaries also entertained romantic ideas about the Chinese mind, doubting what Western civilization had to offer. As Kerr's major opponent Charles Wenyon argued:

> Life generally here [in China] is free from the nervous strain which in the West so often destroys the balance of mind... Owing to the simplicity of life here and the clan system of society, many persons thus afflicted are able to do something for their living, and if not, they freely and safely go in and out among their relatives, and are, with few exceptions, kindly treated.[30]

Echoing the European medical theory of 'diseases of civilization' from the eighteenth century, Wenyon's account posited a direct causal relationship between cultural differences in civilization and social structure, interpreted in evolutionary terms, and the individual's health, especially health of the reasoning mind.[31] While mental illness was a malaise of developed civilization, with its high-strung society and complex mind, the Chinese clan system as a traditional, simple social structure was the matrix for backward civilization and the less sophisticated, less nervous people.

Unsuccessful in defeating such arguments, Kerr had to establish the Refuge mostly with his financial resources.[32] In order to legitimize the Refuge's existence and gain at least symbolic support from his colleagues, he had to formulate an alternative conception of insanity, centered on domestic cruelty, to counter Wenyon's concept of insanity as a disease of civilization. When explaining his own resolve to establish the Refuge, Kerr told his assistants and others a traumatic story: although he had long known of

> the lack of proper treatment by the Chinese of these patients in their own homes, how they were heavily chained, etc... it did not seem possible to take charge of these patients in a general hospital... [O]ne day when he turned an insane woman away, a concubine, the husband took her to the river just in front of the hospital and threw her in.[33]

After the Refuge was founded, themes of family abuse and graphic descriptions of it saturated the Refuge's annual reports and its staff's writings in the globally circulated *China Medical (Missionary) Journal*. For example, Selden wrote:

> If a member of a household becomes insane and unmanageable or troublesome, the common custom is to chain the person to a post or heavy stone in the house so that he or she may not be able to go out into the street or do violence to men or things... Many bear the marks of fetters that have been on hands and feet.[34]

Through their discovery of and intervention into domestic confinement, missionary psychiatrists thereby enacted an Enlightenment project, creating different subjecthoods, especially emplotting the Chinese family as the barbaric other of psychiatric reason. As Chakrabarty points out in his analysis of British colonizers' and Indian reformers' elimination of widow sacrifice, documentation of suffering operated in an Enlightenment discourse, within which universal reason 'was what could release the flow of the compassion that was naturally present in all human beings, for only reason could dispel the blindness induced by custom and habit'.[35] Accounts of the suffering of insane Chinese marked the missionary as the modern self, the universal human, who had the 'capacity to notice and document suffering... from the position of a generalized and necessarily disembodied observer', who was willing to jeopardize his own interest to rescue the victim even when he or she was in no way related to him.[36] Through this intervention the suffering insane also became a universal human, a subject who not only had the same physicality and disease susceptibility as a Westerner, but was also able to incite empathy, was worthy of respect, and, despite being temporarily insane, was capable of regaining reason with the help of humane care. For example, using Emil Kraepelin's categories to diagnose patients, Dr. J. Allen Hoffmann at the Kerr Refuge reported that the 'we have just the same kinds of psychoses here as in the homelands, and the symptoms of the different groups are identical with the symptoms of similar groups at home'.[37] In terms of treatment, one of the Refuge's principles was that 'Though insane, these patients are yet men and women – not beasts'.[38]

While missionary psychiatry humanized Chinese patients, it constructed the Chinese family, symbolized by the chain, the iron cage, and other instruments of constraint, as a patriarchy that jeopardized the foundations of individuality: freedom and life. Kerr remarked, 'A short method of getting rid of the hopelessly incurable has no doubt often been adopted *in a country where the father holds the power of life and death over his family*'.[39] In contrast to the missionary with his capacity of generalized empathy, the patriarch was a local subject, a lesser human, inflicting cruelty on the insane even when she was a blood relative. In this dialogical positioning, the conditions of the insane became 'an index for measuring the quality of a civilization', and the patriarchal family became an index of the oppressive Chinese culture.[40] Thus, in contrast to Wenyon's account that located cultural differences within the individual, the notion of insanity that the Kerr Refuge produced and that soon became the dominant discourse of missionary psychiatry across China situated cultural differences in the household. Because of a universal human nature, Western psychiatry was applicable to the Chinese insane. Because of the oppressive social structure that was symbolized by the family, however, the Chinese mind was always slightly less healthy. Compared to their Western fellow men, the Chinese were more urgently in need not just of psychiatry but also of a social reform that could change and modernize the family structure; better yet, they needed a psychiatry that went beyond curing the individual to discipline and reconstruct family life.

In order to create an evolutionarily backward, morally corrupt, and dehumanizing patriarchy to serve as Enlightenment's other, missionary psychiatry carried out a work of reduction. One aspect of local care practices that was reduced and omitted was the historical and political conditions of domestic confinement. By the mid-eighteenth century, Qing law stipulated rules on 'preventive confinement', requiring that relatives of someone mad manage and restrain that person in a safe room, and that local officials issue locks and chains to the family so that confinement and chaining up could be strictly implemented. If domestic confinement was not enforced well enough and the mad person committed homicide, the law stipulated that the relatives should be harshly sentenced.[41]

Although certainly not every family in late Imperial China locked up any insane member just in order to abide by the law, one can see that political forces entered into and helped configure the household, shaped what madness meant (a potential threat to public safety), and designated what family responsibilities were in terms of managing the insane. Domestic confinement of the insane was in one way a configuration of social concerns of public security as private liability. Despite the law's stipulation, some families furtively unchained the persons whom the local officials saw as potentially dangerous because they needed labor for agricultural work, because they saw the persons as having recovered from madness, or because they did not view chaining as a fit method of care.[42] Therefore, both Kerr's account of families chaining the insane and Wenyon's account of the insane roaming around were partially true to the reality of late Imperial China. And both accounts were gross overgeneralizations, and both also failed to see the historical and political nature of Chinese domestic relations, for instance, how socio-political concerns and legal regulations constituted the public/private divide, and how people resisted and engaged in tactical negotiations with the official spatial demarcation.[43]

This elision of the historical and political conditions of domestic confinement facilitated and concealed missionary psychiatry's strategic alliance with the police and local elites, and this is one reason why this chapter calls psychiatry's Enlightenment project 'colonial'. While the Refuge, in its first several years of existence, only admitted family patients (i.e. patients who were brought by their families), in 1904 a policeman sent in an insane man and asked whether the Refuge would admit the man at the expense of the Police Department. Staff at the Refuge remarked with excitement that this incident was 'a new departure; the first occasion of official recognition'.[44] While missionaries sought to rescue the insane from their domestic chains and to protect them from the intruding public, such as 'inconsiderate outsiders' who made fun of or even harassed the patients, the police and local elites saw the insane as a source of public danger and sought to expel them from the public.[45] Despite their sharply different notions of insanity, they had grounds for cooperation: the containment of the insane in the segregated space of refuge. The police thus handed over to the medical mission some of the responsibilities for confinement that previously had been impressed upon the family, while the missionaries ignored the socio-political conditions of domestic (and hospital) confinement. With this strategic alliance, more people were sent to the Refuge by the police, to the extent that in 1909 half of the patients were supported by officials, and half of this group had been picked up from the street by the police.[46] Faced with this rising proportion of 'police patients', the missionaries again found an opportunity to blame the family. They believed that 'many insane are kept in their houses until they have become a nuisance and until so exhausted that all hope of recovery is lost and are then put into the street for the police to pick up and bring to us'.[47] In fact, the missionaries only observed several cases like this,[48] and we can confidently argue that their belief was constituted by their conceptual lens of the oppressive, but also (as we will discuss later) calculative, family, as well as by their practical and symbolic alliance with the more powerful social actors.

It seems that in its earliest years missionary psychiatry successfully assembled a social network supportive of hospital care by constructing an image of the family and recruiting interested actors such as local elites, governments, and, by the 1920s, medical missionaries throughout the country.[49] However, the unevenly assembled network and the Refuge's spatio-symbolic segregation from local care practices were threatened by many hazards, exacerbated by the way in which missionary psychiatry amputated incommensurabilities and reduced multiplicities in its construction of the other. In an age before mass produced psychopharmaceuticals, staff at the Kerr Refuge saw '*no specifics* for insanity' but only careful nursing, discipline, and removal of the patient from existing conditions.[50] Yet they were constantly frustrated by the medicines that patients' relatives and friends attempted to bring to the Refuge, such as emetics that, in Chinese medical practices, were used to dispel the maddening phlegm.[51] Many visitors also brought food, wine and tobacco to the hospital. Some relatives and friends even insisted on living in the Refuge to accompany the insane.[52] Relatives and friends' gestures suggested not a chain but ties of intimacy binding a collective who cared for each other and viewed their fates as intertwined. On most occasions, however, missionaries saw relatives and friend's medical, material, and affective concerns for patients only as *irrational*, but not *non-rational,* that is, insufficient in but not incommensurable with or potentially disruptive to psychiatric reason. They refused to take account of, let alone compromise with, requests from patients' relatives and friends, choosing instead to maintain their own symbolic, material, and spatial demarcations between the humanitarian refuge and the bestializing household, between enlightened care and superstitious harm. This may explain why family patients did not increase at the rate of police patients, and why China for most of the early twentieth century did not have mass confinement of the insane.[53]

Besides being framed as an irrational subject, the Chinese family was also interpellated as a subject of instrumental rationality: a 'bad' rationality at odds with psychiatry's ideal of liberation. Take for example Figure 1, a photograph from the 1916 report of the Kerr Refuge. In the photo, a new patient lies bound to a pig's feeding trough, the condition in which his fellows carried him to the hospital, while in the background other hospital patients are free from constraints. Previous research on folk practices related to madness in Imperial China suggests that if people suspected madness to be caused by demonic possession, they might then chain the sufferer's body to prevent the demon from harming the patient.[54] The missionary account ignored these cosmological conditions for confinement. With the pig's feeding trough and the rope tying the insane, the missionary author portrayed the Chinese as dehumanizing the insane, treating him as a beast and a waste object to be managed and disposed of using recycled domestic resources (other pictures show the use of a ladder, a chicken coop, and a pig basket). More importantly, by using the word 'resourceful' that connotes economic, instrumental rationality, the author casts the family not just as a cruel oppressor, but also as an agent that calculated every action and the value of everything, including an individual's life, in terms of its own survival. Domestic confinement was thus understood as 'the shortest and most effectual method of treating a psychopathic member' of the patriarchal household.[55]

Yet beyond simply an enemy to fight against, the Chinese family so constituted as a calculative and 'resourceful' agent governing life also gradually became alluring to missionary psychiatry, especially in its handling of the insane's recalcitrant body. Or in Horkheimer and Adorno's terms, 'because that self never quite fitted the mold, enlightenment throughout the liberalistic period has always sympathized with social coercion. The unity of the manipulated collective consists in the negation of each individual'.[56] When missionary psychiatry posited and produced a universal human who could be salvaged from the cultural 'iron cage' and who was amenable to Enlightenment reason, it simultaneously demarcated a norm for the disciplined subject, against which the insane's bodily recalcitrance was minutely calculated, forecasted, controlled, and materialized.[57] While the space of the Kerr Refuge was initially constructed to prevent outsiders from harassing the insane, by 1909, five years after the Refuge willingly took on responsibilities of public security and confinement of police patients, the director decided on building thick doors to prevent the insane from breaking them down and escaping. In a correspondence with the editor of the *China Medical Journal* in 1920, Robert Ross, then the director of the Kerr Refuge, recommended that all general hospitals should be provisioned with at least three articles for handling the insane patient: a bath-tub, a wire restraining frame, and a straight jacket. He also promised to 'gladly supply the dimensions of the above articles as we use them to any who apply'.[58] If we compare Figure 5.2, portraying the wire restraining frame the staff at the Refuge devised for 'humane restraint' of the patient,[59] to Figure 5.3, showing the pig basket the natives used to transport the patients to the Refuge, we see a very interesting parallel in the equipment's shape and use: provided, that is, that we take on the missionaries' perspective and see the pig basket as resourcefully employed tools of constraint. It is likely that missionaries appropriated this bit of 'Chinese wisdom' for their own resourceful use. In any case, the pig basket picture still showed the struggling body of the insane, the relatives-carriers who simultaneously constrained and connected with the insane through the prosthesis, or the spectator who could not close his/her senses to the noise, sweat, fear, and hope of the intimate bond.[60] In contrast, every trace of human connectedness has disappeared from the picture of the wire restraining frame; the recalcitrant body was completely silenced and excluded. When missionary psychiatry characterized the family as an agent of instrumental rationality and a force of objectification, it dialectically held up a mirror to itself.

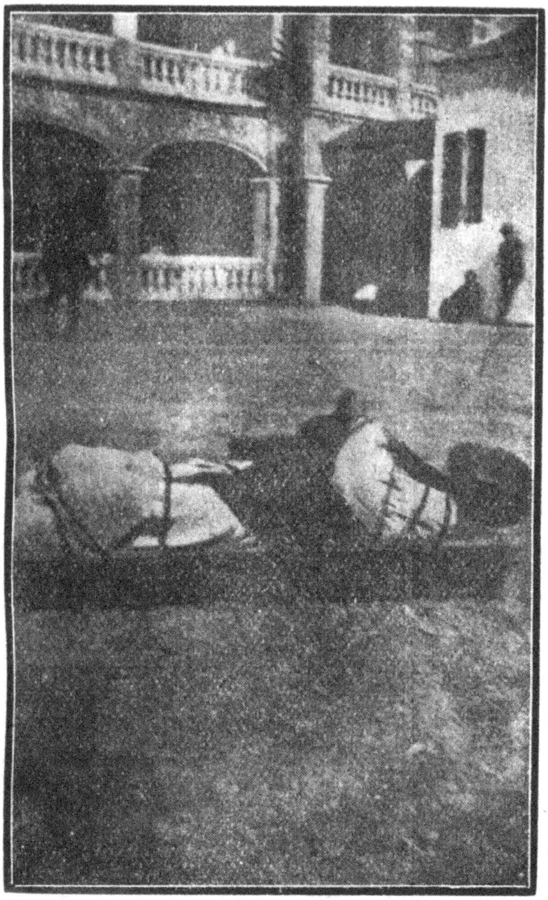

The Chinese are very resourceful. Here is a refractory patient brought tied to a pigs' feeding trough.

Figure 5.1: **Patient Tied to a Pig's Feeding Trough. From the John G. Kerr Hospital for the Insane, Reports for 1916 and 1917 (Canton, China: The China Baptist Publication Society, 1917). Image on the fly page. Courtesy of Special Collections, Yale Divinity School Library**

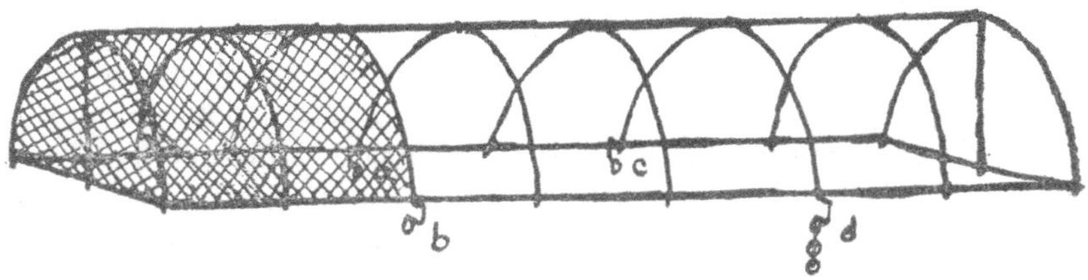

Backbone and ribs partially covered with netting.

Figure 5.2: Wire Restraining Frame. From C. C. Selden, 'III. Treatment of the Insane', *The China Medical Journal* (1909), pp. 373–84, on p. 375. Courtesy of the Center for Research Libraries

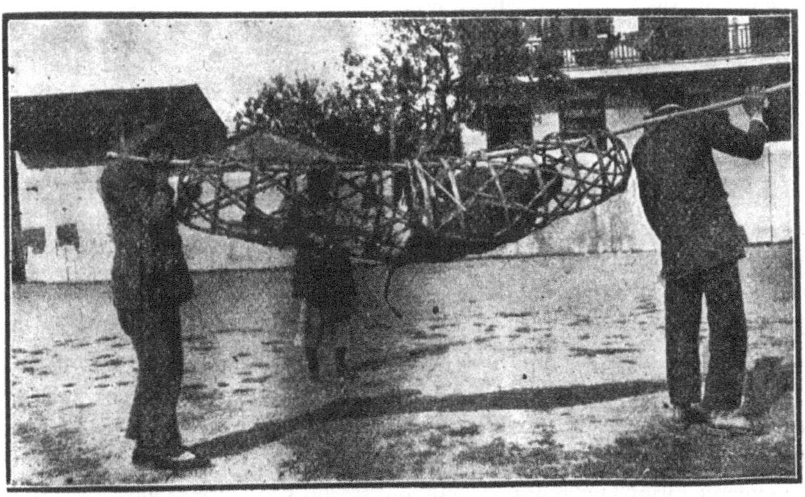

Various patients have been brought in the baskets used for transporting pigs. This one required two fastened together.

Figure 5.3: Patient Transported in Pig Baskets. From the John G. Kerr Hospital for the Insane, Reports for 1916 and 1917 (Canton, China: The China Baptist Publication Society, 1917), p. 12. Courtesy of Special Collections, Yale Divinity School Library

The Chinese Family at the Crossroad of Eugenics and Psychoanalysis

In late 1910s and 1920s, the colonial dialectic of Enlightenment between a supposedly universal psychiatry and its particular, local other, the Chinese family, bifurcated into two new epistemologies of insanity and subjectivity. These continued to position missionary psychiatry tendentiously with different social forces, while shaping psychiatry's future in China. On the one hand, as we will see later, the influence of psychoanalysis came to be felt; on the other, the importation of a eugenics discourse beginning in the 1910s gave impetus to the process by which a value rationality of liberation transformed into an instrumental rationality of managing life and controlling risks. In 1913, the concept of heredity appeared for the first time in publications from the Kerr Refuge, and it was, again, invoked to critique the Chinese family. Noting the prevalence of madness in Canton and the existence of hereditary taint in many patients, Hoffmann argued

> the [Chinese] custom of ancestor worship demands that every male should have offspring. Much as we have advised against it, still it has happened many times that demented patients have been taken out of the hospital to get married.[61]

Using the concept of heredity, Hoffman and other medical missionaries now configured the insane person not as a universal human capable of rationality, but as a biological body carrying and spreading hereditary defects and moral degeneracy.[62] The targeted patient was thus transformed from a sovereign individual to a disciplined body. Moreover, Chinese families, especially those rich enough for early marriage and polygamy, were now figured as instantiations of evolutionarily backward marriage customs and a corrupt social order; these customs could only worsen the heredity of future generations by compelling the sick to reproduce, and the practices awaited elimination by 'the law of the survival of the fittest'.[63] Some later professionals noted in passing that at least in some cases relatives took the patient out of the hospital for marriage 'in the hope of curing the insanity'.[64] But the doctors, again, perceived this hope only as *irrational,* i.e. deviating from the eugenic rationale of containment and sterilization, not as *non-rational*; that is, doctors disregarded the possibilities that relatives might arrange marriage to appease a possessing devil, or to satisfy the patients' yearnings for love, desires that were often seen as pathogenic.[65] Missionary doctors thus sought to rescue society from Chinese families. By preventing families from taking the insane back home, they now endeavored not to bring the patient back to humanity and rationality, but to contain the sexual danger he posed to society.

With a set of institutional techniques that developed around the concepts of heredity and eugenics, missionary psychiatry quickly changed from seeing the Chinese family as its irrational antithesis to regarding the familial reproductive machine as its partner in a synthetic alliance that would manage the insane. In the 1920s, many case reports emerged in the Kerr Refuge's publications enumerating how many members in a single household suffered from insanity.[66] Beyond treating the family as an object of calculation and monitoring, missionary psychiatry sought to turn the family into a subject that calculated and monitored its own internal risks.[67] The Kerr Refuge held two mental hygiene campaigns aimed at educating the public on issues like 'heredity and feeblemindedness', 'segregation of [the] feebleminded', and 'the relation of feeblemindedness to crime, to prostitution, to the spread of venereal disease'.[68] Most importantly, the campaigns addressed the patriarchal family that missionary psychiatry used to deplore in a sympathetic and advisory tone:

> In this land where agricultural methods have been so highly developed along certain lines it is surprising that there is so little evidence of the appreciation of the importance of stock and seed selection. In this land where posterity is so much desired it is surprising that there is so little evidence of the appreciation of the importance of eugenics. Where children are so greatly desired it seems strange to see how little attention is given to the antecedents of the concubine. Among the most enlightened one very frequently finds the concubine who bears children into the family, has been a slave, or even a prostitute, whose parents are unknown.[69]

Interestingly, while knowledge of eugenics and heredity that arose in the US at the turn of the century aimed at erasing the 'depravity' of polygamy that 'fell outside the bonds of prevailing middle-class standards', in China the missionary psychiatrists, most of whom had been trained in the US, no longer sought to defend the middle-class morals.[70] Instead, they urged the Chinese families to heed 'stock and seed selection', to investigate the reproductive history of the concubine:[71] in a word, to be wise patriarchies equipped with an instrumental rationality of sexual and reproductive calculation.

The second development in the epistemology of psychiatry came in the late 1920s, when missionary psychiatrists translated the language of the familial 'iron cage' into a psychoanalytic or quasi-psychoanalytic vocabulary, using this new vocabulary as an etiological framework for critiquing the pathogenic dynamics of the Chinese family. In a 1926 article on mental hygiene, Robert Ross from the Kerr Refuge systematically discussed the 'cause[s] of irritation and strife [in Chinese family life] that we [Westerners] are free from'. These predisposing pathogenic causes included 'the unreasonable authority vested in the mother-in-law', 'the concubinage system' that brought fear to wives and concubines who could not bear sons, and in general, 'the cramping restrictions upon social exchange between the two sexes'.[72] Soon, physicians from other medical facilities started writing more full-blown psychoanalytic discussions of the impact that Chinese culture had on the mind by way of a strenuous family life. For example, Andrew Woods from Peking Union Medical College wrote:

> The sexual life of the Chinese is different from ours in its superficial exhibitions, but obviously has under it the same deep instinctive and emotional forces. They are driven by strong cravings, and these are inhibited by equally vigorous regulative and protective devices on both the instinctive and the intellectual levels. Hence, there are repressions, out of which conflicts arise, causing stormy emotional disturbances.[73]

With the language of psychoanalysis, Woods and other missionary psychiatrists thereby started to depict the Chinese individual as a subject with sexual instincts, and Chinese family life as a field of intensities and inhibitions of desire.

Understanding the Chinese insane in a psychoanalytic register involved a delicate play of universalities and particularities, which, again, hinged on an anatomy of the local family structure. The psychoanalytic discourse saw familial life and sexual exchanges in both Chinese and Western families as suffused with 'erotic coloring', such as longing, fixation, disappointment, and antagonism. This universal eroticism ran counter to the 'average Occidental' view that 'the Chinese betrothal and marriage customs are without emotions', and thereby legitimized the application of psychoanalysis to the desiring Chinese.[74] However, medical missionaries never forgot to locate cultural particularities in the Chinese family. Following the emancipatory discourse that lamented the concubine drowned for her madness, and the eugenics discourse that advised the patriarch to heed the impurity of the concubine's heredity, physicians writing in a psychoanalytic register also turned to pay specific attention to the Chinese concubinage system and its toll on women's emotional life. Woods wrote:

> Jealousy is as fierce in the Chinese as elsewhere when coveted love strays to superior attractions. Herein is *one of the greatest of the drawbacks to polygamy*... it becomes the groundwork of subtler conflicts when its control is disturbed by the pressure of passion.[75]

In this psychoanalytic account, jealousy highlighted women's desire for love and obsession with its objects, casting them as universal libidinal subjects, but this emotion also marked the frustration and repression brought on by the fierce competition, power hierarchy, and demands for propriety that were involved in Chinese polygamy.

The emergence of psychoanalysis in missionary psychiatry brought several new techniques, which produced a new subjectivity of intimacy. Since 'neuropsychosis is a form of reaction which can only be interpreted if the history of the development of the individual is known', analytically oriented physicians called for uncovering patients' past sexual and emotional lives through conversation.[76] In addition, sometimes a medical social service worker was also sent to investigate the intricate history of a patient's family life. Woods reported a case in which a mechanic was distressed by living with his extended family, and particularly by the tension between his equally tyrannical mother and sister-in-law. After discovering this family history, Woods persuaded the patient in 'a reasoning and sympathetic conversation' to remove his nuclear family to another house. The physician placed a social service agent in charge of 'getting into contact with the families, explaining our plans and convincing patients and their relatives'. Finally the patient realized that '[f]ilial obedience had to yield to vital obligations'.[77] With these clinical techniques and social rearrangements, missionary psychiatry for the first time thrust open the door of what it perceived as the sovereign and dysfunctional patriarchy, promoting a change from an extended family that was concerned with ritual propriety to a nuclear family that was concerned with the survival and sexual development of the individual. Through therapeutic conversation and social service investigation, the insane person gained individuality because of his failure to fully identify with an oppressive family and culture, his possession of his own emotional history and sexual truth, as well as his potential to maximize his own libidinal satisfaction by rationally knowing himself and rearranging his social relations. It is no exaggeration to say that, in the psychoanalytic register, the insane became the source and pinnacle of modern Chinese individuality.

Although emancipatory, eugenic and psychoanalytic discourses often intermixed in missionary writings of the late 1920s, these discursive apparatuses later had different fates, which can only be very roughly sketched out here. A psychoanalytic orientation, broadly defined, fostered the birth of psychiatric social service in leading medical institutions, and later led to psychotherapies that focused on the talking cure and mental, emotional aspects of psychopathology. Moreover, the missionaries' use of psychoanalytic theory as a tool of cultural critique was echoed in Chinese intellectuals' attack on the repressive cultural traditions during the New Culture Movement in the mid-1910s and 1920s. For example, in 1929 Pan Guangdan, a US-trained Chinese sexologist, published a famous psycho-biography of the Ming poetess Feng Xiaoqing, in which he used Freudian theory to argue that the concubine Feng's narcissistic symptoms and eventual suicide were manifestations of an arrested sexual development, resulting from maltreatment by the wife and neglect by the husband. Pan used this analysis to advocate for elimination of polygamy, women's rights in choosing marriage partners, and more social awareness of women's toils.[78] As Pan's writing shows, psychoanalysis's 'repressive hypothesis was an effective weapon in challenging the prohibition of sexual effectiveness within the terms of Confucian orthodoxy', and therefore 'it is fervently embraced by modernizing and modernist intellectuals alike for its emancipatory promises'.[79] However, while Pan's writings were taken up in public discussions of family reform, the life of psychoanalysis in psychiatry, both as a therapy and as a tool of cultural critique, was powerfully marginalized by the domination of eugenics, and later on, of behaviorism and dialectical materialism. Within the psychiatric field in China, psychoanalysis enjoyed a brief period of development in the mid-1930s, when Bingham Dai, a US-trained sociologist and analyst influenced by Harry Stack Sullivan and Karen Horney, took up a position at Peking Union Medical College. There he set up a clinic seeing patients and teaching residents psychoanalytically-oriented therapy.[80] Surveying the social situations that precipitated the patients' disorders, he argued that mental disturbances reflected social ills in China, such as concubinage and tensions with in-laws.[81] But after Dai's return to the US in 1939, the voice of psychoanalysis in Chinese psychiatry basically fell silent.

As we have seen, the eugenics discourse rather than seeking to restructure the family, sought to make it assume the doctor's role in monitoring the sexual behavior and hereditary quality of its members, especially the concubine, to prevent the insane persons from injuring 'Chinese society by marriage and the propagation of undesirable offspring'.[82] This discourse thus facilitated missionary psychiatry's active participation in marriage control and other forms of the medico-legal jurisdiction of insanity. For example, the 1923 provisional criminal code of the Republic of China made it illegal for anyone to have sexual intercourse with persons of unsound mind; it required that a psychiatrist determine whether people suspected of insanity were actually so and to provide testimony to the court, while the Police Regulations of Peking stipulated that the insane be detained and accommodated in an asylum.[83] With this intermeshing of medical and legal apparatus, psychiatry in Republican China gradually leaned toward the eugenics discourse, becoming a tool of population control.

'Iron Cage(s)' and the Colonial Dialectic of Enlightenment

As we have seen throughout this chapter, 'the Chinese family' was a singularly important signifier in the development of psychiatry in China at the turn of the century, but one with shifting significations. Understanding these shifts helps us grasp how the globally circulated discourses and practices of humanitarianism, eugenics, and psychoanalysis interacted with local regimes of care and regulation not just to govern individual and collective life, but also to shape what a medical discipline amounted to as a field of thought, practice, and institutions. Moreover, it helps us fathom the seemingly opposing and yet co-constitutive cultural imaginaries of insanity and normality, subjectivity and domesticity, tradition and modernity.

The dynamic configurations of missionary psychiatry and the Chinese family constitute a colonial dialectic of Enlightenment. When missionaries founded the first asylum for the insane in China, their goal was to break the 'iron cage' of what they perceived as an oppressive, patriarchal family, and to emancipate the insane person, casting him as the universal human who was worthy of respect and capable of reason. In other words, designating the family as an ahistorical, essential index of Chinese culture, as its other, missionary psychiatry embarked on an Enlightenment project of transforming traditional, local collectivity into modern, universal individuality. Recognizing only the law of reason, medical missionaries denied the relatives' medical, affective, and cosmological concerns for the insane, as expressed both in domestic accommodations and in family interventions during hospital treatment; or, rather, the missionaries could only see these concerns as insufficient in, but not outside of, rationality. In so doing, they pulled Chinese domestic practices into Euro-American historicity, locating it as backwards on an evolutionary time scale.[84] After amputating the local care practices' incommensurabilities with reason and evolutionary historicity, missionary psychiatry now framed the Chinese family as a calculative agent that measured every member and every action's worth according to the goal of its own survival, and later saw it as a natural unit of sexual reproduction operating under instrumental rationality.

This chapter calls this project of psychiatric emancipation a colonial project of Enlightenment, because, first, it was subject to reason's predicament of objectification, reduction, and alienation, and, second, it was also deeply involved in the intricate networks of power, domination, and regulation in a colonial society. As discussed, missionary psychiatrists elided the fact that domestic confinement had been socio-historically and politically conditioned, partly to assist as central and local governments' displacement of responsibilities for public security onto the private. This elision allowed the police to transfer some responsibilities for confinement from families to asylums, which were then gradually turned into institutions of population control. Moreover, by positing the insane person as a universal human who could be brought to the light of reason, psychiatrists simultaneously demarcated a norm for the disciplined subject, against which they encountered, measured, and tried to tame a recalcitrant body. These growing concerns with discipline and public security, then, turned the image of the calculating agent around, flipping the mirror from the known object, the family, back to the knowing subject of missionary psychiatry. Through this colonial dialectic of Enlightenment, the value rationality of universal, humanizing reason that psychiatry promoted now began to tumble down a slippery slope towards an instrumental rationality of regulating body and managing life.

This chapter also calls the development of psychiatry in China a colonial dialectic of Enlightenment because psychiatry's elision of colonial power dynamics in China enabled it to reiterate cultural essentialism and made for a failed promise of emancipation.[85] Although no single historical continuity can explain the complicated development of psychiatry in China across the extended time span from 1890s to 2010s, nowadays we see ever stronger reverberations of the emancipatory ideal in national mental health campaigns aimed at unchaining and emancipating suffering patients from the constraining domestic sphere. However, this humanitarian utopia is entangled in everyday clinical techniques that intervene in the family, educating relatives to provide psychiatrists reports of patients' psychological conditions and illness histories, to monitor the patients' drug compliance, and to protect them from posing reproductive and behavioral risks to society. In short, as long as they fail to see the cultural colonialism and essentialism involved in designating domestic care practices as oppressive confinement, and as long as they collaborate with government regulations to manage life, contemporary Chinese psychiatrists may risk reproducing the 'iron cages' of civilization.

Acknowledgements

This study was supported by the Andrew W. Mellon Foundation Research Fellowship at Needham Research Institute, Cambridge, UK and the Pre-Dissertation Research Travel Grant from the Committee of Chinese Studies, University of Chicago. I am much grateful to Prof. Judith Farquhar, Prof. Susan Gal, Dr. Howard Chiang, Ms. Tracy Weiner and Amir Hampel, who have critically read through drafts of this paper and provided insightful suggestions. Earlier versions of this paper were presented at the Annual Conference of Association for Asian Studies in Toronto, Canada in March 2012; the Anthropology Graduate Student Conference 'Space-time: Toward an Anthropology of Contemporaneity', University of Chicago Center in Beijing in August 2012; Conference on 'History of Western Medicine in China, 1800-1950' in Beijing in June 2013. I thank the discussants and audience of these conferences for their comments and questions.

6 TROPICAL NEURASTHENIA OR ORIENTAL NERVES? WHITE BREAKDOWNS IN CHINA

Wen-Ji Wang

Introduction

In a survey published on the *British Journal of Medicine* in November 1913, G. Price used missionary statistics to determine the major reasons for why Western residents in the tropics and sub-tropics became invalids. The most common tropical diseases among Westerners in India, Ceylon, China and Japan were neurasthenia and mental disorders. Japan had the worst scenario, with 81.25% of the white invalids diagnosed with neurasthenics. In comparison, the leading illness caught by Westerners in Africa was malaria, and neurasthenia ranked second. Among the 203 cases in China, 25% were affected by neurasthenia and 8.8% by mental diseases.[1] In September 1915, the *China Medical Journal* used Price's data to emphasize the arduous life of the missionaries stationed in the country. The high prevalence of neurasthenia was mostly attributed to their tremendous responsibility and heavy workload.[2] Similarly, Frank Oldt, an American medical missionary in Canton, stated in 1919 that nervous disorder posed the greatest health risk among foreign populations in China.[3] In 1920, William Lennox of the Peking Union Medical College conducted a statistical study on the health of missionary families in the country and showed that nervous breakdown ranked fourth among the most frequently occurring illnesses, and nervousness was a key cause of miscarriages.[4]

Since the early 1900s, tropical neurasthenia and other related disorders have been a focus of attention in the field of tropical medicine. After its first appearance in the Philippines, tropical neurasthenia was discussed in medical journals in every major Western language.[5] In 1913, Sir Richard Havelock Charles, president of the Medical Board, India Office, adopted an imperialist perspective and reported that neurasthenia was the most serious impediment to the immigration and procreation of the 'northern peoples' in India. As a consequence, 'European struggles during the first, dwindles and degenerates during the second, and becomes extinct, as such, during the third or fourth generation'.[6] A 1920 report by the Dutch East India Company stated that 111 out of 189 sick cases (58.73%) were afflicted with psychosis or psychoneuroses.[7] Tropical neurasthenia was mentioned in other publications as well. In 1925, the Bishop of Singapore asked readers of the *British Medical Journal* about the cause of insanity and nervous breakdown among Europeans because the 'tropical colonies and dependencies of the empire are of great importance to us, both in producing wealth and in providing honourable careers for our young men'.[8] The next two to three years were marked by further discussions on the topic, with letters coming in from the West Indies, South America, West and Central Africa, Ceylon, India, China, Canada, Australia and even Northern Russia.[9] Tropical neurasthenia, 'colonial psychosis' and other related disorders were also mentioned in contemporary textbooks in tropical medicine in the 1920s and 1930s.[10] In his authoritative book, *Manson's Tropical Diseases*, Philip Manson-Bahr suggested that, based on the colonial administration, the damage caused by tropical neurasthenia far outweighed that of other tropical diseases.[11]

The above examples demonstrate that tropical nervous and mental disorders have been widely discussed in the early twentieth century. However, compared with other tropical diseases, only a few historical studies are available on the subject. Dane Kennedy has focused on the colonial representation of the tropics. He observes that the heated discussion about the breakdown of the white nervous system showed, first, the endurance of environmental determinism after the discovery of germ theory and, second, the contemporary concern about the feasibility of Western colonialism. The behavioral, mental and physical pathologies of the colonizers indicated the impending collapse of the moral and physical boundaries between them and the natives. Thus, the medical attention provided and the measures introduced to combat the problem aimed at consolidating racial categories.[12] Notwithstanding that several contemporary medical practitioners expressed apprehension about the desirability of permanent migration, Kennedy posits that the opinion of medical practitioners was not a critique of imperialism per se, but illustrated the manner by which colonial medicine influenced colonial affairs.[13]

Warwick Anderson's study underscores the transformation of theoretical models of tropical neurasthenia in colonial Philippines. Before the 1920s, American physicians discussed the damaging effect of tropical heat and sunshine. Thereafter, the Freudian theory of sexuality and psychical conflicts became increasingly dominant. The lure of sexual promiscuity, the need of single adults to remain abstinent and other sex-related problems made 'philippinitis' or 'brain-fag' a common complaint among the colonizers. Within some twenty years, the social perception on tropical neurasthenia has transformed from being a noble act of self-sacrifice for the Empire to an inclination that was often faulty in character. Despite their theoretical difference, Anderson argues that the goal of the medical discourses on tropical neurasthenia was to cultivate the mind and body of male colonizers to fight against enemies within and without. The concepts of colonialism and Western civilization remained intact, considering that the disease was an outcome which may be attributed either to the treacherous environment or individual unconsciousness.[14]

Whereas Kennedy and Anderson attempt to unveil the colonial implications of medical discourses, Anna Crozier's more recent study highlights the close connection between tropical neurasthenia and its original clinical conceptualization in American and British medical cultures. 'Home-grown preoccupations' of modernity, gender and class resonated in British East Africa. Crozier's second observation is more related to that of Kennedy and Anderson. The popularity of the diagnosis is attributed to its practicality as a tool for the regulation of the colonial personnel: '[T]ropical nervous diagnoses were used as a means of policing the colonizers and trying to control and homogenize behaviours to a model of acceptability'.[15]

Sloane Mahone's analysis shows that 'mal-adaptation' was a common fate shared by the colonizers and the colonized in East Africa in the early twentieth century. In addition to the frequent accounts of neurasthenia among Europeans, the modern psychiatric framework expanded so that the African mind and culture were pathologized as well. Constant contact with the colonizers caused many local elites to succumb to nervous ailments. Likewise, African religious activities and even political acts of rebellion were considered psychopathological in the view of colonial doctors.[16]

Based on the above, it can be seen that tropical neurasthenia was subjected to divergent interpretations during the first half of the twentieth century. A similar case can be found in colonial Taiwan. Yu-Chuan Wu's account of the development of psychiatry in Taiwan during the 1930s and 1940s emphasizes the conflicting ideologies surrounding the disease and the role of colonial medicine in reinforcing racial differences. Neurasthenia was often considered a sign of individual and racial degeneration in Japan but, in the perspective of colonial psychiatrists, its psychosomatic symptoms were the result of the nostalgia on the part of their transplanted compatriots. These medical officers embraced the psychological model that rendered tropical neurasthenia as an 'illness which was comprehensible, deserving sympathy or even respect, and more importantly, treatable'. Accordingly, their neurasthenic patients were not degenerates but self-abnegated vanguards of the Empire.[17] In the same vein, Wu's other study on tropical neuroses investigates the manner by which the Japanese and the Taiwanese were regarded differently in colonial discourse.[18]

The debates surrounding the possibility of successful white acclimatization were 'part and parcel of a wider conversation congregating around matters of colonial praxis and imperial health'.[19] The studies mentioned above have thoroughly examined the social and cultural implications of medical and scientific discourses from the context of colonialism, particularly the role of these conversations in reshaping white identity and safeguarding racial boundaries. In light of the existing studies, the present chapter reviews the medical discussions about the so-called 'tropical' nervous and mental breakdowns of Western expatriates in China in the late nineteenth and early twentieth centuries, particularly the ways in which the problem of acclimatization was subjected to different models of explanation. The present study particularly focuses on the heterogeneity in terms of medical knowledge systems, as well as the different social concerns involved in the debates. Moreover, considering that a noticeable proportion of the discussion on the nervous and mental instability of white inhabitants in China were written from a *missionary* rather than a *colonial* perspective and, as an extensive part of the country was not under direct Western colonial rule, the following analysis investigates the feasibility of utilizing the analytic framework developed through the colonial context to explain the situation in China, which was then under the influence of several 'informal empires' and Western medical systems. As Anderson cautions, 'China's role in the colonial drama of the nineteenth and twentieth centuries is too ambiguous or marginal to insert it readily into the analysis of the medical dimension of imperialism'.[20] Using tropical neurasthenia as an example, the present chapter explores the complex relationship among colonial medicine, missionary medicine and the development of medical sciences in the country.

Shattered Nerves in Tropical China

Nervous and mental breakdown among Western residents in China from the late nineteenth century to the 1930s was a theme often discussed in contemporary missionary documents, personal accounts, biographies and medical reports. Several well-known missionaries, including Dr. Peter Parker, were believed to have experienced forms of mental disturbance.[21] In the early 1890s, cases of 'mental illness', 'melancholia' and 'nervous weakness' among British 'white troops' were recorded in China.[22] Various causes had been suggested for generating 'nerves', namely, strenuous work, insanitary environment, stringent climatic conditions, diseases and the social depravity of the locals.[23] Similarly, researchers have observed the pathogenic effects of tragic events, such as the loss of loved ones or the gruesome experience during the Taiping upheaval and the Boxer Rebellion, and religious fanaticism.[24] Lottie Moon, the Southern Baptist missionary who would later suffer from emotional depression, wrote an account in the 1880s that was characteristic of the era:

> The life here [Pingtu City, in rural Shantung province], as we Western people consider life, is exceedingly narrow and contracted. Constant contact with people of a low civilization and many disgusting habits is a trial to one of refined feelings and tastes.[25]

Climate was the most prominent among the predisposing factors. As recounted in a report by David Duncan Main of the Hangchow Medical Mission in 1894, the 'unhealthy climate' of mid-China, particularly its 'continued heat', caused malaria, headaches and 'general depression' among foreign missionaries and made them a 'feeble folk'.[26] In 1901, Edward Henderson, who had previously worked as the municipal surgeon and a general practitioner in Shanghai for over three decades, commented about the effect of tropical heat on the European constitution. Heat resulted in the 'general enfeeblement of the nervous and muscular systems'. Thus, he followed the advice often made regarding tropical hygiene and suggested that 'the European ought not to be allowed to spend more of his young life in the tropics than can be helped'.[27] In the viewpoint of the above commentators, the ancient country was in great need of salvation; however, taking residence in this country was an extremely debilitating experience. As such, a missionary report noted in 1920 that 'China is a relentless discoverer of weak points'.[28]

Decades after neurasthenia had become a fashionable diagnosis in the West, this illness began to be listed as one of the frequent nervous and mental diseases afflicting foreign expatriates in China around the beginning of the twentieth century. The disease spread, but not as widely as expected when considering its pervasiveness in contemporary Western societies.[29] Bromide therapy was used in Shanghai in the late 1890s to treat cases of morphine addiction, neurasthenia, nervous disturbance and acute mania.[30] Neurasthenia became the focus of attention in 1909 when Hugo Weber, former assistant sanitary inspector, petitioned the Council for the Foreign Community of Shanghai for the full amount of superannuation after resigning on the basis of ill health. When Weber requested for a 'change of climate' after he attributed his neurasthenic symptoms to climate and excessive work, four medical doctors (including W. B. Billinghurst and Millais Culpin, whose views will be discussed shortly) were summoned by the Council to verify his claim. Their testimonies regarding the authenticity, severity and prognosis of Weber's condition demonstrate the familiarity of the local Western medical practitioners with the disease.[31] Similarly, neurasthenia was coupled with the condition of staying away from one's homeland to market patent medicines. In 1910, a Mr F. L. Harrison from Tsingkiangpu, Jiangsu Province, praised the heavily promoted Pink Pills for Pale People by Dr. Williams, which saved his wife from indigestion, headaches and neurasthenia. He highlighted the value of the medicine in his household, particularly because they were living 'far away from the ordinary comfort and conveniences of European civilisation'.[32]

With the broadening discourse on 'tropical neurasthenia' in the European and American colonies, China soon turned into another venue for the debate on the illness. Despite the sanitary reforms introduced in the country, China was still considered by the medical authority in the 1920s as an impossible place for white men to settle in because of its trying living conditions, which resulted in nervous breakdowns among adults and lack of 'mental and physical energy and buoyancy of spirit' among children.[33] 'Tropical neurasthenia' may be a new clinical category, but the framework through which the illness was discussed in China was not entirely new. Studies focused on the influence of predisposition, local climate, environment, political situation or social practices on the occidental nervous system. For example, in his comment on Sir Havelock Charles's paper in 1910 on the factors affecting Europeans in the tropics, John Preston Maxwell of the English Presbyterian Church at Amoy agreed with the importance placed on screening out individuals with a family history of 'nervous unsoundness'. In addition, his clinical experience in southern China showed that residents who had previously had kidney problems 'rapidly became neurasthenics'.[34] In the view of another missionary observer, the 'peculiar electrical conditions' in northern China had the tendency to 'affect unfavorably the nervous system of many foreigners'.[35] The abovementioned article by Price from 1913 noted that the primary reason behind the high incidence of white neurosis in northern China was its dry weather and excessive sunshine, which resulted in the increase in mental activities to the extent of nervous irritability or breakdown. The violence involved in the political and religious turmoil worsened the problem.[36] In response to Price's commentaries, Duncan Whyte of the English Presbyterian Mission Hospital at Swatow proposed the 'over-stimulation of the optic nerve by glare' as a cause of neurasthenia. After two years, the editor of the *China Medical Journal* utilized the statistical data provided by Price again to explain the high percentage of acute mental diseases and neurasthenic disorders among foreign missionaries. Climatic conditions and 'political disorders accompanied by mob violence' played a role in the onset of the disease; however, the underlying causes of nervous exhaustion in every missionary field were excessive work and the immense responsibility at work.[37] Arthur H. Smith, the editor of *A Manuel for Young Missionaries to China*, noted that the nervous system was the most sensitive bodily system 'to the change to China'. Medical examinations showed that the strain was often caused by the dryness of the atmosphere.[38]

Apart from providing opinions on the etiology and symptomatology of tropical breakdown, some scholars suggested methods for the prevention and treatment of the disease. Price urged missionaries with a nervous disposition and family history should not be allowed to go abroad – a suggestion that was often repeated in similar contexts.[39] A comment published by the *China Medical Jour-*

nal quoted a medical authority to characterize the 'non-missionary' residents who were able to 'stand up against the trials of life in the tropics':

> The man wanted is one 'with his head well screwed on, an even temper, not over intellectual, one who can take an interest in things around, not unduly introspective ... capable of bearing exposure to the sun, one who will practise temperance in all things, with self-control and common-sense'. Many are prepared to say that the last is the most desirable quality of all.[40]

Furthermore, the importance of taking regular furloughs or reducing the interval between furloughs to prevent the occurrence of nervous breakdowns and similar diseases was stressed by medical missionaries residing in China.[41] William W. Cadbury of the Canton Hospital elucidated this point by stating that 'long term of [missionary] service predisposes to nervous breakdown'.[42] Considering that the issue of the frequency and length of furloughs was consistently a topic of interest among foreign missionaries and their home mission boards in terms of both their recuperating effect and 'the immense investment of time and life' involved, abbreviating the term of service should not be dismissed as a mere medical advice.[43]

Similarly, other prophylactic measures against the climatic effects often found in contemporary tropical hygiene textbooks and medical reports were recommended for the Chinese context. In 1926, Walter B. Billinghurst, a former doctor of the British Consulate and the High Court in Shanghai, wrote that he had treated most British cases of mental and nervous disorders in the city. The symptoms included memory loss (or 'tropical amnesia'), irritability and suicidal tendencies. Recognizing the roles of 'intellectual, aesthetic, and emotional influences' in causing mental imbalance, Billinghurst stressed the failure of cortical circulation, particularly the over-excitation and fatigue of cortical cells. Thus, Billinghurst suggested that Europeans should acquire the Chinese custom of taking naps in the afternoon to enable the cortex to be fully rested. Hats, sunglasses and late-afternoon sports were likewise recommended.[44] After studying two severe foreign cases near the Nanking area, British physician Andrew S. McNeil attributed nervous irritability and collapse to metabolic dysfunction triggered by the relentless sunshine and mugginess.[45] Thus, he recommended dressing in Chinese fashion and adopting local eating habits and measures to avoid 'the tropical sun'.[46]

Neurasthenia has been known in the history of psychiatry for its considerable elasticity as a medical category.[47] The reports discussed above illustrate that the discourses on tropical neurasthenia in China had multiple sources. Thus, numerous social issues had been associated with the diagnosis. First, the discomfort about the ability of white races to be acclimatized in foreign environments had a long history, and this idea had been incorporated into different medical and scientific ideas during the course of the nineteenth and early twentieth centuries.[48] Similarly, the climatic determinism of diseases was often intertwined with social, cultural and economic explanations,[49] a fact that can likewise be observed in the present study. Furthermore, the anxiety underlying the aforementioned commentaries on tropical neuroses was similar to that made in reference to other tropical diseases in China during the same period.[50] As a derivative of the Westerner's apprehension with unfamiliar environments that has been in place for more than a century, tropical neurasthenia easily entered contemporary medical parlance. Second, Crozier observes in the context of East Africa that the Victorian language about nerves[51] and the catch-all idea of neurasthenia were incorporated into the already flexible framework of analysis. Interestingly, in most of the cases, it was not civilization, but the want of it, that exhausted white physical and nervous systems in the tropics. Third, and more importantly, the sometimes 'ethnographic' depictions of the physically strenuous environment and social depravity of China further enhanced the price paid by Western adventurers to maintain their status and perform their duty. Moreover, the extensive involvement of missionaries in the discussion elevated the image of a martyr into that of a champion of Western civilization and progress. In this sense, medical studies on neurasthenia combined with contemporary missionary discourse in China to generate 'a narrative of Christian sacrifice, suffering, death, and resurrection'.[52]

Two more ideas are also worthy of notice. For contemporary commentators, the degenerating capability of the Middle Kingdom and that of other foreign milieus appear to have no qualitative differences. The discourse that was originally used to explain colonial experiences in India, Africa, the Philippines and Australia was applied in a country where foreign powers supposedly had only 'informal' influence. Owing to the similar intellectual background and living conditions, medical commentators with Chinese connections were keen to join the debate on tropical hygiene, even from the periphery, as far as the clinical construction of white nervous breakdown is concerned.[53] The fact that the pieces of advice for prospective missionaries being assigned to non-Western surroundings[54] and the narrative of self-sacrifice were very similar in the context of imperial influence serve as a testament to the translating and transmitting power of tropical medicine and civilizing Christianity. Nonetheless, what stands out in the case of China is the numerous references made to the internal political turmoil and so-called 'mob violence', of which the local foreign community had little control.[55] Therefore, the tides of anti-Christian, anti-imperial hostility and social upheavals in the rapidly transforming country lent a political bent to the medical discourse.

Finally, these commentaries on white breakdown in China were all provided by doctors who had no neuropsychiatric background.[56] These doctors had the tendency to concentrate on the physiological effects of climatic, social and political influences on the nervous system, partly because of their medical training. Similarly, Kennedy observes that neurasthenia in itself was an indistinct and convenient disease category that served to bolster climatic interpretation.[57] However, given that no consensus had been achieved in terms of the etiology and symptomatology of tropical neurasthenia,[58] different models of explanation coexisted in China. The next section turns to another system of constructing and resolving challenges that affected the survival of the white man in the Orient.

White Prestige, Repressed Desires, or Failures of Adaptation

Apart from the climatic-physiological model dating from the 1910s, a few Western medical practitioners in China considered difficulties in acclimatization as the result of psychological pressure or psychical conflicts. This development was primarily influenced by the international rise in popularity of psychological explanations and treatments of nervous disorders during the same period.[59] For example, starting from the mid-1910s, the *China Medical Journal* reviewed several treatises on psychotherapy, including suggestion, hypnotism, Carl G. Jung's analytical psychology and psychoanalysis.[60] The psychological manner of thinking gradually entered the foreign medical community in China; this worldview was therefore employed to illustrate the influence of the mind on the body, as well as the mechanism of nervous and mental disorders such as neurasthenia, which had been enervating numerous Western immigrants.[61] In terms of their academic backgrounds, these psychological discourses on white nervous and mental breakdown in China were heterogeneous, and had different focuses of concern, which is discussed in greater detail below.

The influence of religious healing on medical treatment could be observed given that a considerable number of medical practitioners in China were missionaries.[62] In a 1910 article on the value of psychotherapy, Harry B. Taylor of St. James Hospital, Anking lauded the Emmanuel Movement for its contribution to restoring bodily, mental and spiritual health. Taylor further demonstrated that nervous symptoms induced by excessive work, climate, lack of spiritual stimuli and the stress of living among strange people and conditions could be controlled through suggestive psychotherapy. The American physician illustrated his point with a case report on a diligent foreign nurse with a nervous predisposition. After several months of treatment, the patient was relieved of neurasthenia, asthenopia, lack of control and insomnia.[63]

Discussions of nervous breakdown extended beyond the confines of scientific and medical journals. In 1923, the *North-China Herald* used the clinical results of a squadron leader in the British Royal Air Force stationed in India to show the difficulty of maintaining mental equilibrium in China.[64] Without mentioning the effect of tropical climate or environment described in the original study, the Shanghai-based English newspaper underscored the psychogenic factors in unsettling the occidental mind. The pressure of being under 'constant observation', as well as 'the desire to maintain the prestige that ['the white races'] feel their position or their nationality carries with it' had the same effect on expatriates who resided in China:

> It is not so much the amount of power which is entrusted to them, as the feeling that often they are the final court of appeal in matters relating to their missionary or business work, that there are few to whom they can come for helpful counsel, and worst of all the knowledge of what things are in China to-day, when there is often no power behind them to back up their authority, that brings about the nervous breakdowns that are so common.[65]

Interestingly, what appeared to be a criticism of the lack of metropolitan support was in fact a remark frequently made in similar contexts. The erosion of foreign influence was attributed to the surrounding 'swarming masses of China' and to the lack of assistance from the *Chinese* authorities. Akin to the observations of Anderson and Wu in colonial Philippines and Taiwan, it was the eagerness to showcase white superiority in an unfriendly milieu that brought about its travesty.

Psychoanalysis was introduced in the field of tropical neurasthenia in China during the late 1910s, and this psychological science gradually became an important framework of analysis.[66] After enumerating the aetiological models of neurasthenia and hysteria, Frank Oldt urged to look into 'more fundamental and less widely recognized conditions'. Despite his reservations about the Freudian sexual theory, Oldt concurred that 'the sexual factor is an important cause, if not the most important, of the nervous troubles which affect so many of the foreigners living in China'.[67] Compared with their compatriots living in their home countries, single people living in the East lacked the means to release their repressed desires. 'Imagine the strong, insistent, overmastering desires; consider the sensitive, over-trained consciences, and is it surprising that neurotic symptoms appear?' Married couples did not fare better because sexual abstinence sowed the seeds of neurosis. The United Brethren medical missionary advised their readers that sex is 'a pleasure, a preserver of health and character, a preventive of queerness, crossness, jealousy, nervousness, and hysteria' if practiced properly.[68]

As Oldt concentrated on the sexual elements expressed in the writings of Freud, other researchers focused on the psychogenic factors in nervous breakdowns. During the 1930s, Millais Culpin, Professor of Industrial and Medical Psychology at the London School of Tropical Medicine, argued that the so-called 'tropical neurasthenia' was in fact the mild psychoses or psychoneuroses being experienced by residents in the tropics. Given that mild psychoses were defined as the 'failures of adaptation dependent...on predisposition' and could be caused by several factors in either temperate or tropical climates, 'tropical neurasthenia' became a questionable diagnosis. The patient often used climate as 'a physical scapegoat for his trouble'. After working as a senior surgeon at the British Hospital in Shanghai from 1907 to 1913,[69] Culpin realized in the 1930s that what he had previously diagnosed as physiological diseases were in fact psychoneuroses, which he now called 'anxiety states' in the Freudian sense. Shanghai was often called 'a nervy place' because several of its foreign residents had a feeling of uprootedness. 'Life is luxurious, recreation was abundant but artificial, and people expected to go home 'on leave' about every three years'. In contrast, the permanent or 'poorer' European residents were rarely susceptible to nervous disorders.[70] The future president of the British Psychological Society even stated that this 'air of unsettlement' rendered Shanghai rife with 'tropical disorders', which made the condition of the city worse than that of northern Queensland, where Culpin used to work as a schoolmaster in his youth. Several Chinese residents in Shanghai were also afflicted with psychoneuroses because of this new way of living.[71]

'The Irresistible Call of the East'

The most systematic academic discussion on tropical nervous and mental disorders in China was presented by the American psychiatrist James Lincoln McCartney. Born in 1898 to an established Methodist doctor in Chungking, McCartney received his medical training at Rush Medical College, University of Chicago. He briefly returned to China after his internship on the American East Coast and his experience with famous psychoanalysts William A. White and C. G. Jung.[72] From 1925 to 1927, McCartney practiced in Chungking, Hankow, Kuling, Shanghai (St. Luke's Hospital) and Beijing (Union Medical College Hospital) and conducted a series of surveys on the neuropsychiatric conditions that plagued these cities. During the second half of the 1920s, he published several articles on the development of neuropsychiatry in the country as well as other medical cases in Chinese and American medical and scientific journals.[73]

In his papers, McCartney identified psychoanalysis as the solution to the plight of Westerners living in China. In 1926, he clarified in the *China Journal of Science and Art* that the so-called 'Oriental Nerves' were not caused by climate, diet, or economic conditions. Given the massive size of the country and the varying climate across the regions, the spread of such disease across the country explained away the relationship often made between climate and 'tropical' neurasthenia. Following Freud, McCartney assumed that the main cause of neuroses was the psychical conflict between the repressed desires of an individual and the cultural demands of his or her environment. However, the experience of the foreigners in China exacerbated the situation, such as the tendency of the Chinese to procrastinate, the constant gaze to which foreigners felt themselves subjected and the heavy responsibilities they had to carry. Dire poverty, child labour, illiteracy, local superstition and 'the degraded sociological state of China's majority' had 'a certain galling effect on the Occidental mind'. The Chinese society was so engulfing that:

> [t]here is the ever present feeling that one is surrounded by the swarming masses of China; a veritable sea which salts everything that falls into it, for China is the only country in which Jewish communities have entirely lost their identity and become absorbed into the general population.[74]

Visiting countries with different customs and habits could further exacerbate the instability of non-mentally prepared individuals. As McCartney further explained:

> the possibilities for the stimulation and gratification of the sexual side of the psychic Occidental are more numerous in the Orient, and the continued flaunting of the erotic makes its impression on the mind of the Occidental. If he evades it, it callouses his nature, if he succumbs to its wiles, it erodes him; wither of which may throw him into a morbid mentality.[75]

Moreover, when unmarried young adults moved to China to forget their painful experiences, their experiences in the new yet trying environment deepened their feelings of self-contempt. Their moral standards were lowered considering the absence of the companionship of their compatriots. These factors enhanced the desire of maladjusted foreigners to escape from their reality. The conflicts between the repressed desires and the demands of reality were often converted into nervous symptoms.

The article of McCartney, 'Oriental Nerves', directly borrowed many concepts and sentences from the psychoanalytic study of American Navy Commander Joseph C. Thompson on the tropical neurasthenia in Guam,[76] particularly from the sections that discussed the urge of individuals to fly from reality and psychical conflicts. Such plagiarism was noteworthy in the sense that McCartney considered psychical reactions, such as the feelings of alienation and frustration, as common phenomena in the tropics. Whereas the all-pervasive concern of Western displacement turned China into another 'tropical' country, the tendency of psychoanalysis to universalize human experiences made the missionaries in China and the armed forces in an American possession trapped in a similar predicament. Nevertheless, McCartney emphasized other points. 'The *irresistible* call of the East'[77] damaged the occidental mind, but there were other cases of successful acclimatization:

> The man or woman who succeeds in China and avoids getting Oriental Nerves is the person who approaches the new environment with a spirit of cheerfulness and a charitable attitude towards the people with whom he or she plans to live and associate, which attitude is only gained through an understanding of the people. Men who have succeeded

in China, and women who have remained the social attraction they are, are those who have worked with the current, while at the same time lending the full strength of their personalities and characters in helping to bring about better conditions.[78]

McCartney argued that individuals who had command of the native language seldom expressed dissatisfaction or exhibited nervous instability. In other words, the enervated European and American sojourners tended to develop weak will-power, questionable characters and a shallow understanding of their reality. He further emphasized that Chinese businessmen were honest and reasonable. Therefore, people should 'understand and respect the customs and practices of the country when doing business with the Chinese'. At the end of the article, McCartney suggested some handy, common tips for the prevention of nervous diseases, such as taking morning tea in bed, taking short naps after lunch, drinking afternoon tea and playing sports.[79]

The 'newer' way of conceptualizing the hardship of white displacement as offered by McCartney was not a clean break from the older model. His allusions to an exotic yet dangerous Orient were familiar to those contemporary readers who were preoccupied with the 'relocation costs' of migration.[80] Moreover, the image of a nervous system that was physiologically irritated and exhausted by everything alien was incorporated into the discussion of psychogenic mechanisms. The remarks of McCartney were also intriguing because his representation of China was not as derogatory as that of other commentators on tropical diseases. The social reality of China was mind-shattering for some individuals, but the development of nervous and psychiatric illnesses hinged on the function of the white nervous, psychological and moral systems. The favourable attitude of McCartney toward China was also expressed in the 1927 survey of the Chinese military medicine, in which he spoke highly of traditional hygienic measures. 'Regarding food...modern hygiene has little to teach the Chinese while he abides by the principle of eating and drinking nothing that has not been thoroughly cooked, is moderate in his meat eating, and temperate in his meals'. Turning all the rubbish into compost was what 'the modern hygiene has the least to teach and the most to learn from the Chinese'. The new, bacteriologically informed sewage system was only among the 'crude imperfections'. The prevalent opium smoking habits of Chinese soldiers was less harmful than the alcoholism frequently observed in Europe. McCartney concluded that, if 'true scientific spirit were introduced into China, she would become perhaps a model of sanitation, because the methods of living of the people are essentially good'.[81]

The view of McCartney on white breakdowns was further expressed in his two articles on psychogenic headache. His first clinical report singled out headaches as signs of psychoneuroses. According to Freud, neurasthenia was an organic neurosis that was linked to sexual excess. Moreover, many psychoneuroses might be caused by 'the flight from reality'. In this sense, headache was merely a symptom through which the unconscious desire of an individual could be partially compensated.[82] In his second article, McCartney used the Freudian theory to explicate the mechanism of psychogenic headaches. After the treatment, which included the interpretation of dreams, R. T., the 16-year-old daughter of a missionary, realized that her abnormal love for elder women was related to her childhood experience and to her narcissism. Psychoanalytic treatment eventually ended her youthful passion, and her amorous feelings for the opposite sex began to emerge.[83] The devastating effects that China exerted on Western personalities that were mentioned in the previous articles of McCartney did not appear in the two abovementioned articles because of the subject matter or the nature of these journals.

Not long after his return to the United States, McCartney presented his study of neuroses to a different audience. He began his 1928 article, 'The Call to Foreign Missions: Its Effect on Unstable Personalities', by noting that the ability of *colonial* migrants to withstand harsh foreign environments became an important issue as the religious, educational and economic powers of Western countries continued to increase. For instance, under the influence of religious enthusiasm, young missionaries looked for 'a life of martyrdom' and 'the mysterious mission field appeals to the unstable or psychopathic personality'. After describing the seriousness of tropical neuroses, McCartney reemphasized the idea of psychogenesis, suggesting that 'the foreign customs and habits may be the factors that bring on the neurosis, but they are not the *cause* of the neurosis – the *cause* lies within the individual, the difficult situation being at most a precipitating factor'.[84] He added that 'neurosis – or, if severe, psychosis – is a flight from reality and an endeavour on the part of the individual to substitute a self-produced product of psychic fantasy for the unbearable reality that he is actually in a foreign environment'.[85] Morbid missionaries might be sent back home, but were eager to return to what McCartney referred to as the 'thraldom of their fate'. 'The very factors that appeal and entrance are the same that undermine the psychic being'.[86]

From the above description, one could observe that a new aetiology of nervous disorders began to emerge as psychoanalytic knowledge travelled to 'the tropics'. As Anderson has noted, according to the psychodynamic model, the relocation became perilous not because of the physical collision between white bodies and 'the tropics', but because of the psychical conflicts within the agents of Western expansion.[87] The frequent usage of 'psychoneurosis' and 'anxiety neurosis' in Anglo-American medical literature about the psychiatric problems in colonial and tropical contexts reflected the increasing emphasis on neurotic predisposition, which was in contrast to the 'conscientious, hard-working, earnest' images of expatriates that were pictured in the climactic and physiological models.[88] The extreme climatic environment was often ruled out as the primary cause, as well as the term, 'tropical neurasthenia', despite still being frequently used in colonial settings.[89] The arguments of Oldt, Culpin and McCartney were clearly part of this newer international intellectual development.

Individualizing and psychologizing the problem of white immigration inevitably involved moral evaluations. McCartney argued in his analysis that the so-called unrefined customs and the destitution of the Chinese society were detrimental to some individuals, but identified unstable personality as *the* cause of physical, mental, cultural and moral maladjustments. This inextricable link between moral judgement and clinical diagnosis was acknowledged in historical studies on tropical psychiatry, and our study of white breakdowns in China provided another example.[90] After Culpin had presented his findings at the Royal Society of Medicine in 1933, Lord Malcolm Watson, the Scottish malaria expert who used to work in the Malays for 28 years, commented that patients afflicted with tropical neurasthenia were not 'wasters'. These young patients should not be discriminated against because of their brave actions for the Empire. Therefore, the diagnosis of 'neurasthenia' became questionable in the military context, especially with the implication that patients had been sexually involved with native women. The remark of Watson clearly reflected his cognizance of the stigma that was associated with neurasthenia in the psychoanalytic sense.[91] David Forsyth, an English psychoanalyst who was analyzed by Freud himself, explained the reason that 'had led the patient to select a life abroad instead of remaining at home as did the vast majority of young men'. The neurasthenic cases handled by Forsyth in Britain tended to produce 'some neurotic or temperamental infirmity before going abroad'. These patients often displayed a negative attitude toward life and their inferiority complex drove them to live less challenging lives in a 'more primitive state of society'. Their shyness, especially in the presence of women, prompted them 'to find relief in tropical stations remote from white women'. In other words, these neurasthenic young men tried to find an easy way out of the toils of their lives and their internal conflicts by going abroad.[92]

The above analysis shows that the psychological discourses to which we may refer as 'tropical psychoanalysis' did not constitute an integrated body of knowledge. As psychoanalysis began to exert an international influence from the 1910s, its theory and practices were modified to comply with the local contexts and requirements. McCartney argued that an individual should compose and behave himself or herself to avoid personal disintegration while living with different kinds of people. Given that tropical neuroses were caused by unconscious psychical conflicts, internal transformation was essential to mental soundness. Moreover, a sympathetic understanding of the alien culture was imperative, apart from the enforcement of a rigorous screening process by military and missionary societies.[93] McCartney argued that the 'tropics' remained exotic and often triggered pathological reactions in unstable persons, but were no longer places of utter torment and destitution as in the view of climatic determinists. McCartney and Forsyth were well versed in psychoanalysis and both observed that neuroses indicated a certain degree of personality faults, but their opinions on some aspects differed from one another. Forsyth argued that the Western overseas expansion was a form of neurotic escapism. Although McCartney disliked some behaviours of his compatriots in the Orient, such discontent did not necessarily reflect his critique of imperialism. The 'Call to Foreign Missions' was framed within the contexts of expansionism and colonialism. Missionaries often became morbid in foreign lands, but the process of acclimatization might also be a trial of character, especially for the sake of rejecting the undesirables.

By considering the psychological discourses on white nervous breakdowns in China as a whole, one could examine homogeneity and heterogeneity in terms of their concerns. There was a collective attempt to use local foreign nervous cases to expand the nascent psychological knowledge in psychiatry. Oldt examined the role of medical missionaries in maintaining tropical hygiene in Christian households, whereas the local English newspapers underscored the psychological pressure that the expatriates had to endure according to an 'older' tradition. Taylor advocated for the further cooperation of clergymen and physicians and treated white breakdowns as a clinical and a spiritual matter. Culpin and McCartney focused on the self-inflicted sense of uprootedness and passed moral judgement on temperamentally indisposed and culturally insensitive individuals. The diversity in these psychological discourses and in the images of transplanted Westerners was too wide that no single framework, either maintaining white authority or managing racial boundaries, could explain the complex issues involved.

Conclusion

Although tropical neurasthenia in China had attracted limited medical attention, a few tentative conclusions about this disease could be inferred. Such limited attention might be attributed to the special role of China in Western expansion and imperialism. Despite its sizable foreign presence, especially in the treaty ports, the majority of the country was not under direct colonial rule as in the cases of British Africa and India or American Philippines.[94] Under the condition of 'semi-colonialism' or 'incomplete colonialism', the practical problem of regulating *colonial* personnel, as discussed by Crozier, might be a challenging but not a pressing one.[95] The medical discussions on mortality and morbidity were part of an ambivalent concern about the presence of Western elements and the fear of corroding white identity in an ancient civilization, as pointed out by the 1923 comment of the *North-China Herald* on the desire to maintain a

Western prestige. However, given that many neurasthenic patients mentioned in this chapter were not colonial officers but were mostly missionaries and businessmen, nervous and mental breakdowns were also practical concerns facing the members of the local foreign community. The constant demands of medical missionaries to shorten the interval between furloughs highlighted their interest toward practical and vital matters, a request that might not be fully appreciated by their colleagues in Britain or in the United States and might be occasionally criticized by their non-missionary expatriates.[96] Moreover, the illnesses and even the death of missionaries became great concerns for the home churches, given the considerable time and effort that were spent in mastering indigenous languages and building up local connections.[97] In this regard, tropical neurasthenia created a discursive space in which the material, physical and psychological costs of white displacement could be actively negotiated among different agents of the Western influence. This non-'imperial' or 'colonial' dimension in medical provision added to the increasing historical efforts in providing a less static view of the development of medical services in colonial and tropical contexts.[98] As Michael Jennings remarked in his study about missionary medicine in Central Africa, the ideological and evangelical concerns were never 'the only driving forces behind the development and expansion of the mission's response to disease both amongst themselves and within the wider community'.[99]

However, this does not imply that the missionary medicine and 'secular' Western medicine that were practiced among the foreign communities in China were qualitatively different from colonial medicine. Students of science studies and historians of science have recently argued that knowledge could travel across the boundaries of space, period and disciplines.[100] This chapter demonstrates that the medical discussions on the breakdown of Westerners in China were part of the current debates on the possibility of white settlement in tropical regions. The problem of white migration was not only discussed in different disciplinary contexts, but was also spread beyond colonial boundaries. Culpin was Professor of Industrial and Medical Psychology at the London School of Tropical Medicine when he commented retrospectively on the 'anxiety states' that were found in 'nervy' Shanghai.[101] The experiences of Europeans living in rural Queensland, metropolitan Shanghai and industrial Britain were collected and examined to further 'the investigation of the incidence of temperamental and psycho-neurotic symptoms in the working population' at the Industrial Health Research Board.[102] During the Second World War, McCartney served as the Lieutenant Commander of the United States Navy Reserve. This time, he combined the 'older' climatic-physiological model – the enervating effect of the *tropical sun* – with the psychological model to explain the nervous exhaustion of 'blonde' American military personnel in the Pacific.[103] His earlier psychiatric work on morbid missionaries in China was discussed to illustrate his modified view on tropical irritability. The prior experiences of Culpin and McCartney in China were later incorporated into the knowledge of other places, including that of their home countries.[104] Different Western medical systems, in this case tropical medicine, colonial medicine, missionary medicine, industrial medicine and military psychiatry constantly interacted with one another in a strategic manner.

The Western medical practitioners in China agreed on the severity of white breakdowns, but they disagreed on their causes and continuously debated their cultural and political meanings. This lack of consensus partly resulted from the different subfields in which these doctors were trained. Several theories emerged to explain the causes of the disease, even from within the climatic-physiological model itself. The vastness of China and its geographical and cultural variations hindered researchers from framing the situation in a generalized fashion. The underdevelopment of neuropsychiatry, particularly dynamic psychiatry, among the Western medical communities in China limited the psychological understanding of the maladjusted whites.[105] Furthermore, the few Anglo-American neurologists and psychiatrists who were practicing in China preferred to provide medical and philanthropic services to the native population or to explore their nervous, mental and cultural systems scientifically.[106] Their views, if any, on the current debates about tropical breakdowns were yet to be discovered. The emergence of the psychodynamic paradigm reflected the richness of medical culture in Republican China. However, such paradigm was too weak to replace the climatic model of white breakdowns, such as in the case of the colonial Philippines. Given the different psychiatric systems that existed within the country during the period, no consensus could be reached on the classification and explanation of neurasthenia.[107] Therefore, the diverging medical discourses on white nervous breakdowns in China in the late nineteenth and early twentieth centuries had as much to do with the international expansion of tropical medicine and dynamic psychiatry as with the development of medical sciences within the foreign community of the country.

Acknowledgements

Earlier versions of this chapter were presented at Workshop on Medical Culture in nineteenth and twentieth-Century Chinese East Asia: Comparative Colonial Medicine and Beyond (The Chinese University of Hong Kong, June 2009) and the Fifth Conference for the Asian Society for the History of Medicine (Ajou University, Suwon, October 2010). I thank the participants of the conferences for their helpful comments. I am also grateful for the insightful suggestions of the referees of this chapter and the editorial work of Howard Chiang. The research was subsidized by the National Science Council (NSC 98-2410-H-010-001-MY2, NSC 100-2628-H-010-002-MY2).

7 PATHOLOGIZING MARRIAGE: NEUROPSYCHIATRY AND THE ESCAPE OF WOMEN IN EARLY TWENTIETH-CENTURY CHINA

Hugh Shapiro

Before the twentieth century, medicine in China traced disruptive behavior by women to biological or reproductive function, to menstrual disorders, or intense emotions such as anger and fright. Mucus accumulations (*tan* 痰), too, could explain conditions such as confusion, bouts of madness, or sustained derangement.[1] However, in the early twentieth century, a nascent neuropsychiatry in China began tracing female mental health problems to the stress of the marriage system, to women's vulnerable status, to pathos in the home. Clinical observers began rethinking the self-injuring actions of women, such as swallowing poison or stabbing one's body with needles. To be sure, self-harm was still classified as a suicide or suicide attempt. Yet analysis of self-destructive actions looked to the misery of the patrilineal household and woman's untenable position within it. These shifts in medical reasoning are seen in the writings of European and American doctors working in China and in the case histories of hospitals where physicians consciously resisted the approaches of foreign medicine.

Ameliorative institutions in cities such as Beijing and Shanghai assiduously recorded the tormented histories of female patients. These hospitals, both wittingly and unwittingly, became part of marriage avoidance strategies pursued by women in trouble. The broader context of these etiological shifts is the totalistic attack on received 'traditional' culture and biting criticism of the treatment of women inside of marriage. Framing the new thinking about marriage as a pathologized system must begin with the near impossibility of extrication from it and the dearth of options for women in distress. Within this context, psychiatric institutions became one among several refuges for marriage escapees.

Few Routes of Escape

Conflict within the patrilineal household drove women to kill themselves more than any other reason in circa 1920 Beijing, according to Sidney Gamble's renowned survey.[2] For women living in north China, ways for escaping marriage – available paths of defiance – were conspicuously limited. In China's deep south, by contrast, in the relatively affluent Canton Delta, women resisted marriage or fled sexual bondage in 'extravagantly unconventional' ways.[3] 'Compensation marriage', one striking practice, enabled women with resources to obtain the social benefits of marriage while avoiding sexual contact with the husband, altogether evading residence in the virilocal home.[4] *Mui tsai* (*meizai* 妹仔), indentured servants who sometimes became concubines, physically represented the woman in sexual, reproductive and ritual duties.[5] Women might also avoid marriage by entering 'vegetarian halls, Buddhist nunneries', or by joining 'the houses of sworn sisters'.[6] The revelatory work of Watson, Topley, Stockard and Jaschok convinces us that these avoidance strategies were contingent on economic autonomy and upon the distinct cultural milieu of this prosperous silk producing region that acknowledged these strategies as legitimate.

In the absence of avoidance institutions, a woman might simply run away. Doing so, however, was extremely dangerous. Police detained 'run away women' (*tao nü* 逃女), as authorities in Chahar did in 1935 to Ke Dashen, a female identified only by name.[7] The Chahar authorities requested that the Beiping Public Security Bureau locate the woman's family, promptly, as she would be held until someone would make the two hundred fifty-mile trip to retrieve her.[8] Being on the run put a person out of place, inappropriate and socially disruptive and runaways caused anxiety both for municipal authority and society's mainstream.[9] In the 1870s, a young woman wandered away from home after fighting with her mother-in-law and husband. Drifting aimlessly, standing blankly on a bridge in an unfamiliar neighborhood, the group of strangers gathered to watch, labeling her 'insane' within only a few moments.[10] Fleeing was understood as only a slight alternative to suicide. So quips a character in the 1929 social novel, *Haishang huo diyu* (Shanghai: The Living Hell): 'She doesn't look as if she is in the mood to commit suicide', thus 'she is probably planning to run away'.[11]

Flight from marriage (*tao hun*) did become a common idiom during the 1910s, 1920s and 1930s, despite its danger and limited promise.[12] Widely consumed middlebrow journals, such as *Shenghuo* (Life), encouraged young female readers to be as Ibsen's popular heroine Nora, to run away from unwanted betrothal or to leave troubled marriages. As its publisher Zou Taofen counselled, '[w]hat you may try under the circumstances is to flee from home'.[13] Yet married women remained stymied, even within the new discourse deriding marriage. In the debates of educated youth, whether to accept arranged marriages or break with the family, marriage was framed as an institution oppressing both sexes.[14] Men too were victims. As much as women fleeing abusive husbands or miserable marriages, mainstream discourse described modern husbands abandoning traditional wives.[15] Feminist and Communist writings in the 1920s lambasted the institution of marriage, condemning it as 'lifelong imprisonment for women', a condition distinguishable from prostitution only by the length of service.[16] Thus, when male political leaders divorced or abandoned their lesser-educated rural wives, this act might be couched in the language of humanitarian social reform. By being deserted, the rural woman was thus emancipated from oppressive marriage.[17] Yet a wife deserting a husband remained atypical. A wife leaving a husband was so rare, disturbing or humiliating that it could drive the abandoned man into an asylum for the insane (*fengren yuan* 瘋人院), as in Lao She's 1934, *Xisheng* (Sacrifice).[18]

While divorce did become more accessible for urban women in the 1930s due to legal reform, obtaining one remained arduous.[19] Progressive legal reform also inadvertently closed a loophole for women seeking refuge with their natal family, providing husbands with a new 'legal tool to force their wives back home'.[20]

Legal reform raised expectations among women seeking divorce in the 1930s, yet conservative judgments often disappointed these hopes: the 'courts promoted a modern form of conjugal patriarchy' that hindered wife-litigants' 'right to divorce and to bodily freedom'.[21] And in the countryside, divorce remained rare.[22] It could also be deadly: to thwart divorce, husbands kidnapped, raped, mutilated, or murdered their wives and former wives.[23]

Families could also nullify a divorce, without violence. Take the case of a battered woman who had managed to divorce her husband in 1933 Beijing.[24] The husband's mistreatment of his wife began three days after the wedding ceremony. After sex, the husband convinced himself that his wife was not a virgin. Then, he heard gossip that soldiers had robbed her during one of the Zhili–Fengtian Wars, in 1922 or 1924.[25] Before the marriage, for his erratic behavior, construed by his family as paranoia, the husband had been in and out of medical institutions in Beijing, including the French Hospital and the old asylum for the insane, the Gaogong An Jingshen Bingyuan.[26] What distinguished the husband's habitual abuse that day was that he struck the wife's head with a wooden object, badly injuring her and causing profuse bleeding. The man's father was a warden of a prison in a provincial capital and perhaps understood the shifting legal landscape of the 1930s.[27] The husband's family punished him and sanctioned a divorce, after which the woman moved back with her natal family. However, it came to light that she had been pregnant at the time of the savage beating to her head and four months after the divorce, she gave birth to a son. Both families thereupon denied the divorce. The woman remained living in her natal home, but both families acknowledged the woman and child as belonging to the husband's family. Women who succeeded in obtaining a divorce through the courts still remained exposed to its de facto reversal by family intervention.

Part of the problem was that the nascent autonomy of the 'new woman' in China bred discomfort for the modern man. This ill-ease is apparent in the both literary criticism and the new journalism of the era.[28] Even media devoted to women's issues, *Funü zazhi* (The Ladies' Journal), for example, was written largely by men and was 'primarily aimed at a growing male readership'.[29] Progressive writers subjected China's 'new woman' to 'a moralistic regime of patriotic virtue', exposing latent tensions between an emerging nationalism and the escape of women from inequality.[30]

Flight or departure from marriage was dangerous not solely because husbands and families might react with violence. Society militated against it. In 1938 Shanghai, a sympathetic observer lamented the hopelessness of prostitutes attempting to flee bondage. Prostitutes in flight were beaten by enforcers, captured by police, or punished by the courts. Gail Hershatter elucidates the critic's indictment: 'state power intervened to legitimize and perpetrate the conditions of servitude in the brothels, overwhelming the capacity of women and their families to escape'.[31] In early twentieth-century China, the scope of female action had shifted, but as Joan Judge explains, 'the cultural value that set these parameters – feminine service – remained constant'.[32] Despite fundamental shifts in other aspects of life, the cultural milieu enveloping women's dealings with men changed slowly. A generation later, in 1951, a riot erupted when Communist cadres announced to a crowd in the city stadium that an abused woman was divorcing her husband under the PRC's new Marriage Law. Getting to its feet, the crowd threw stones and threatened 'to beat her to death'.[33]

Without access to resources, without social tolerance, without a responsive legal culture, women could hope for few routes of escape, tangible or symbolic. Martyr-revolutionary Qiu Jin articulated this position before her execution in 1907, an observation reiterated in Lu Xun's 1924 essay, 'What Happens After Nora Leaves Home?' Without 'money', Lu Xun answers, without 'economic rights' (*jingji quan*), Ibsen's Nora, who walked out on her marriage, would starve to death or be forced into prostitution.[34]

Marriage and Psychic Disturbance

Domestic conflict and female dementia were tightly woven into the imagination during the Republican era (1912–49). Lectures delivered at the Beijing Police Academy used this scenario in teaching recruits how to anticipate trouble. 'If you see a woman running with hair all disheveled, her behavior is suspect...Normal women comb and wash their hair and dress up'. Such aberrant behavior, the lecture concludes, 'is a sure sign that she is worried and angry...this is some kind of madness'.[35] Scratching the head while walking quickly also signified the madness of women. Family conflict lay at the root the hypothetical woman's dementia. 'She has felt the anger of her in-laws'. Or:

> She and her husband had a fight. Or her husband is not successful enough. He does not understand her anxiousness and helplessness. Or she has somehow lost face. Her family has been too strict with her and there has been a row.
>
> That sort of thing.[36]

By tracing female madness to anguished domestic conflict, the police were merely formalizing a commonly held notion in lay society. To Liang Qichao (1873–1929), among the most influential thinkers of his time, the internecine conflict between women in the household bred noxious social ills.[37] Pan Guangdan – translator of Havelock Ellis, Freudian practitioner, sociologist, eugenicist – set his 1927 psychological study *Feng Xiaoqing* within the enmity of women locked in sexual competition.[38] Mirroring this criticism was a diffuse yet widely articulated social belief: that the madness of women originated from psychological pressures endured inside the conjugal family.[39]

European and American physicians working in China broadly attributed female dementia to the pathos of the patrilineal family. Their published clinical record holds especial criticism for polygamy.[40] These analyses coalesced around three frictions: hatred between wife and concubine, discord between wife and husband and conflict between daughter-in-law and mother-in-law.

Among John Kerr's first patients at his Canton asylum, from 1898, were the 'second wives' of officials and wealthy men.[41] Kerr's successor, Charles Selden, published in 1913 an overview of the polygamously married woman. He described the 'grief and shame' of being 'childless', the 'sorrow' at losing the husband's affection, the 'jealousy' of the 'interloper'. 'Then', Selden observes, 'comes the interference of the husband for the second wife against the first. Is it strange that unstable minds are upset?'[42] In 1920 Guangzhou, Dr. Robert Ross writes that 'much diseased thinking gathers' from 'friction in the household economy', not least of all from conflicts arising from the 'domineering mother-in-law and her treatment of her daughters-in-law and female dependents'.[43] The 'wife who has borne no male child' also endured multiple threats.[44] Dr. James McCartney, in 1927, reiterates these points as the source of 'much pathological thinking'.[45] In 1929, Dr. Andrew H. Woods, who led neurology at the Peking Union Medical College (PUMC, 協和醫院) from 1919 to 1928, describes the '[i]ntolerable situations in domestic life' which originated with the junior women of the household being 'cruelly overworked and imposed on' or when principal wives were bypassed for younger concubines in the event of old-age or childlessness.[46] This sexual competition, Woods posits, provoked 'sexual perversion': during menstruation, married women practiced 'objectionable methods of securing sexual orgasms for their husbands', to prevent the men from turning to 'a secondary wife or concubine'.[47]

Juvenile insanity, in these deliberations, was the product of an abusive family system that tolerated female slavery. Writing in 1920, Dr. Ross observed children in Guangzhou 'sold in brothels' who are 'so terrified that they become deranged'.[48] From the lower Yangzi area, McCartney wrote in 1926 that children sold into slavery often succumbed to 'a neurosis first, which goes on to a psychosis'.[49] In 1931 Yunnan Province, a twelve year-old girl developed a 'nervous condition' after being sold six times.[50]

Denunciations of the family system by foreign doctors might skeptically be viewed as part of the pervasive indictment of life in China among the foreigners in the early twentieth century. Yet doctors practicing what today we refer to as traditional Chinese medicine at an asylum in Shanghai, with different training and orientation than Euro-American counterparts in China and abroad, made analogous diagnostic connections between about female madness and marital disaster.

Shanghai Special Hospital for the Insane

In treating female patients, physicians at the Shanghai Special Hospital for the Insane, concentrated their analysis on domestic strife.[51] These doctors also worked under a hospital charter requiring the use only of 'treatments and medicines of the country' (*chunyong guoyi guoyai* 純用國醫國藥).[52] An institution for the insane, the Special Hospital also housed displaced women, which can be seen on various levels. The Hospital's Board of Directors included members of the powerful criminal cartel, the Green Gang (*Qingbang*) and officials of the Nationalist (*Guomindang*) Government. Crime-cartel lord, Du Yuesheng, was Vice-Chairman of the Board (*Fu dongshizhang*), patrician crime-boss Huang Jinrong was the Board's first member and Xu Shiying was Chairman.[53] Female dependents of the Green Gang leadership were at times admitted to the hospital on a permanent basis (*liu yuan*). More typically, though, married women who had suffered trouble at home ended up in the Special Hospital. Here, the analysis of the Special Hospital's staff resonates with Lu Xun's critique: married women alienated from the conjugal family lacked economic means. Many of the poorest women during this period were those who had been isolated from their families and being poor hastened a diagnosis of insanity. Patients of this hospital often simply had no place to go and these 'pauper lunatics' were generally diagnosed as mad. In Elaine Showalter's words, it was the 'social services available to women' that made 'them ill'.[54]

The precipitating factors identified by the medical staff of the Special Hospital, viewed as a whole, catalogue the pressures endured by women in patrilineal households. Culled from several hundred case histories, the analyses of the attending physicians are here organized into seven scenarios regarding the sources of female madness: 1) marital discord; 2) husband taking a concubine; 3) husband having an extramarital affair; 4) conflict with family; 5) lack of inheritance; 6) husband disappeared; 7) sense of failing in domestic role. Below are representative examples from each category. In the hospital's case histories, patient age and official residence are listed first. Recorded etiologies, such as pent-up rage, loss of the soul, or *tan*-mucus accumulations, are the observations of the physician, unless otherwise noted.

1. Marital Discord

Twenty-four year-old, Pudong. Unhappy relations with her husband, exacerbated by his transmission of syphilis to her (*fufu bumu, qiechuan you meidu*). The hospital first cleansed her blood, remedied the accumulated *tan* expectoration and then treated the madness.[55]

Twenty-eight year-old, Shanghai. Husband was not attracted to her (*buwei fu suoxi*).[56]

Twenty-seven year-old worker in cigarette factory, Haiyan. Conflict with husband; lost interest in life; jumped in river, rescued by river police (*shuizai; yu fu ganqing buqia*).[57]

Twenty year-old, Shanghai. Married to an imbecile, became depressed, soul escaped from body (*jia chunfu, shenhun shining*).[58]

2. Husband taking a concubine

Thirty-six year-old, Shanghai. Because husband took a concubine (*yinfu quqie*), her pent-up rage eventuated in madness (*qifen zhidian*).[59]

Forty-five year-old, Shanghai. After husband took a concubine, she was overcome by an oppressed and despondent sensation (*qimen youyu*), her spirit became confused (*shenzhi cuoluan*), eyes clouded (*yanmu hunhua*) and she leapt from a window, injuring her leg (*tiaochuang shangtui*). The patient explained that the four walls had closed in on her and that she had mistaken the window for the way out (*sibi zusai, wuyi chuang wei chulu ye*).[60]

3. Husband having an extramarital affair

Thirty-year old, Anhui. Because her husband was having an extramarital affair (*yinfu you waiyu*), her pent-up rage caused her to become insensate (*qifen zhichi*), also manifesting in the spitting of blood (*luoxue*).[61] After one week of treatment, her spirits were restored to good health and the blood spitting ceased (*jingshen shuangjian, luoxue yizhi*).[62]

Thirty-seven-year-old, Shanghai. Due to her husband having a lover (*yinfu you waihuan*), her sorrow combined with rage and an inflamed abscess formed on her chest (*beifen jiaoji, xiongpang qi jiekuilan*), a result of the internal imbalance of cold and heat (*hanre*). Her spirit became confused (*shenzhi hunmi*).[63]

4. Conflict with family

Twenty-two year-old, Pudong. The patient arrived to the hospital in a state the doctors described as crying and laughing madly (*diankuang kuxiao*). After three days her spirit began to clear (*shenzhi shiqing*). A calmer patient described her irrational state (*chi*) as having arisen from 'fighting with her family and being cheated' (*jiating douqi, you zao qipian*).[64]

Forty-five year-old, Wuxi. Due to unhappy relations with family, the patient's spirit (*xinshen*) was disturbed (*yin jiashu bumu, xinshen buning*). After several days of treatment, her 'spirits were restored' (*jingshen huifu*) and her 'brain cleared' (*naojin qingchu*).[65]

Twenty-nine year-old, Haiyan. Following marriage, she immediately grew conscious of problems in her relationship with the mother-in-law (*poxi zhijian*), until there was no hope of obtaining love from the new mother (*buji zimu zhi qin ai*). Despondent and miserable (*yiyu guahuan*), her spirit became disturbed (*xinshen shining*). The doctors treated her liver, the system associated with anger,[66] 'calmed her spirit, regulated her menstrual function and then soothed her spirit' (*zhiyi pinggan, anshen, tiaojing, shuqi*).[67]

5. Lack of inheritance

Forty-three year-old, Zhenhai. Her first husband died, leaving no inheritance (*fugu fasi*). Her subsequent paramour (*pinfu*) fell ill.[68] Unable to provide support, he abandoned her (*yiqi*). In the hospital, when in her delirium (*chi*) she grew suicidal she was put under special watch (*yanjia fangfan*). Following two months of treatment, she was discharged.[69]

Thirty-four year-old, Wujin. When her husband passed away, the husband's lover usurped the family assets (*qifu guhou, caichan wei pinfu bazhan*).[70]

Thirty-one year-old, Nanjing. Born in Sichuan Province, she moved to Nanjing and became married as a concubine to a Mr. Wu (*jia wei qie*). His death devastated her, driving her to madness (*diankuang*), kowtowing uncontrollably to everyone she encountered (*koushou buyi*).[71]

6. Husband disappeared

Twenty-nine year-old, Jiading. Because her husband enlisted in the army and never returned, her thoughts became disoriented (*yinfu toujun bugui, sixiang chengchi*).[72]

7. Sense of failing in domestic role

Thirty-one year-old, Yin County. Failed to perform the duties of housewife properly. She was admitted to the hospital for lavish living, squandering money and ignoring her husband's dissuasion (*xingxi shehua, huihuo chengxi, fu quanzu buting*).[73]

Most of the remaining diagnoses fell under biological function, such as menstrual dysfunction and the weakening trauma of childbirth. Postpartum madness (*chanhou chengdian*) was another commonly articulated female-specific disorder.[74] In the analysis of physicians of Shanghai's Special Hospital, the source of distress was the depletional quality of birth (*chanhou tikui*).[75] The act of delivery left women in a 'condition of depletion' (*xu*) that was 'indistinguishable from serious illness'.[76] The 'woman's vulnerability at [birth] was also thought of literally as an abnormal bodily openness', Charlotte Furth explains, 'a weakening of the functioning systems that usually warded off outside invasion. Opening herself physically to expel the child, not only did her pelvic ligatures stretch, but 'all her joints are loosened' and 'all her pores are opened'.'[77] The cases of female dementia that occurred outside of the home and unrelated to marriage, hint at the narrow social territory available to women once away from the household.

Women who followed a spouse abroad, or to other parts of the country, constitute the first category of illness occurring away from the home. The medical narrative focused on the innate dangers of travel and foreign influences. For the thirty-sevenyear-old who accompanied her husband to South-east Asia on business, her deranged state was conceptualized as a lack of adjustment to the local environment (*bufu shuitu*), literally being 'unaccustomed to the water and earth'.[78] Localities were interpreted as intrinsically superior and inferior, beneficial or injurious, as determined by the soil, air, food, customs, indigenous peoples, miasmas and *qi*.[79] In the Hospital for the Insane the toxicity of local *qi* was pertinent only in the diagnosis of women.

The next type of case occurring outside of the home described women disconnected from 'human society', picked up from the street in destitute states by the police. Their names and background largely remain unknown. In one anonymous case, the hospital tersely logged '*Jiangbei ren*', a pejorative term for people from north of the Yangzi River.[80] Other details regard lack of cooperation by the patient and, for example, the subsequent medication of patient by hiding drugs in the food and tentative clinical results.[81]

The prostitute represented the final type of patient whose illness was attributed to factors outside of the realm of domesticity.[82] These cases describe physical abuse, high rates of sexually transmitted infection and premature death. These records expose the nightmarish experience of certain classes of sex workers during this period.[83]

Psychobiology

The neuropsychiatric ward for which the most detailed case histories of the period exist and the ward to which many female patients from the city asylum would be admitted, was operated in the PUMC. Throughout much of the

1930s, this ward was run by Dr. Richard S. Lyman. Richard Lyman first arrived to China in 1931 at the invitation of Dr. F. C. Yen, Director of the National Medical College of Shanghai.[84] Lyman lectured at the Medical College until 1932, when he departed for Beijing to become Chief of Neuropsychiatry at the PUMC.[85] Having trained under Swiss-born Adolf Meyer at Johns Hopkins, Lyman embraced Meyer's psychobiological methods and viewed patient condition as much formed by latent syphilis as by unpredictable life events.[86] At the PUMC neuropsychiatric ward, he brought to bear the Hopkins paradigm, setting up a system of case history production aimed for the totalistic mapping of patient experience. A premium was placed on patient expression and the ward went to considerable lengths to capture what patients uttered, sometimes sober, sometimes under sodium amytal, such as the training of bi-lingual stenographers who could record patient statements in Chinese and the observations in English by the foreign or foreign-trained medical staff. The result: a detailed chronicle of the patient's world shot through with intimate details largely based on the patient's own description.

Even with this system in place, to realize his research vision, Richard Lyman sought a group of patients more diverse than the cases of neurasthenia populating his ward and consuming his time. Lyman recognized in the city's psychopathic asylum an opportunity to expand his patient base, as had his predecessor, Dr. Andrew H. Woods. In the mid-1920s, Woods had negotiated with the municipal authorities, making progress towards cooperation between the PUMC and the city's asylum, but this was derailed by the political uncertainty of 1928.[87] To Lyman's disappointment, the police, which ran the asylum, restricted his visits to two per week and limited interviews with patients to fifteen minutes. The patient's family was also permitted to sit in on interviews. When Lyman re-opened negotiations with the police in 1933, the worldwide economic Depression raged. Because of economic hardship, a host of factors exacerbating the pervasive insecurity of the city and the financial burden of maintaining the asylum, Lyman persuaded the asylum in 1933 to cooperate more closely with the PUMC.[88]

Under the new regime, PUMC physicians no longer visited the asylum to examine patients. Instead, asylum patients were transferred from the asylum via automobile to the psychiatric ward of the PUMC, where they remained for a minimum of one week, or upwards of several weeks or even months, as per the discretion of the PUMC doctors. Multiple admissions of asylum patients to the ward were not uncommon.[89]

This patient population enjoyed no legal or social basis for refusing the analysis they encountered at the PUMC. Patient acquiescence, or refusal, to the physician's orders directly affected diagnosis, treatment and the chance for discharge. Likewise, some patients calibrated their responses to questions or modified their behavior in the wards to prolong their stay in the ward, avoiding that which waited for them on the outside.

For its part, the police-managed asylum gained access to the resources of the PUMC, including medical attention for indisposed inmates. Lyman prevailed upon the police to stop using beggars from the 'Beggars Home' as asylum attendants, as the beggars would often leave their posts 'time to time to resume their calling'.[90] After October 1932, the 'administrative and technical staffs' were all supplied by the PUMC.[91] The asylum was refashioned into a 'psychopathic hospital' and the police retained control. The police continued to admit people to the Psychopathic Hospital for a broadly defined 'disruption'. Instead of carting them off to jail, the police used the asylum as a palliative to over-crowded prisons, or as a cudgel for meting out justice on the street. In addition to reducing its burden, the police claimed that by sending people to the asylum it was providing scientific solutions to social problems.[92] Conceptualizations of deviance as disease resonated with criminological theories of the day.[93]

This collaboration between Neuropsychiatry at the PUMC, the Police and the Psychopathic Hospital resulted in China's preeminent neuropsychiatric ward treating the indigent, displaced and alienated of North China. During the 1930s, downwardly mobile patients, often detained or arrested by the police, some fleeing violence, others poverty, were transported from the asylum to the PUMC. The relationship of neuropsychiatrist to Beijing and its hinterland was utterly transformed.

Violence Against Women and Sexual Competition

Bleak images of domestic violence pervade the record. In 1935, a seventeen-year-old cut her own throat with a kitchen knife, unable to face the habitual beatings of both in-law parents. The father-in-law began the beatings after she refused his advances. The mother-in-law, suspecting what had transpired, joined in the beatings. A neighbor discovered the patient's neck wound and stopped the bleeding with chicken skin.[94] Another case from 1935: a 'second wife' checked herself into the psychiatric ward, to escape her husband's concubine whom the patient claimed had already driven the principal wife to her death.[95]

Upwardly mobile families also used the hospital to resolve complex domestic conflicts. One convoluted yet representative example dates from 1940, from a Tianjin household.[96] The family head, Mr. Zhang, age forty-seven, started as a policeman on the Pinghan Railway,[97] working his way up to an official position in the Tianjin police, eventually prospering in the fruit business. The principal wife, age forty-three and uneducated, adjusted to the life of luxury and retreated into the Buddhist sutras. The first concubine, age forty-seven, had been married once before at age nineteen, to a man who ran away not long after the marriage. She then entered a brothel and met Mr. Zhang while working as a prostitute. He purchased and married her. During treatment for an unnamed illness, she became addicted to opium. Mr. Zhang spent six days a week in her room, though their relationship no longer involved sex, due to the woman's lack of interest. She managed the household. Mr. Zhang had purchased the second concubine, age twenty-nine, from an indigent family in 1934, for the purpose of birthing a son. As the other wives, she did not. After this failure, the second concubine was mistreated, sank into a depression and idled the days away sleeping and eating. Because she acted on 'impulse', she earned the label 'insane'.[98]

The third concubine, age twenty-two, came from an impoverished family. She was cousin to the first concubine. The first concubine had convinced her husband to marry her cousin, thus solving two problems: first, her cousin's poverty; and second, she prevented the husband from marrying someone else, someone she could not control as she believed she could the younger cousin. After the marriage, the third concubine gave birth to a boy. According to the husband, the new mother's attitude suddenly changed from obedience to arrogance and this junior concubine started looking down on her cousin, the first concubine. The first concubine then told Mr. Zhang that, her cousin, the third concubine had some sort of relationship with one of his co-workers. The husband responded by transferring the worker and demanding that the third concubine behave properly. The second concubine claimed that the younger concubine had not given birth at all, but had obtained the boy through adoption. The third concubine responded by swallowing her gold ring in a suicide attempt (and then apologized for subsequently giving the ring to her indigent sister).[99] As a solution to the mounting discord, the husband proposed that he divorce the third concubine, supporting her until she could find a younger man to marry. However, the suggestion shocked the third concubine into a stupor and abandoning the plan, the husband brought her to Beijing for treatment.[100] The third concubine was seen in the PUMC Neurology Outpatient Department and then admitted to its psychiatric ward. After three weeks, she regained composure and was discharged by request of her husband. Staff neurologist, Dr. Feng Yingkun (*Y. K. Feng* 馮應琨), concluded: 'reactive depression to situational factors'.[101]

Leaving Husbands and Evading Male Pollution

In the 1930s, women of moderate means began using the PUMC neuropsychiatric ward to leave their husbands. They simply showed up, stating their intention of abandoning their marriages. In 1938, a twenty-five year-old self-proclaimed 'modern woman' demanded that the PUMC admit her; she could no longer bear her old-fashioned mother-in-law during her husband's prolonged absence.[102] Her husband remarried while she experienced a hospitalization that physicians reported as pleasant, one that included regular sedation.[103] An estranged thirty-year-old announced in 1940 that she was ill and that the illness could only be cured by divorcing her husband. She then planned to concentrate on the opera.[104] At the Kerr Hospital in the far south, in the early 1920s, Charles Selden observed that despite the recent establishment of a rescue home expressly for women fleeing slavery, many fugitives took refuge in the hospital compound. They routinely remained for more than a year until safe residence could be secured elsewhere.[105]

Some patients, sometimes quite young, managed to use the new medical institutions to avoid marriage and sexual relations altogether. Miss Song, for instance, born in 1916, grew up in Beijing among people with chronic sexually transmitted infection. Since childhood, she had nursed an anxiety about being infected.[106] When a cousin pressed for marriage in 1935, the eighteen year-old Song succumbed to a range of ailments, which hospital internists could not diagnose. Her condition did not relent and the family admitted her to the Beijing's Psychopathic Hospital.

For observation, Song was transferred to the Neuropsychiatric ward of the PUMC, where she underwent a battery of psychological tests. The psychiatrists were impressed by her brilliance. In a series of essays she expounded her vision of chastity. Marriage was ruinous due to the probability of sexually transmitted infection and the exhaustion of pregnancy.[107] She wrote in the language of Social Darwinism. Her essays on the virtues of remaining single were inducted into the PUMC library.[108]

Song 'would be an unusually good subject for a real psychoanalysis', observed Dr. Lyman, as 'our talks with her in the hospital appeared to have shown that she can be reached effectively along these lines'.[109] At the end of two years of analysis, Song had debated her examiner on Freud, pondered behaviorism, absorbed the psychology textbooks he supplied and secured a summer job in the hospital's Social Service Department.[110]

Patient Song succeeded in using the hospital to evade both marriage and sexual contact. Her preoccupation with infection and her determination to remain unwed suggests a shift in the meaning of feminine virtue. The cult of feminine purity – the obsession with woman's chastity – had been strictly upheld by male prerogative. By the 1920s, the ethos of virginity, reconfigured as a survival strategy against infection, describes a transposition of values: from that of providing for male pleasure, to defending against male pollution. This period of China's Enlightenment, of cultural transformation, is rightly characterized by the new atmosphere surrounding the relations between women and men. Yet uninhibited expressions of sexuality – seen in the media, in the public icon of Dr. Sex, in such fictional archetypes as Miss Sophia – do not obscure equally radical departures: the freedom to refrain from these relations.[111]

Hospital staff understood that they controlled precious resources: food, medicine, shelter, medical treatment, small amounts of disposable cash. Such assets could save a person in vulnerable moments of desperation, when completely exposed, with no options, exhausted, hungry, sick. Hospitals offered sanctuary from violence, due to politics, debt, or bad luck. They offered stable retreat from untenable marriages. They offered disenfranchised wives and abused daughter-in-laws shelter from domestic conflict. In these hospitals, we also witness deep transformations in how physicians understood women's mental health: a shift driven by new thinking about women's compromised position within families and within marriage, rather than physiology, reproductive function, or emotion.

8 GONE WITH THE *WEST WIND*: THE EMERGENCE AND DISAPPEARANCE OF PSYCHOTHERAPEUTIC CULTURE IN CHINA (1936–68)

Geoffrey Blowers and Shelley Wang Xuelai

Although psychological ideas from the West that anticipated the development of modern psychotherapy began to permeate China from the beginning of the Republican era, psychotherapy as both a theory *and* a practice did not take root until the 1930s. When it did, it was because, it is argued here, of a conjunction of interests involving psychologists, literati and a new generation of doctors sensitive to their patients' mental health, working symbiotically in the fields of publishing, writing and practicing new ideas about persons caught in states of mental distress. This activity was concentrated in Beijing, Shanghai and Nanjing, although it later spread to Chongqing during the Sino-Japanese war. On the one hand, many scholars, doctors and psychologists were writing about these new ideas and disseminating them through the popular discourse of a monthly magazine entitled *Xi Feng* [West Wind]; on the other, several practitioners were taking these ideas and incorporating them into their everyday practices. These activities then resulted in further publication and dissemination, contributing to, in effect, the spread of psychotherapy from written ideas in theory to a method for treating patients in a clinic. An overlap was found amongst the names of those who contributed to both activities. They were Huang Jiayin 黄嘉音, the chief editor and publisher of *West Wind*; Su Zonghua 粟宗華, one of the leading psychiatrists of China and an important writer of articles in *West Wind*; Ding Tsan 丁瓚, a Communist, but also a passionate analyst and psychotherapist, who co-founded the Chinese Psychological Institute and introduced medical psychology to China; and Cheng Yulin 程玉麟, one of the earliest Chinese psychiatrists who set up the first public psychiatric hospital in Nanjing and who also contributed articles for *West Wind*. These scholar-practitioners had a twofold aim: to educate the public and their fellow professionals into accepting new ideas about self-improvement culled from Western sources and, through their experiences of treating clients coming for help, advance an understanding of what possibilities there were for helping people deal with problems they couldn't solve for themselves.

This chapter charts the activities of these four individuals, who worked in two distinctly different political climates and with varying degrees of political commitment. Initially, they embraced new theories from the West through an open publishing platform serving to disseminate ideas for self-improvement. They were also able to travel to Europe and America for training and to receive it locally from qualified professionals coming from those regions. Subsequently, these avenues of opportunity became closed off and they had to continue as best they could under the most trying of circumstances. In spite of their enthusiasm and devotion to their goal of developing psychotherapy on behalf of their fellow countrymen, it brought them to unfortunate ends, in spite of their efforts to work within and adapt to the repressive orthodoxy imposed by the Communist Government at the end of its first decade. The demise of their activities was a result of a number of political events that impacted significantly and crucially upon them and brought their careers and in some cases their lives, to an early end. The chapter closes by considering the question of whether the collaborative culture of the period under review generated by intellectuals of differing professional stripes was more collaborative than present day psychotherapeutic training in China, which, since the late 1970s, has been revived.

Promising Beginnings

In 1936 a new monthly journal, *West Wind*, in large part given over to articles about mental health, commenced publication. Its publishers were two brothers, Huang Jiayin 黄嘉音 (1913–61) and Huang Jiade 黄嘉德 (1908–92), who were both educated at St. John's University (Jiayin in history, psychology and journalism; Jiade in English literature) and the literary celebrity, caricaturist and writer, Lin Yu-tang 林語堂 (1859–1976). As a journal of cultural life, *West Wind* placed a lot of emphasis in its contents on mental health and psychological education, perhaps due to the strong personal interest in psychology of its publisher, Huang Jiayin, who also published texts of abnormal psychology and developmental psychology.

According to Wen-ji Wang, in his review of *West Wind*, more than 170 articles related directly to psychological diseases, mental health and psychiatric problems appeared between 1936 and the journal's demise in 1949. This did not include those appearing its sister journal, *West Wind Supplement*, also run by the same group. As with other already established monthly magazines devoted to culture, such as *Dong Fang* [Oriental Magazine], *Xin Qingnian* [New Youth] and *Xinli* [Psyche] – the latter being the first journal devoted entirely to psychology studies – the form of these articles varied from original pieces, through translations taken from Western magazines and journals, to 'reports' on intellectual trends and activities overseas. Also included were 'special topics' written by invited experts or psychological professionals, a 'forum for freedom' comprising articles from readers and 'solicited essays' open to the general reader. Among these, was a volume named 'psychology education' which indicated how much *West Wind* focused on mental health issues.[1] Many of its articles were chosen by the editor, Huang Jiayin, who was already versed in psychology as a member of the Chinese Mental Hygiene Society, engaged long-term with the promotion of mental hygiene, as well as being the deputy director of the 'Shanghai Mental Health Promotion Association'. As Wen-ji Wang noted from Huang's own article, 'Talk about Mental Hygiene with Dr. Su Zonghua', Huang saw his task as raising awareness of the need for mental hygiene in China as an interim measure 'before a real professional journal starts up'.[2]

West Wind's readership also attracted a new generation of medical doctors educated abroad and at Peking Union Medical College (hereafter PUMC), the most prestigious and best financed teaching hospital in China, financed by the Rockefeller Foundation through its China Medical board.[3] Prior to 1932 there had been no academic psychiatry in China to speak of and, according to one of the Rockefeller Foundation's Presidents, it was 'the most backward, the most needed and potentially the most fruitful field in medicine'.[4] A psychiatry program was begun in 1932 and, one year later, until 1938, Dr. Richard Lyman, a neuropsychiatrist from Johns Hopkins, directed the department of neuropsychiatry and provided opportunities to train outstanding Chinese doctors and psychologists in psychiatry and psychotherapy. Notable amongst them was the psychiatrist Su Zonghua (1904–70), who had graduated from and then worked at Shanghai Medical College and followed Lyman to PUMC before going to Johns Hopkins in 1935. Also invited to join him were Ding Tsan (1910–68), a graduate of National Central University who, as a young psychologist, later practiced psychotherapy in Peking and Chongqing and became a passionate exponent of psychotherapy in China; and Cheng Yu-lin (1905–93), a psychiatrist who later set up in Nanjing the first public psychiatric hospital in China in 1947 after the Second World War and also invited Ding to direct the psychological unit of the hospital. All of them contributed articles to *West Wind* and enhanced its prestige as it moved from being initially a vehicle showcasing in translation articles of mental health conceived and written abroad, to articles written by Chinese scholars and practitioners about a variety of problems confronting the population – as well as allowing non specialists with an interest in these problems to voice their concerns.

Su's articles included 'Talk about Sensibility and Emotion', 'The Attitude that we should have to Psychiatric Disease', and 'Opinions to Our Mental Health

Activity'.[5] Ding wrote a number of pieces in a regular column *Mental Health and Youth Culture*, amongst them, 'Why I am a psychoanalyst', 'Culture and Psychological Abnormality', 'A Brief Discussion about Unification of Thought and Sensibility', 'Mental Health Work in the Military', 'Animosity in Dispersion', 'Training the Young to meet an Emergency' and 'Anxiety', which showed his passion and concern for youth, in terms of prevailing ideas about psychopathology, war and social problems.[6] Some Western psychiatrists who worked in China at that time were also invited to contribute. Fanny Halpern (1899–1952), an Austrian Jewish psychiatrist working in Shanghai Medical College in 1933 (having trained under Julius Wagner Jauregg and Alfred Adler) gave many talks on mental health and its needed reforms, one of which was published in *West Wind*. Also, Dr. Olga Lee, a Swiss mental health worker in Peking Union Hospital left her working diary in a private school for counselling practice and it was eventually published as 'Talk about a Mental Health Experiment'. In addition to these, Huang Jian-hou, wrote 'A Talk about Psychotherapy' and 'The Work of Self-esteem Maintenance'; Liu Lun-ci wrote 'A World of the Insane: The Life of My Career'; Wu Zhen, who worked in the social work department of Peking Union Hospital, emphasized the need to develop case skills by writing 'Techniques in Case Work', 'Piece Together Those Who are Broken up', '10 Years' Experience in Medical Social Work' and 'Skills in Interviewing'.[7] According to Wen-ji Wang, these writings represent a high level of expertise due to the professional background of their writers, though they were writing in a non-professional magazine, yet helping to spread ideas and foster an awareness of mental hygiene throughout China.

The Dearth of Practice

In spite of the plethora of articles extolling practical advice and wisdom about mental health, there was little momentum initially for putting these ideas into practice. Halpern wrote of the practice of psychiatry and neurology as they existed in China in the 1930s:

> these two subjects had hardly been taught in Central and South China; neurology only very briefly in connection with internal medicine, psychiatry [was] not at all included in the medical curriculum. Nowhere in Central China was there a psychiatric division or a hospital for the insane. Psychiatric patients were held, without any treatment, in an asylum in the old 'Chinatown' of Shanghai (St. Joseph's Asylum), the restless cases lying on the floor by the means of iron wristbands and chains fastened to the walls. Numerous mentally ill people lived in private apartments together with their relatives and children. Psychiatric nursing, psychiatric hygiene, psychotherapy and so forth [were] unknown terms.[8]

Hart Westbrook of the University of Shanghai, in a letter to Professor Gesell of Yale, described Halpern:

> Dr. Halpern was influential in securing the interest and funds from a wealthy Chinese for the establishment of a hospital for the insane and other mental cases at Minghong, near Shanghai, several years ago. And last year she was the moving spirit in enlisting various clubs and organizations of Shanghai in the appointment of a Mental Hygiene Committee for Shanghai. This Committee has become a Sub-Committee of the Committee on Psychiatry of the China Medical Association and with her assistance has carried on a course in Psychopathology ... for the training of laymen ... to assist us in voluntary service in the Mental Hygiene Clinics which we hope to open this autumn under Dr. Halpern's direction.[9]

In spite of these developments and having been trained under Adler in Vienna, she did not accord psychoanalysis high priority, seeing a more pressing need to improve general psychiatric facilities. Halpern was Professor of Neurology and Psychiatry at the National Shanghai Medical College (affiliated to Jiangsu Medical University) in 1933, replacing Richard Lyman, who had gone to Peking Union Medical College to head the department of neurology and psychiatry there. It was Lyman who invited Bingham Dai back from America to teach psychology and psychotherapy to young doctors. Dai, whilst studying for a PhD in sociology at Chicago, had been selected to take part in a year-long seminar on culture and personality at Yale, sponsored by the Rockefeller foundation. He was recommended for psychoanalytic training by Harry Stack Sullivan, was supervised by Leon Saul who himself was in analysis with Karen Horney. Dai thus became the first psychoanalytically trained Chinese psychotherapist.

Dai's stay in China was a brief three years but during this period he 'saw patients, trained the residents and staff in psychoanalytically oriented psychotherapy and gave supervised psychotherapy at the Peking Municipal Psychopathic Hospital'.[10] He also selected a small group of doctors and gave each of them a ten-month period of training in self knowledge – 'similar to the training in a psychoanalytic institute but not quite the same'.[11] While we cannot be sure, it is most likely that one of those doctors was Ding Tsan, who began working in the department of psychiatry and neurology at PUMC from 1936, since we learn from his biography that it was from this time his interest in Freud and psychoanalysis began.[12]

Ding Tsan had been one of the major contributors to *West Wind* in its 'Special Subject' column, contributing eighteen articles, several of which are cited above.[13] These articles were based on his own experience of study, research and clinical practice in Peking and Chongqing. Later, most of these articles and some others based on the speeches he made to the public, particularly those to students in schools and universities, were published in two books, *Mental Health Essays* and *Mental Cultivation of Youth*, which became his most important academic work before 1949.[14] His *Mental Health Essays* begin with 'How to Initiate Mental Health Work' (a speech he gave to an academic forum in the Central Health Experimental College); next came his development of medical psychology (*Yishi Xinlixue*) in speeches given to the united weekly assembly of Central Hospital, the National Shanghai Medical School and the National Central Senor Nursing School. He also reviewed and summarized 'The Current Situation of Mental Health in the Modernization of Our Society' and discussed 'The Relationship Between Mental Health Work and Cultural Amelioration' and how to 'Build Up our National Philosophy and Spirit from the Point of View of Mental Health'. Ding was always highly concerned for the mental health of youth, as we find amongst these essays: 'Mental Problems of Children in War Time' and 'Aimless Wandering in Adolescence'. Other essays dealt with his concern for sexual differences: 'Between the Two Genders', 'Understanding Problems between Males and Females', 'Sex Education in Childhood' and 'Between Father and Son'. Ding also took an interest in some of the more common attitude problems of the society of his day, such as 'Neurasthenia' and 'Feelings of Inferiority and Arrogance'.

The written speeches were aimed at young people and the general public. They were not, as Ding himself said, 'serious academic theses with research reports or systematic theories with terminology, but were the expression in extremis of what people needed and wanted urgently to know'.[15] But by writing popular pieces he also claimed to be meeting the needs of psychologists, health-professionals, nurses, caregivers, social workers and children's guardians, which would benefit their work in their practice. In one of his academic discussions in Central Health Experimental College in Chongqing, he expressed his intention of becoming active in the field of mental health which led him to set up an experimental lab and a mental health division in that Central Health Experiment College, which later evolved into the Chinese Psychological Institute after 1949.[16]

Ding's studies carried out on children's behavioral disorders are revealing not only of his scientific approach to psychological problems but are suggestive of his regimen of treatments for dealing with them. Ding and his team undertook many surveys of children and young people, using psychometric testing methods on groups, alongside individual case studies, to determine what were the most commonly occurring behavioral disorders amongst them. Much of this work was done when the entire Government and the Universities relocated to Chongqing during the Sino–Japanese War. Common disorders found in children included loss of emotional control, teeth grinding, timidity, being scared of the dark, tearful, rebelliousness, lack of concentration and a tendency towards fighting.[17] In Ding's view, these disorders arose as a result of an emotionally unstable early life, possibly due to an unhealthy family background. In order to correct these problems, he advocated the guidance of the child's emotional life. He also felt that a systematic introduction should be given to parents about how to guide their children through their emotional difficulties. While he acknowledged the importance of biological, mental and social factors in correcting children's behavioral problems, he laid more emphasis upon the latter two factors, for he disagreed with the prevailing tendency of his day that it was sufficient to label them as 'problematic' or as 'little baddies' (*wan lie* 顽劣) and thereby separate them from other children. Instead, he tended to instruct them in how to better cope with life's exigencies, rather than focusing on 'correcting' bad behaviour. He also found working with children in groups and educating the general public through lectures, discussions, forums and workshops were better for helping children deal with their problems more positively, rather than by individual counseling.[18]

Ding Tsan was also a pioneer of medical psychology and introduced the concept of psychosomatic medicine to China in his speech entitled 'The Development of Modern Medical Psychology', given in the Central Hospital, National Shanghai Medical School and National Central Senior Nursing School United Ceremony.[19] In this speech, for the first time, Ding outlined the importance of applying psychology to the field of modern medicine. Citing Jung, he asserted 'psychology is a must for medicine, because psychopathological factors coexist with our somatic diseases, particular with chronic diseases' and 'no doctor could achieve what he does achieve in his life practice without having some knowledge of the techniques of psychotherapy and psychoanalysis'. In appealing to his audience of students and young professionals to take note of their patient's personalities and how they impact upon their illnesses, Ding linked medical psychology to Freud.

His work in this field originated at PUMC and focused upon individual treatments and prevention and public health education – a line of work he was to continue in Chongqing during the Sino–Japanese war. In the period in which he was writing for *West Wind*, Ding was a strong supporter of Freud and his psychoanalytic theory and practice, although Fan Tingwei, a current Chinese psychologist, has tended to think he was more influenced by the pragmatic psychology of Adolf Mayer's theory and the neo–Freudian training he received under Richard Lyman and Bingham Dai. However, Ding Tsan's passionate commitment to Freud can be seen in his own writings. In one of his essays on the relationship between psychoanalysis and medicine described above, he claimed that

> from my six years of experience of practicing psychotherapy, I have to say I feel very sorry for any misunderstanding and criticism of Freud's psychoanalysis. Freud's theory is not only about 'sex' as some have twisted it; it is not rhetorical talk; it is not about occult dreams or armchair imagination; every thread of his theory was based on his own everyday clinical practice, in case after case ... it is truly 'case based'.[20]

He also pointed out in the preface to another of his books that Freud's psychoanalysis is an important facility for people to know about in order to gain insights from a scientific perspective.[21] He went on to say that though some of Freud's classic works had been translated and popularized in China, further developments in those theories were largely unknown in China. Other essays dealt with 'Freud's Influence on Sociology', 'Freud's Contribution in Theory and Practice of Social Work', 'Freud's Influence on Western Thought and Culture' and 'The Limits of Freud's Theory'.

Ding also wrote about his psychoanalytic training at PUMC.[22] According to his own account, he was under the supervision of a 'foreign teacher', who seriously warned him not touch any books on psychoanalysis before and during the period of his training, when Ding asked him for a list of books that he could read about psychoanalysis. Instead, he was asked to spend one hour a day lying down on a couch, like his clients and train his ability to think freely (freely associate). His teacher sat beside him silently without offering any interpretation. Within a month he found himself able to think more freely, though at the beginning he found it hard to think of anything during that one hour. Then his teacher started to occasionally interpret some thought of his and of course explained it using some psychoanalytic terminology when they encountered it. In this way he found himself having 'a totally different understanding of himself'. And in his later reading of books on psychoanalysis, he found how 'easier and familiar' he had become with those theories.[23] Fan Tingwei thinks this 'foreign teacher' must be Lyman though more likely it was Bingham Dai 戴秉衡, whom Lyman had invited to teach psychoanalysis to his young staff at PUMC.[24] Dai has recalled his time of teaching in PUMC in a letter that states 'a group of half a dozen young staff were selected to be trained by me in psychoanalysis, who planned to set up the first Chinese Society of Psychotherapists' (which didn't happen, due to the outbreak of the Sino–Japanese War). Two of them went to the US with Dai himself; 'one of them stayed working in the communist government, playing a role in the mental health area until he passed away'.[25]

The training Ding undertook at PUMC nurtured his success in his later practice. During this time while working at both the hospital and in other clinics in Peking, he successfully analyzed two cases. One of them concerned a young lady who suffered from visual and auditory hallucinations of periodically being visited by a devil. Ding noticed that the girl had serious religious convictions and several failed relationships with men. Ding also observed that this woman's attitude to this 'devil' was one of tolerance. Instead of being eager to alleviate her symptoms, she preferred to 'leave it to God' in spite of Ding's offer of help. In writing up this case Ding, following the psychoanalytic theory in which he had been trained, pointed out that this 'devil' existed in everyone's mind, 'attached to our body', but which went under the more generally accepted name of desire; or as Freud named it – the id. Ding eventually concluded that the girl's problem arose from her denial and repression of this desire, which led to a perverted satisfaction from periodic seduction and abandonment by the devil figure itself.

Ding based his interpretation on the historic case of the Loudun possessions in which several Ursuline nuns claimed to have been seduced by a devil, later identified as Father Urbain Grandier, who was convicted and burned to death.[26]

The other case he described in detail was based upon a letter he received from a woman who consulted him over her guilt at being unfaithful in her marriage. Enquiring into the woman's background brought further facts to light. Her grandmother had had 'several' relationships living with men in different cities, a not uncommon practice in northern China at that time. After her father's death, her mother lived with a 'much younger' military officer. One day, her mother disappeared suddenly, leaving a message to her daughter's 'step-father' to look after her daughter, but also asking him to marry the daughter. For the next few years, the step-father paid her school tuition and generally supported her, eventually becoming her husband. She found married life a painful and unhappy experience due to differences in the culture and lifestyle of her husband. Ding used the case as an exemplar of Freud's theory of projection and repression – the projection of the woman's desire to get rid of the current marriage and wanting to run away made her feel guilty; at the same time her hatred towards her mother for abandoning her had led to the repression of her desire to run away. This conflict of repression and desire manifested itself in symptoms of panic and fear that led her to write to Ding asking him whether her desire to be 'disloyal to her marriage was a family trait'[27]

The Demise of *West Wind* and the Fate of Huang Jiayin

By 1946, Huang Jiayin had set up his own Family Publishing House with his wife, Zhu Qi, an esteemed translator in her own right.[28] That same year he became the editor of the *Shanghai Evening Post and Mercury* (supplement) and had briefly been editor of *Shun Pao* (1940–1). His other published works in psychology and mental health included *Wanderings: Meandering in Abnormal Psychology* (1950), *Cases of Counseling in Prevention and Treatment of Children's Psychopathology* (1951); *Psychoanalytic Case Reports in the treatment of Children 's Abnormal Behavior* (1952); and *The Girl Who Thought She was the Queen: A Case Report of Abnormal Psychology*, co-authored with Su Zonghua (1951).

However, Huang Jiayin's life after 1949 seemed tragic and short. With the founding of the People's Republic, the Communist government severed all ties with non-Communist countries. Attention became focused on Russia in the early part of its first decade and psychology followed Pavlov's work very closely. The new blueprint, inspired by the work of Vygotsky, Luria and Leont'ev, made dialectical materialism the central philosophy underlying all permissible psychology which had to be practiced according to two principles: 1.) Psychological phenomena are a product or function of the brain, 2.) Mind, that is consciousness, was a reflection of outer reality. As such, it was a historically and developmentally formed mental product. Consciousness was seen as the supreme force governing human behaviour, unchallenged by (and therefore granting no status to) competing forces such as the preconscious or unconscious. With China's turn to Russia after 1949, this ideology became practice in many educational fields, leading in a short time to the effective shutting down of research and development predicated upon ideas developed from Western psychology and culture. As Hsueh and Guo in their history of psychology in China pointed out, much of this ideological shift took place against the background of the Korean war and the internal social movements (*sanfan wufan*) attacking corruption and state and businesses, in which Western forms of market practice based upon capitalism were seen as underlying the corruption problems that beset the country.[29] As such, private businesses had to close down. It was in this social context that *West Wind* had to terminate publication.

Huang had used the magazine as an informative and informed voice of ideas generally foreign to China. Its content ranged over many details of American cultural life, the family, student campus life, American car culture, memorization methods, foreign food and sanitation, Western table manners, notes on international cities and how to study overseas. Its aim had been to introduce 'Western' lifestyle and culture to a readership that could learn, compare and judge its offerings from the viewpoint of its own traditions and culture and thereby adopt a modest and respectful attitude without being either adulatory or rationalistic. Not content with bringing aspects of foreign cultures into print, Huang Jiayin had become a newfound enthusiast for ideas on mental health, which first came to his attention in his undergraduate studies at St. Johns and then in the pages of his own magazine. His enthusiasm did not diminish after he was forced to close it down.

In the new political climate Huang Jiayin's Family Press did not last much longer either and shut down in 1953. However Huang Jiayin kept active in publishing and journalism by joining the Shanghai Translator's Association in 1951 and later worked part-time for Wen Hui Bao as chief editor of its literary supplement. He focused more and more on psychotherapy and started his own practice in a private community facility – Hongqiao Psychiatric Rehabilitation Hospital, which had been opened by Su Zonghua in 1944 and which ran until 1954.[30] His psychotherapy practice became successful and established his reputation for which he was later able to present details of his cases in an academic conference. Prior to the shutting down of his printing press, he published the results of his therapy in 1951 in a book entitled 'Psychotherapy 300 Cases'.[31]

Given the political climate, it is all the more surprising that this book came into print at this time and, now that it has been rediscovered, we learn from its pages that Huang Jiayin appeared familiar with both the theory and the practice of psychoanalysis.[32] Although he makes the obligatory claim that his psychotherapy is based on 'dialectical materialism', in order to distinguish it from the critique of mentalism, and denied it had any similarity with a 'psychoanalysis of the bourgeoisie', Huang Jiayin's actual work with his patients as recorded in the case histories in this tome is all the more remarkable. His clients suffered diverse problems and ranged in age from nine to sixty. Although a few of them had only three to five sessions with him, making it impossible to build up a relationship, most contracted for a larger number of sessions, usually from six to twenty, the longest being fifty-six.[33] Huang Jiayin's therapy focused on building relationships with his patients, analyzing the reasons for their illnesses, improving their perceptions of illness, through education and persuasion, techniques he had probably learned from the psychiatrist Su Zonghua with whom he had earlier published a case study and who often referred patients to him. [34] Huang Jiayin also mentioned in his book that he most frequently used the talking method to 'comfort, encourage, divert the patient's attention away from his problems, even promise a positive outcome, to effect improvements in the condition'. Sometimes his solutions involved getting the patients to change their work habits or effect changes to improve their social life, all done to 'eliminate the symptoms and alleviate the patients' pain'. Before beginning therapy, he would advise those in his care to first undergo a medical examination in order to demonstrate to them that the origin of their condition was not somatic. Working in this way he soon came to the conclusion that the causes of most of his patient's problems were not reducible to a single factor but likely involved several factors making it important, he claimed, to collect information on his patients' childhood and early life experiences, as well as the life events experienced prior to the triggering episode.

Huang Jiayin was not much interested in politics and was no shouter of slogans. But for appearances sake, he attended the Chinese Democratic League in 1956 and later, as a nonvoting delegate, the National Committee of the Chinese People's Political Consultative Conference (CPPCC) for a while, perhaps trying to remain active even in this new political environment, according to his motto 'everyone should contribute his part in doing something to serve society'.[35] Nonetheless, the fact that Huang Jiayin was still practicing psychotherapy in China at this time made him politically suspect and he was soon branded a Rightist (*You Pai*) for his conservative views. This was because, during the '100 Flowers' period where intellectuals had been encouraged to voice any concerns they may have had about developments during the first 8 years of the People's Republic of China (hereafter PRC), he had advised the setting up of clinics for more psychological counselling for its citizens, against the prevailing view of the Chinese Communist Party that counselling was unnecessary because its citizens could not have been unhappy.[36] In August 1958, Huang Jiayin and his family had to move out of Shanghai and the only work he could obtain was as an 'office boy' in a local school in the desolate northern-west region of Ninxia, in Gansu Province; later, he was subjected to forced labour along with other Rightists, under the political slogan 'recast their spirit and world view'. Huang Jiayin died there after three years at the age of forty-eight, although the circumstances of his death are shrouded in doubt.[37] It was widely accepted that he died of extreme depression and resentment in jail, but one of his students recalled him being executed in a criminal reform farm.[38] Yet another account suggests he was put to death for having 'committed malicious murder'.[39] Whatever the actual circumstances, his wife only knew of his death eight years after his disappearance and one of his sons committed suicide on hearing the news.

The Fate of Ding Tsan

If Huang Jiayin had died an ironic death, advocating a desire to help the new Republic with forms of therapy which he felt could invigorate a discontented population and then resisted recanting even under the most trying of circumstances in the camps, Ding Tsan's demise appears all the more ironical as, unlike Huang Jiayin, he had been a early advocate and staunch supporter of communism. As a young man he had been politically active and joined the Communist party in 1927, prior to attending university, at a time when there was deep rooted unrest and suspicion amongst differing factions of the Kuomintang (although he later lost contact with the party and his membership lapsed in 1930). Unlike Huang Jiayin, he had come from a poor family in Jiangsu province and was appreciative of their struggle to obtain for him an education. He graduated from National Central University with a degree in psychology and started work at Peking Union Medical Hospital (hereafter PUMH) in their neuropsychiatry department, during which time he also underwent ten months psychoanalytic training based upon Freud's ideas. But with his concern for the welfare of the young he put some of his ideas into practice by giving talks and opening mental health counselling centres in the community such as the First Beiping Health Centre, a clinic in Yu Ying High School and another in the Renli Carpet Factory.[40]

During the Sino–Japanese war he worked as a volunteer for one year at the front, then transferred to western China in 1940; at first teaching in Chongqing College of Social Education. Later, he took on the work of setting up a mental health division in the Central Health Experimental College (the former body of the Chinese Medical Academy of Sciences). Subsequently, in 1944, he opened the first laboratory of mental health and medical psychology in China, which had affiliated clinics and counselling offices. Through these facilities, he was able to undertake systemic work on psychological research, practice, teaching and public education during which time he and his team went on to complete more than 4000 psychometric assessments and 120 cases of counselling. His two books, *Mental Health Essays* and *Mental Cultivation of Youth*, appearing in 1945 and 1947 respectively, were based on these practices and those at PUMH.[41]

After the war, Ding Tsan joined Dr. Cheng Yu-lin in setting up the first neuropsychiatric specialist public hospital in Nanjing attached to Nanjing Central Hospital, to which, funded by WHO and UNRA, Dr. Karl Bowman and Ms. J. Picherella had been sent as advisors in 1947.[42] One of their recommendations was to send several young doctors to the USA for training, Ding Tsan among them. He went as visiting scholar for one year, studying at the University of Chicago while doing psychological research at Michael Reese Hospital.[43] Whilst in America, Ding also travelled to other cities, connecting with and recruiting outstanding scientists for the new China.[44] He set up the 'Chinese American Overseas Scientific Scholar Association', forging links and persuading Chinese overseas students to return and work for China in the future (the so-called 'front unit' work). In August 1948, Ding travelled to London, Paris, Copenhagen and Geneva making visits to institutions in connection with his research, as well as to connect to Chinese scientists in the hope of persuading them, too, to ultimately return to China. The work he had done in forging alliances with Chinese abroad was to bear fruit for Ding, who became one of a handful of scientists called upon by Zhou En Lai to construct a new Academy of Sciences, the PRC version of Academia Sinica which began in Nanjing in 1928 but transferred to Taiwan after 1949.

However, the lapse in his party membership, only reactivated in 1948 in Hong Kong on his way back to China from Europe, made him a target of some suspicion soon after he assumed a senior position within the very academy he helped to set up. In 1953 his party membership was abrogated and he lost his position as the deputy chief secretary of the Chinese Academy of Sciences.[45] In building the Chinese Academy of Sciences, it had been Ding who had insisted that it also contain within the umbrella organization an Institute of Psychology. But because of his political problems in the early 1950s, he had been forced to renounce his previous convictions of the value of Western psychotherapy and the Institute of Psychology suffered an enforced downgrading to a psychology office.

There was a brief period of respite, however, during which he initiated a new form of therapy that came to be known as the 'speedy synthetic method' (*kuaisu zonghe liaofa* 快速綜合療法). This was a comprehensive therapy that included use of drugs (insulin, Novocain, herb medicines) and physical treatments (acupuncture, electric shock, techniques for inducing artificial sleep) to help students at Beijing who were diagnosed as suffering from neurasthenia (*shenjingshuairuo*), the limited but allowable diagnostic category. It was generally applied to groups of patients at a time who were lectured on its benefits and it boasted a high rate of success for the removal of headaches and sleeplessness. The therapy was quickly applied to other populations and was found useful for the treatment of other diseases such as peptic ulcer, hypertension and schizophrenia.[46]

Although some suspected the motives of the government in supporting this development (in that it helped to get many people worn down by the harshness of the Anti-Rightist or Criticism movement back on their feet) it had implications for forms of therapy which became permissible.[47] To begin with, it broadened the concept of therapy to include psychosocial processes. While talk of the unconscious was avoided, it allowed discussion and application of the functions of consciousness using suggestion (*an-shih* 暗示) and reasoning (*shuo-li* 說理) and, even though it disregarded individual differences in effects of the treatment applied to groups, forms of therapy in groups was possible.

In spite of this initiative, the Institute had a very tough time from the late 1950s onwards and psychologists had to subject themselves to severe disciplinary reform.[48] Often accused of lapsing into idealism and not sufficiently taking account of the biases in their research by subjecting it to a 'class analysis', their work was criticized for being too centred on outdated and politically incorrect Western theories. Eventually, in the cultural revolution of the 1960s, the whole field of psychology suffered an assault by Yao Wen-yuan, one of the Gang-of-Four, whose harsh critique led to its shutting down and the destruction of the Psychology Institute. Ding Tsan, throughout this period, was one of the major targets of these criticisms; long suspected of working for the Guomindang government, he was subjected to restricted movement and publically vilified. Also, his medication for cardiovascular disease and hypertension was deliberately delayed, leading to his death soon after these events in 1968.[49]

The Faring of Su Zonghua

Among the first generation of psychiatrists, Su Zonghua (1904–70), was one of the first to apply psychotherapy to psychiatric patients. Born in Hunan Province, he studied medicine in Xiang Ya Medical School in 1924 and later transferred to the National Shanghai Medical School (affiliated to Jiangsu Medical University), where Lyman and Halpern, respectively, headed the department of Neurology and Psychiatry. In 1932, after graduation, he worked in Peking Union Medical Hospital where, under the influence of Richard Lyman, he was encouraged to specialize in psychiatry and, in 1935, went to Johns Hopkins University and, later, Harvard University, where he specialized in neuro-psychiatric medicine in the functionalist school of psychiatry under Adolf Meyer. In 1938, to serve his nation during wartime, he returned to China to work in his alma mater, the Shanghai Medical School, as both a teacher and a practitioner and later became its director. With the outbreak of the Sino–Japanese War, the whole school and hospital moved out of Shanghai, but Su stayed in Shanghai and started his own private practice by setting up a psychiatric rehabilitation hospital (Hongqiao) which opened its doors in 1944 (and which was to remain open for 10 years). Su's reputation rose during this period and he became the top psychiatrist of Shanghai. Academically, he edited the first Chinese psychiatric monograph in 1951, *A Survey of Psychiatry,* which used Chinese cases and clinical data. Huang Jiayin practiced and collected data in Su's private hospital and published his own text, 'Psychotherapy 300 Cases', in 1951. In 1954, when private property and businesses were outlawed in China, Su Zonghua brought his Hong Qiao Hospital and staff with him to the Shanghai Municipal Psychiatric Hospital and worked there as its director. He was appointed dean of this hospital in 1956; he successfully ran it and combined it with several other psychiatric prevention centers into the umbrella organization known as the Shanghai Chief Psychiatric Treatment and Prevention Hospital, which played an important role in the development of psychiatry in China in terms of clinics, teaching, research and prevention.

Su's reputation was based on a number of achievements, not only his having produced the first textbook, which used local clinical data and cited Chinese cases, he was also the first to use electroshock therapy for the treatment of major depression and the first to apply the antipsychotic drug, chlorpromazine, in clinical cases. He even undertook lobotomies for the treatment of refractory (drug resistant) schizophrenia. Apart from his work in clinical intervention he is remembered for his 'Shanghai model' of community building: forging links between the hospital and the family as a firm basis for preventive psychiatry. Even in the period of his early private practice in Hong Qiao Hospital in the late 1930's, he was analyzing patients by himself.[50] The psychiatric patients, when necessary, were offered or encouraged to take psychotherapy given by psychologists and by Huang Jiayin. His analytical orientation was developed though his association with his former American teacher. This fact was one of the reasons why, in 1957, he was criticized.

His growing reputation brought him to the attention of several high profile people who were to become his patients and thereby raise his own celebrity. Chief amongst these were the Shanghai movie actress Zhou Xuan; Mao's wife, Jiang Qing; and Lin Zhao, a young talented student from Beijing University, who first stood out when she questioned Mao's political policy in ruling China and one after another of his political movements.[51] She was jailed in Shanghai several times for her statements and eventually executed. But on the second occasion of her incarceration she was sent to Su Zonghua for examination and he returned a diagnosis of 'psychiatrically abnormal' (*Jingshen Yichang*) which Lin Zhao's sister believed was Su's way of trying to protect her.[52] Nobody knows whether Su was using his expertise to explain why this girl was so unusual in freely expressing her own thoughts against the current political climate, or whether he was trying to save her by putting her into the custody of a psychiatric hospital instead of allowing her to be being tortured in jail, since Su told others later that 'Lin was a unexpected talent' after he interviewed her.[53] Su himself was accused of covering up for her anti-revolutionary crimes and therefore was criticized during the cultural revolution and died soon after, in 1970. However, the criticism and vilification of this talented psychiatrist had started as early as the 1950s. Dr. Jin De-chu recalled that, after reading his teacher's confession article 'My re-understanding of Dr. Mayer's psychophysiology', he rhetorically asked 'early in 1956, under what kind of stress and force did our professor labour to surrender with both his hands up?'

Although, politically, Su was challenged for using Meyer's theory in his case analyses in his practice, the criticisms were stepped up when he later confessed his political point of view. In the 1960's, this persecution forced him to stop any clinical work and administrative duties in the hospital and he was required to attend meetings where he received critical censure. He was also earmarked for an 'isolation review' (*Geli Shencha* 隔離審查) and was later consigned to labour as a cleaner of outpatient room.[54] Su Zonghua died of cancer in 1970 at the age of 66.

Conclusions

Psychotherapy in China as a practice had only a brief period of less than thirty years in which to develop before being forced to shut down in the political climate of the mid-1960s. The handful of people who could lay claim to furthering it came from fields as diverse as psychiatry, psychology and literature and each had begun that interest through writing in a common platform: *West Wind*. The articles, appearing alongside the contributions of others, were often written in a popular style and showed a progressive shift of direction and of intention and purpose. Initially informative, they brought knowledge of psychology from Euro–America to raise awareness of developments abroad and how they might be of benefit in helping solve the social problems of China. The target was a general readership but also one made up of doctors, nurses, caregivers, social workers and children's guardians. From being informative, the articles progressively became prescriptive and shifted from a reliance on imported theoretical ideas to educating the readership to become problem solvers in a common quest. What remains distinctive is that adaptation to cultural expectations would appear to have been in educational rather than clinical contexts initially. Doctors and students are the first to be sensitized to their patients' needs and to be instructed on the benefits of these new forms of treatment; parents are encouraged to see their children as having problems of adaptation, not be seen as problem children. Later, as the demand rises, the number of cases reported increases and new hospitals and clinics begin to open. However, the work is hampered by massive eternal upheavals: the Sino–Japanese War bringing on a forced relocation of hospitals, schools and laboratories, even the journal, to the interior, followed by a civil war and then the formation of a new republic in which the ideological turn to Russia brings forth a condemnation of many of the assumptions upon which the psychotherapeutic interventions are predicated. Seen against this backdrop, the work of the people reported here seems all the more extraordinary – and tragic. The ideologies shaping mental health policy in the early years of the PRC were seriously in conflict with those of individualized psychotherapy. Trying to continue that line of work and even extol it at risk to themselves proved fatal in the case of Huang Jiayin, detrimental to professional and disciplinary development in the case of Ding Tsan and a serious loss of prestige to Su Zonghua, to say nothing of the flight of Cheng Yulin, with so many others, from the mainland to Taiwan.

Against this bleak picture one must take account of the struggle of psychologists and psychiatrists themselves to develop their ideas within an increasingly constraining political orthodoxy which ruled out notions of individual persons as having individually bounded psychological problems, such thoughts being dismissed as 'bourgeois', and instead confining therapies of improvement to groups. In this context, the speedy synthetic method might be considered an achievement, although more details would be required to make a better-informed judgment of its efficacy over the political motive of rejuvenating a population laboring under increasing restrictions on freedom. In any event, by the time of the cultural or proletariat revolution launched by Mao in 1965, anarchic students were encouraged to overthrow the authority of intellectuals (whom Mao distrusted), leading to psychology and many other disciplines coming under attack. A crucial moment in this period was the leading editorial written by Mao's Minister of Propaganda, Yao Wenyuan, drawing seriously into question the results of a study on colour and form preferences in children by Chen Li and Wang Ansheng for much the same reasons that had motivated the criticisms of psychology during the Anti-rightist campaign: the experiments abstracted from the lived realities of people in actual social contexts and were not therefore legitimate objectives of research.[55] This line of thinking, quite unfounded, denied the possibility of there being any common or universal features of the mind that were worthwhile objects of study. Yet Yao's criticisms fueled the flames of a growing attack on the discipline as a whole, forcing it to be shut down by 1966, with the banning of its books and journals and the ceasing of its teaching in universities and research institutes.

Only since 1978 has psychology emerged in China with a new agenda, largely free of previous ideological constraints. The Government has recognized that, with its booming market economy, it is encountering social problems for which psychological services are now very much needed, particularly in the areas of Counselling (now a government approved job category), Human Resources and Health Psychology. Consequently, some Chinese doctors and psychologists have been receiving psychoanalytical and psychotherapeutic training from specialized interest groups outside of China since the mid-1980s. This training has involved exchanges with Chinese doctors spending periods abroad for study and research, as well as analysts and psychotherapists from other countries visiting China for short periods, running workshops and seminars, supervision sessions as well as conferences. Currently there are groups from Germany, Norway, France, Japan and the United States each with its own orientations within increasingly diverse and specialized psychological practices. It thus remains to be seen how integrated these sets of ideas will become into broader therapeutic practices relevant to the host culture but the training of diverse groups with increasing specialties might be one consequence of this current activity.

In contrast, one can look back to the period of the 1930s and 1940s and see, in spite of the smaller numbers of people involved in these practices, that a greater level of integration and harmonious cooperation existed between people of different intellectual training who also took it upon themselves to contribute to, and maintain, a broad popular front in the education of the general public and related health professionals through writing in a common platform – a singular journal devoted to this end. One can only ponder the question of how far this might have developed had psychotherapy not been forced to shut down.

Acknowledgements

In researching this chapter, the authors acknowledge the support given by the Research Grants Council of the Government of Hong Kong.

9 A CHARTED EPIDEMIC OF TRAUMA: CASE NOTES AT THE PSYCHIATRIC DEPARTMENT OF NATIONAL TAIWAN UNIVERSITY HOSPITAL BETWEEN 1946 AND 1953

Harry Yi-Jui Wu

Introduction

In the early years after the Second World War, the island of Taiwan saw a rapid growth of psychoneurotic patients across different ethnic groups. This hidden 'epidemic' remained covered until the case notes of the Department of Psychiatry at the National Taiwan University Hospital were unearthed recently.[1] The causation of these disorders among the suffering individuals is assumed to be dissimilar. The emergence of this phenomenon could be grounded on the external reality of the post-war societal turmoil, the altered aspiration of psychiatric services, and most importantly, the psychiatrists who found themselves accountable for the betterment among those who sought their help. This chapter, as the first attempt to study the case notes kept by the Department of Psychiatry at the National Taiwan University Hospital (NTUH), aims to unpack the contextual meaning of such a mental disorder epidemic through analyzing this clinical archive.

Psychiatry in early post-war Taiwan experienced the re-institutionalization of the discipline during the handover period between two political regimes, in large part due to the social upheaval that caused mental instability in this context. Under these circumstances, psychiatrists managed to diagnose individuals who sought help from the newly established National Taiwan University Hospital. Facilitating the process were a newly acquired linguistic resource of psychiatry, and a newly learned medical technology to treat the unsound minds.[2] Apart from psychotic patients who already existed at a relatively unchanging rate, the sudden increasing epidemic of psychoneuroses marked the professional interests of psychiatry. The ideology of Taiwanese psychiatrists played a significant role in accounting for such disorders.[3]

Informed by what had been long considered the mainstream approach to the history of medicine, historians employed an institutional approach to probe into various themes and issues of the medical sciences.[4] In recording the history of psychiatry, due to the voiceless nature of psychiatric patients and the limited accessibility of patient records, historians tended to amplify the role institutions played in regards to the management of psychiatric subjects, thereby ignoring the subsistence of mental patients, including how they behaved, what they thought, how they looked, and in what ways they were perceived, whether it be objective or subjective. This was until Roy Porter's call to retrieve 'the patient's voice' from a wider choice of accounts that actively frame the discovery of psychiatry, or psychiatric disorders.[5]

Contrary to the institutional approach, other scholars are concerned about the constitution and transformation of physical bodies and individual identities through technological practices. In clinical settings, the application of diagnostics is a practice of medical technologies, which are neither independent of the agency of medical practitioners, nor of the individuals on whom the technologies are practiced.[6] Such practices are located at the 'intersections' between the action of diagnoses and the social worlds of both clinicians and patients. In keeping with this spirit, by using a hospital's case notes, this chapter attempts to picture the context in which certain psychiatric diagnoses were placed onto suffering individuals (or even communities) in a particular timeframe. Combining the institutional approach and that accentuates the role of agencies, this analysis of the NTUH case notes reveals how an epidemic of psychiatric disorder was documented and constructed.

Case Notes as a Source of the History of Mental Disorders

The study of case notes regarding the history of psychiatry is a fresh area. Apart from disclosing various aspects of psychiatric diseases, they can overcome the limitations of one-dimensional perspectives raised by experts and the inadequacy of numerical rationality represented by statistical methods. Case histories have been employed heavily in the field of psychoanalysis, which are unfamiliar to historians and clinicians. These stories are told from patient's viewpoints and therapist's outlooks, and the detailed dynamics between the two are examined. Such an approach, however, does not explain the psychology of larger cohorts, which have gradually vanished with the development of modern psychiatry. Psychiatric patients began to disappear as hospitals and laboratories dominated newly emerging medical cosmologies.[7]

Case notes are the medical records that are systematically documented upon a patient's outpatient visits or admission to hospitals. Historians have recently reiterated the significance of these documents as a means to revealing fuller aspects of psychiatric diseases. They have been used for the understanding of the ways in which madness was institutionally constructed,[8] and to understand the various interpretations of doctors on certain disorders, but they are also useful in constructing the picture of particular mental disorders.[9] Some are significant regarding the ways in which case histories were constructed through negotiations between doctors and patients.[10] Research of hospital case files shows the clinical experiences of inmates in psychiatric wards, and how clinicians' engagement with patients have transformed psychiatric theories.[11]

A newly developed approach has endeavoured to analyze hospital case notes in a systematic manner. Employing either quantitative or qualitative methods in a colonial or postcolonial framework, many of these approaches have developed problems related to altered theories of psychopathology, cluttered psychiatric language usage, and constantly shifting disease classification systems.[12] For the history of psychiatry in East Asia, the analysis of Akihito Suzuki, two decades before the Second World War, of patients in Ohji Brain and Komine Hospitals, was probably the first and only attempt in employing case notes. He indicated the complexity of Japanese psychiatry during that period, as mostly concluded by Japanese medical historians, as opposed to pure 'Westernization', and emphasized the role of therapist power in radically transforming the meaning of hospitalization in these hospital contexts.[13] Following analysis, the work of psychiatric classification passed to the historian to roughly lump together cases assumed as belonging to several categories according to current fashionable diagnoses. This process might obviate certain unique cases, contradicting the original intention of case histories.[14] These systematic or sporadic efforts to redraw the profiles of psychiatric patients through case notes have shown the disadvantages and limitations of such attempts.

This chapter examines the characteristics of an institution, the effect of certain sociocultural factors on its psychiatric practice, and the composition of its patients by analyzing the patient notes archived at the Psychiatric Department of the National Taiwan University Hospital (NTUH). These case files, documented between 1939 and 1953, were donated by Professor Hsien Rin 林憲, a pioneer of transcultural psychiatry at NTUH, to the research program of the History of Hygiene at Academia Sinica. Originally from Professor Rin's private collection, they survived being discarded during re-institutionalization after WWII and were kept in his office until May 2009.

Chinese Psychiatry before the end of WWII

To contour the general picture of psychiatric practice while the case files were recorded, a brief introduction of psychiatry in Chinese societies and the establishment of the Psychiatric Department at NTUH is necessary. Psychiatry is a young medical speciality in the Chinese-speaking world that was not adequately developed until the second half of the twentieth century. From the mid-nineteenth century to the early-twentieth century, missionaries or colonial enterprises introduced psychiatry to Chinese cities, either as part of the modernization process, or as benevolent charity work. For example, in Canton, John Kerr (1821–1901) established the first hospital for mental illness in China in 1898.[15] In Hong Kong, Victoria Mental Hospital was built with a 130-bed capacity.[16] In Beijing, a specialized institution for the mentally ill was built with the aid of the Rockefeller Foundation.[17] Regardless of the theories and practices on mental illness in traditional Chinese medicine, these institutions were sporadic efforts diffused during the development of Western medicine in Chinese-speaking areas.

Development of psychiatric science at national levels in East Asia should be examined in view of the modernization of nation states and their colonial expansions. In East Asia, the most prominent example is Japan. In the late 1860s, the regime of the Meiji emperor attempted to reform Japan, introducing Western culture, technology and legal and medical practices to catch up with the more powerful countries in the West. German psychiatry was introduced to Japan and the University of Tokyo was the first hub to accommodate this newly launched medical discipline. In Japanese colonies such as Taiwan and Manchuria, psychiatry was included in the syllabi and was largely shaped by the descriptive school of Emil Kraepelin.[18] Psychiatry in the colonies was mainly a service for emigrants from Japan. Similar to most colonies during the pre-World War II period, a range of psychiatric diagnoses was derived to serve the health and power of the colonizers. In colonial Taiwan, the epidemic of tropical neurasthenia, hypochondriasis and the hypotheses on the personality of indigenous people were the most classic examples.[19] Toward the end of the Second World War, no other countries in East Asia, apart from Japan, had developed their own national version of psychiatry.

Mental health issues attracted attention after the Second World War, both at international and local levels. In China, the renowned demographer Ta Chen 陳達 emphasized the need to examine those among the Chinese with mental and physical deficiencies. Ta Chen argued for the need of population studies in China, not only because of incomplete and inaccurate data left behind by a series of wars, but also for mutual understanding to attain 'international peace of a permanent order'.[20] Because of continual instability in mainland China, Ta Chen's appeal was not realized until the late 1950s when an epidemiological survey was attempted.[21] In the mid-1960s, however, all psychiatric activities were suspended due to the Cultural Revolution.

Re-Institutionalization of Psychiatry in Taiwan

In contrast to the situation in China, where psychiatric activities were suspended after the end of the Second World War, psychiatry in Taiwan was reinstituted and developed continuously as a new discipline in the name of Chinese psychiatry. In August 1945, after Japan's defeat, Taiwan broke away from a half century of colonization. Under the authorization of Douglas MacArthur's General Order, Chen Yi 陳儀, the Chinese delegate, was escorted by George Kerr to Taiwan to accept the surrender of the Japanese government. Chen Yi was commissioned to organize an interregnum to govern Taiwan as a province of what was then the Republic of China. Most public institutions established during colonization were handed over to the Nationalist Chinese government, including the governor's offices, banks, the tobacco and alcohol monopoly bureau, railway systems, educational institutions, hospitals and other infrastructure systems.[22] For the medical system, handing over Imperial Taihoku University and its affiliated hospitals was most important.[23]

The Chinese Nationalist government took over the Japanese institutional properties, despite the shortage of labor and financial resources. To facilitate communication with the Japanese, the Chinese Nationalist government employed the only native Taiwanese professor at the Medical School at the time, Tu Congming 杜聰明, and the only native Taiwanese lecturer, Bosei Lim 林茂生. They were the only two higher teaching staff at the College of Humanities at Imperial Taihoku University who were familiar with the Japanese administration. Tu Congming was the first Taiwanese to receive a Doctorate of Medical Science from Kyoto Imperial University during Japanese colonization. He became the first Taiwanese professor in Japan's imperial university system. Bosei Lim was the first Taiwanese to receive a Doctorate in Philosophy. In the 1920s, he studied with John Dewey at Columbia University in New York. In his dissertation, he criticized the Japanese educational policy to assimilate the colonized in Taiwan and emphasized the importance for students to develop individual autonomy based on liberalism.[24]

Medical sciences at Imperial Taihoku University were substantially better developed than other disciplines, of which the Chinese Nationalist government was immediately aware. This was because, during Japanese colonial times, native Taiwanese intellectuals were prevented from taking advantage of higher education and eventually entered the public administration system. This is the reason the two Taiwanese members of the adoption committee Tu Congming and Bosei Lim were appointed professor and a lecturer, respectively, although they held equivalent degrees. Taiwanese who performed better academically chose to study medicine to become freelancers and exempt themselves from regulation by the Japanese government. A career as a physician became the most popular aspiration among the

Taiwanese.[25] According to statistics, among the personnel still working for Imperial Taihoku University at the end of the Second World War, more than 2,000 were medical school graduates, including 140 people awarded doctorate degrees, mostly from universities in Japan, whereas there were only sixty-four scholars in total, from the domains of humanities, legal studies, agriculture and engineering.[26]

Mental health issues in Taiwan had long been downplayed or presumed unimportant by the Chinese, including the Chinese Nationalist government. Because the Chinese race is of such an ancient origin, it had attained an unusual degree of stability so that the incidence of mental and physical deficiency among the Chinese was relatively insignificant. During the pre-war period, there was a controversy as to whether mental illnesses existed among the Chinese. Whereas missionary doctors believed that insanity prevailed to a considerably lesser extent in China than in Europe, others affirmed the very real existence of Chinese mental illness, although they were thought to take different forms from Western ones.[27] Even if modern psychiatry had been popularized in the Chinese-speaking world, fundamental Chinese thought regarding health beliefs and practices continued to exert important effects on symptom manifestations and health-related behaviours of Chinese patients.[28] Such attitude was reflected in the words of a government official, who expressed the non-necessity to Tsung-Yi Lin of funding the psychiatric services of the National Taiwan University hospital.[29]

Tsung-Yi Lin 林宗義, son of Bosei Lim, was the first native Taiwanese physician to pursue the study of psychiatry before the Second World War. Understanding the nature of the Han Chinese (漢民族), an ethnic group native to China who were the main population in Taiwan, was one of the main motives of Tsung-Yi Lin as he discussed furthering his specialty training with his father.[30] Like other distinguished Taiwanese students during the Japanese colonization, Lin pursued higher education in Japan after graduating from Taihoku High School (台北高等學校). One reason for this was that there was no systematic psychiatric training in Taiwan. While in Japan, between 1939 and 1946, he spent three years studying medicine, receiving two years of specialty training in general medicine in psychiatry at Imperial Tokyo University, and another year at Matsuzawa Hospital (松澤病院).[31]

For most Taiwanese intellectuals, the blows of the post-war situation on the island shattered their imagination of China. On 25 October 1945, Tsung-Yi Lin saw his father in a photograph sent to Tokyo, in which Bosei Lim was welcoming the retrocession of the Chinese Nationalist government dressed as a *magua* (馬褂), a kind of long coat that represented Chinese culture. In the photo, his father was wearing an 'excited, confident, and robust' facial expression.[32] This cheering and hopeful atmosphere did not last long. In the communications between father and son, Lin discerned the disillusionment of his father and gradually realized the worsening situation in Taiwan, including the ill treatment and discrimination of the Chinese toward the Taiwanese, a lack of constructive plans and cultural discontinuity caused by the ban of the Japanese language.

Tsung-Yi Lin returned to Taiwan on 30 May1946. On the day of his arrival, using the metaphor of 'black heaven and dark earth' (*hei tian an di* 黑天暗地), Bosei Lim described the current situation in Taiwan in contrast to his excitement only a few months earlier. 'Has the quality of Chinese people deteriorated?' was the first question Tsung-Yi Lin asked his father. This question represents the gap between how the Chinese were imagined by most Taiwanese and how they were in reality, which also left an anticipatory remark in his mind for his later inquiry. On the same day, he took three suggestions from his father on how to conduct psychiatric research in Taiwan: 'First, take the approach from social and cultural perspectives; second, integrate with other disciplines; third, consolidate connections with international academics'.[33] Bosei Lim's suggestions not only reiterated his concerns on his son's choice, but also showed his anxiety regarding the isolation of Taiwan in the context of post-war international relations.

The aftermath of war provides rich soil for psychological trauma to emerge among clinicians and the general public. The blows perceived by these young psychiatrists were crucial for them to recount their own trauma and that of people who sought help from them. However, such trauma was unable to come to terms until clinicians acquired and became familiar with the language and diagnostic tools of modern psychiatry. After Tsung-Yi Lin returned to Taiwan, he observed that the Taiwanese had difficulty admitting that the Chinese, who had completely different language habits, took the most power in government, and he was reminded of his father's experience of disillusionment some years before. He also found it difficult to communicate with colleagues and patients without learning Mandarin. Tsung-Yi Lin was also confronted by his own identity crisis because he was not treated as fairly as those Chinese who were newly immigrated to Taiwan.[34] His experience was shared among the Taiwanese and could be found in various personal accounts. The war, the change of language policy and the shift of culture all had an effect on the psyche of the Taiwanese people. Wen-Shing Tseng 曾文星, one of Lin's students, found the Taiwanese people to be confronted with the effect of economic collapse and social turmoil immediately after the war. In the mean time, he was reluctant to transform his national identity and to adjust to the Chinese language and culture.[35]

Trauma after the Second World War: War, Immigration, and Ethnic Conflicts

In the early post-war period, psychiatrists in the newly re-institutionalized psychiatric department directly attributed psychopathological mental illness to various devastating post-war events. After the end of the Second World War, psychiatry in Taiwan underwent a wholesale re-institutionalization, including staffing, services provided, objectives, psychiatric education and theories. Dr Naka Syuzo and most of his colleagues were repatriated immediately after the end of the war. Tsung-Yi Lin, a Tokyo-educated Taiwanese psychiatrist, returned to Taiwan in 1946. The only remaining Japanese psychiatrist, Ryosuke Kurosawa 黑澤良介, who worked for the Chinese Nationalist government as a consultant, returned to Japan in December. The next year, Tsung-Yi Lin became the director of the newly institutionalized psychiatric department at National Taiwan University Hospital. Under Lin's leadership, psychiatry in Taiwan developed in a completely different direction.

Upon his arrival, Lin immediately observed different manifestations of mental illness among the Taiwanese population. Because of his personal cross-cultural experiences, Lin realized that he had to develop his own syllabus with comparative cultural psychiatry as the central focus. Together with his newly recruited students, he conducted statistical surveys regarding psychiatric representations of various populations in Taiwan.[36] Lin's door-to-door fieldwork not only laid the foundation of his methodology in epidemiology, but also caused the World Health Organization (WHO) to take notice of him. He led the mental health section of the WHO regarding its cross-national studies in social psychiatry.

The epidemiological research of Lin and his students won international attention later in the mid-1950s; however, psychiatric services at NTUH were a completely different story. With imperfect theories and limited resources, this newly established medical speciality had to provide care and treatment for a drastically increasing population of psychiatric patients. Before Lin returned to Taiwan in 1946, he spent the entire wartime in Japan, during which he received his general medical and psychiatric trainings. He spent two years studying psychiatry at the University of Tokyo and one year interning at Matsuzawa Hospital.[37] Because of such a short training experience, Lin more than once refused the invitation to take up the directorship of the psychiatric hospital at NTUH. Ryosuke Kurosawa remained with the NTUH administration until the work left behind by the original staff was handed over. Upon Lin's return to Taiwan, patients were still being admitted to the wards.

The psychiatric department led by Tsung-Yi Lin was not large enough to form its own school of thought or practice. With only one person officially trained as a psychiatrist, Lin's department was seen as a hall ruled by one man's voice. To some extent, Lin and the practice of his students were influenced by current fashionable psychiatric schools of thought, such as the international diffusion of Freudian psychoanalysis, the international mental hygiene movement during the interwar period and the remnants of Japanese colonial psychiatry. Traces of these schools can be found in various types of diagnoses in patient notes. Lin's psychiatric insight was heavily influenced by his supervisor, Yushi Uchimura

内村祐之, who specialized in cultural psychiatry. However, his own vision of Taiwanese psychiatry derived from the differences between the Taiwanese and Japanese cultures he observed upon his arrival in Taiwan. Because of these differences, Lin's version of cultural psychiatry was relatively incompatible with the colonial approach of Uchimura; Lin cultivated his insight in epidemiology and emphasized the need to study what caused the differences in prevalence and manifestations of psychiatric disorders among various populations in Taiwan. The educational syllabi at the psychiatric department of NTUH included two intact textbooks, which survived the fire caused by the war: one was edited by Oswald Bumke and the other by Carl and Frederik Lange.[38] The development of ward services, treatment and education curricula were all subject to Lin's directorship. As a result of the break in tradition with the original Imperial Taihoku University Hospital and the limited resources to develop the department, different schools regarded psychiatry in the new NTUH as lopsided and occasionally confusing.

The NTUH notes cover records of outpatient visits and admissions. Apart from the small number of patients remaining after Japan's defeat in the Second World War, most patients in the notes were those who sought help in the context of post-war social and political turmoil. Such patients included those experiencing immigration and ethnic conflicts, Chinese public servants who recently relocated from Mainland China to Taiwan, Japanese salary men who remained on the island and local Taiwanese people who became increasingly fearful after witnessing the February 28 Incident in 1947. Diagnosed mainly by Tsung-Yi Lin and the students he personally trained, these case notes show the complexity of 'psychological trauma' as it was conceived in the conflicting cultural context of post-colonial Taiwan, the transformation of this general concept during psychiatric paradigm shifts and the controversial and subjective nature of related medical diagnoses.

Statistical Analysis of NTUH Psychiatric Department Notes

From these recently unearthed patient notes, this study excluded wartime records held at the psychiatric department of NTUH to unify the historical context of analysis. From 1945 to 1953, there are 5,185 records including admissions and outpatient visits. Unfortunately, no admission records were preserved from 1951 or 1952. Before 1949, the year the Chinese Nationalist government was officially established in Taiwan, the original Japanese version of case notes was still in use. Racial categories included Inlanders (内地人, meaning Japanese), Hokkien, Cantonese, Indigenous People, Koreans, Chinese and foreigners. In this analysis, Taiwanese include Hokkien (福建人), Cantonese (廣東人, recognized today as Hakka, 客家人), and Indigenous populations. After 1949, patient notes were printed in Chinese instead, with the heading of the NTUH Department of Neurology and Psychiatry (*Guoli Taiwan Daxue Shenjing-Jin-*

gshenke 國立台灣大學神經精神科). Racial categories were abandoned; in their place, ancestral homes (*jiguan* 籍貫) were recorded. For analysis, Taiwanese includes those who were recorded as Taiwanese (*Taiwan Ren* 台灣人), the Taiwan Province (*Taiwan Sheng* 台灣省) and Native Provincials (*Bensheng Ren* 本省人). Immigrants from the mainland were documented according to the provinces they emigrated from or, simply, as mainlanders (*Waisheng Ren* 外省人). In the following paragraphs, outpatient visits include those who called on the hospital more than once.

Following the previous paradigm established by Japanese psychiatrists and the educational background of Tsung-Yi Lin, who was head of the department at the time, the diagnostic theories and treatments of mental illness were profoundly affected by the legacy of Japanese psychiatry, whose roots can be traced to German influences during Japan's Meiji period. Patient records at Imperial Taihoku University (renamed National Taiwan University after 1945), however, were highly informed by the prevailing racial science before and during the Second World War and consisted of the descriptive psychiatry style of Kraepelin and dynamic (psychoanalytical) psychiatry. Race was categorized in the first page of each patient record and the impression of diagnosis and the etiology (*yuan yin tui ding* 原因推定) of the illness were jointly given. The fashion of assuming the causation of mental illnesses, which was heavily influenced by psychoanalytical psychopathology, is no longer seen in phenomenological- and neurobiological-oriented modern psychiatry.

During the early post-war period, the language habit of psychiatrists gradually transformed from the Japanese-German to the English-Chinese system. The case notes show that German, Japanese, English, Chinese and Romanized Taiwanese languages were used intermittently. According to Tsung-Yi Lin, the immediate post-war society was 'total chaos' (*yipian hunluan* 一片混亂).[39] After the Japanese people returned to their homeland, the Taiwanese people could not quickly adapt to the administrative and technical workings that the former population had left behind. People with completely different languages and habits from Taiwanese populations unexpectedly took over all public sectors. According to Tsung-Yi Lin, the chaos was reflected by the 'odd triangle relationship' involving Taiwanese, Japanese and Chinese immigrants.[40] Lin was not the only psychiatrist or intellectual who experienced difficulty with language barriers and identity crises.[41] Under these circumstances, Lin began to learn the Mandarin language. He took notes in Romanized Taiwanese (*Tâi-ôan Lô-má-jī* 台灣羅馬字), a transcription system for Taiwanese Hokkien, to complete the 'present illness' sections on forms in order to faithfully present current symptoms of patients, particularly when transcribing their verbal communication.[42] Lin continued to use a combination of Japanese, German and Chinese for noting disease progress and treatment, until the 1950s, when English became the dominant language in the notes.

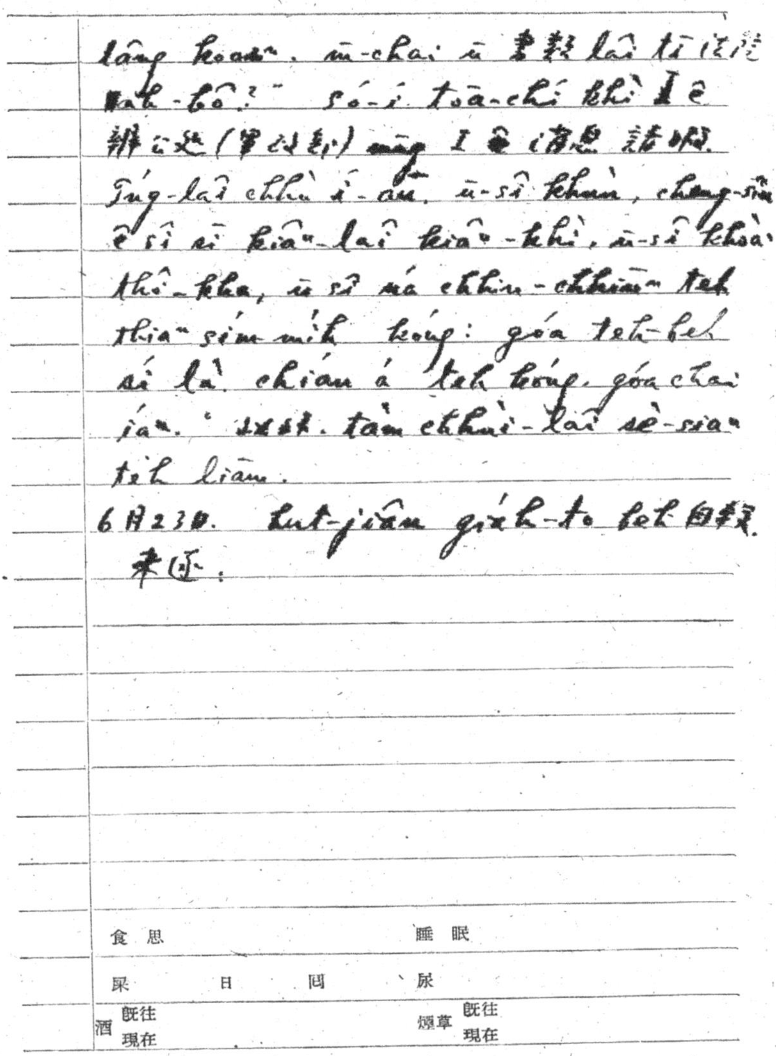
食思 睡眠
屎 日 回 尿
酒 既往 現在
煙草 既往 現在

Figure 9.1: Note of Present Illness from National Taiwan University Hospital Psychiatric Department Case Notes (1946), no. 100. This note documenting 'present illness' in the case of an attempted suicide was written in Romanized Taiwanese in order to accurately present the narration of the patient's mother.

The statistics in Figure 9.2 show the increase of outpatient visits from 1945 to 1953. In 1947, the number of outpatients doubled from those in 1946, whereas the number of admission services decreased. Many patients came to the hospital because of the horrors experienced during the February 28 Incident and its aftermath and were mostly diagnosed as having a Psychogenisch Reaktion. The number of outpatients surged in 1950, but the number of admissions did not reflect an obvious change because of the limited expansion of admission services. People who called on outpatient services were mostly Chinese immigrants relocated by the Chinese Nationalist government. Most of these patients worked for the military, public sectors, and schools. Many of them were diagnosed as having psychoneurosis (anxiety state) and Neuröse. Figures 9.3 and 9.4 show a steady increase in the number of Chinese immigrants in admissions and outpatients. Chinese immigrants accounted for more than 50% of total outpatient visits after 1950. In these notes, cases of functional psychosis (schizophrenia and mania-depression psychosis) remained stable in quantity. This echoed the later research outcome of WHO, which stated the prevalence of schizophrenia is universal. However, if it was not historical events that inflicted mental illness in patients, it was psychiatrists who attributed the suffering of those patients to these events.

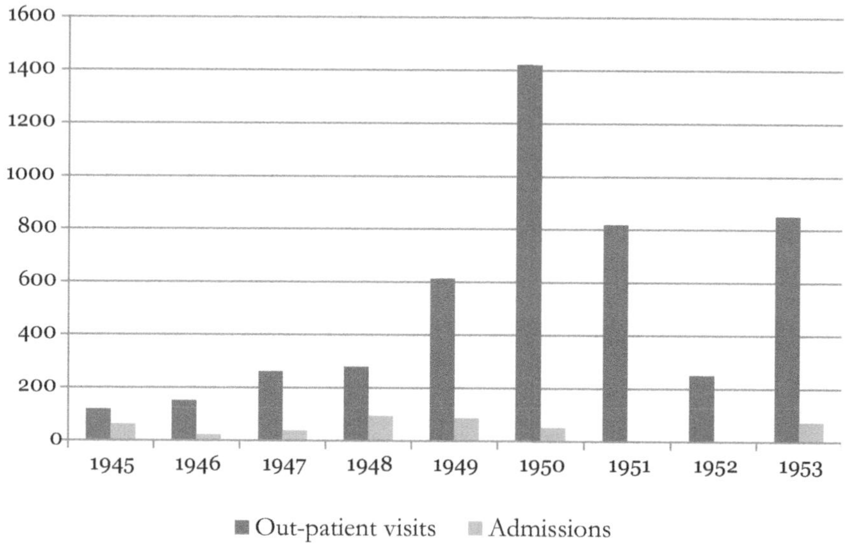

Figure 9.2: Numbers of Outpatient Visits and Admissions.

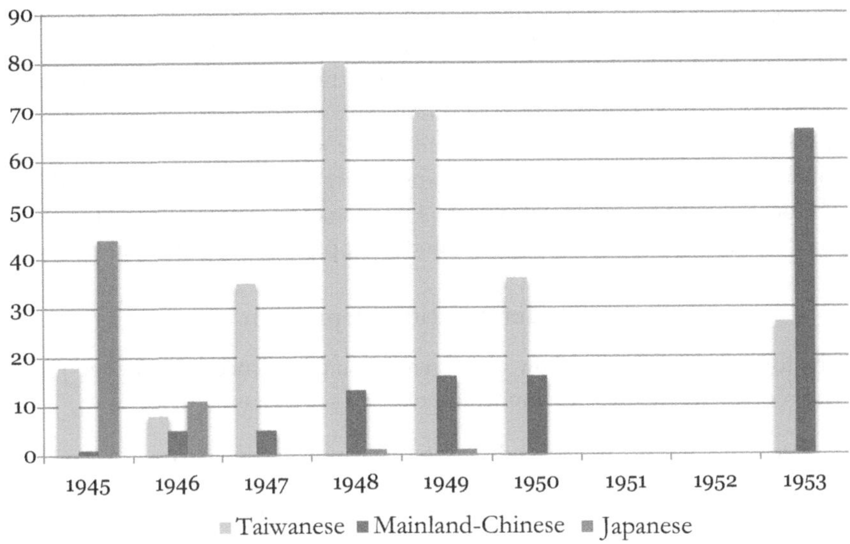

Figure 9.3: Numbers of Admitted Patients, with Racial Distribution

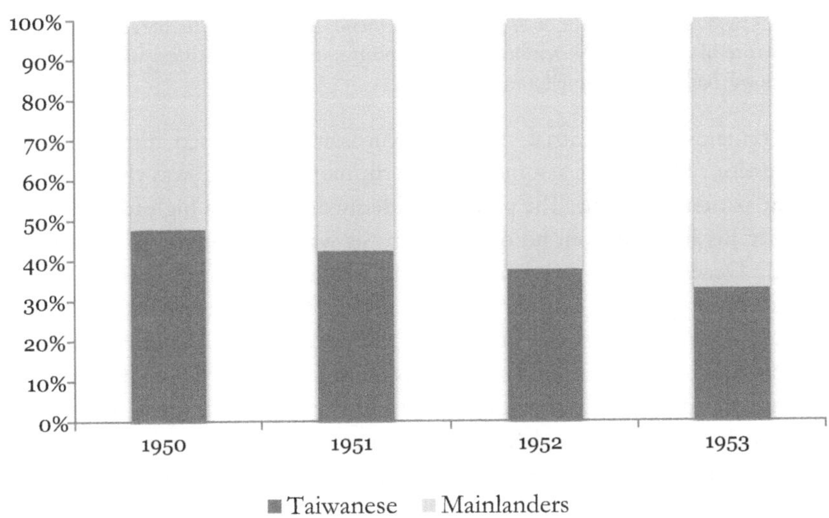

Figure 9.4: Statistics of Taiwanese and Chinese Immigrants (Mainlanders) among Outpatients

During the period in which this set of case notes was preserved, the defeat of Japan, the takeover of the Chinese Interregnum, the February 28 Incident, the establishment of the Chinese Nationalist government and the wave of Chinese immigration all affected society, the emergence of psychiatric patients and the manner in which psychiatrists diagnosed people who sought aid from them. The following section discusses cases of non-psychotic disorders that were recorded as obviously caused by specific life events. Functional disorders such as schizophrenia, hebephrenia, delusional disorders and other psychotic disorders are excluded.

War Termination Depression

The following case shows how a traumatic event influenced patient symptoms and reoriented the doctor's impression of the disease causation:

> After the end of the Second World War, a special case register showed a 57-year-old Japanese salary man (會社員). He had been living in Taiwan for three years (since 1942) and visited the psychiatric department because of 'Schlafstörung' (sleep disturbance) and 'Brustbeklemmung' (chest tightness). According to the patient notes, he began to consider many things and felt uneasy after the end of the Second World War. He felt tired when making contact with other people. His chest tightness appeared in September. He was admitted to the Governor-General of Taiwan Psychiatric Home (台灣總督府精神病院養神院) for treatment. After being discharged ten days before his revisit on November 7, his symptoms, including tiredness and depressed mood, had not been ameliorated.[43]

The remaining psychiatrist, Ryosuke Kurosawa, diagnosed him as having a depression. He further assumed that 'termination of war' was the main cause of the patient's ailment. The patient suddenly developed a high fever; however, despite his ill condition, no other diagnosis was made other than depression. On 22 December, the patient died. In this case, the patient obviously died from deteriorating physical conditions characterized by uncontrollable fever. Nevertheless, the psychiatrist did not pay further attention to the patient's medical conditions, but concentrated only on his mental infirmity before the underlying disease was discovered a few days before his death. This tragedy demonstrates the shock of the Japanese defeat in the war not only to the patient, but also the doctor, whose preoccupation with the impact of defeat led him to overlook life-threatening physical ailments.

The February 28 Incident and Psychogenic Reaction

The February 28 Incident was the first event, after World War II, that caused widespread psychological distress for the Taiwanese people. Long before Taiwanese psychiatrists in the 1980s remembered and retrospectively interpreted its legacy, the instantaneous effect on the Taiwanese people was shown through mental symptoms. Many of the diagnoses of these patients that appeared in the medical case files were 'psychogenic reaktion [sic]', which is a 'psychogenic reaction' with partial German spelling. Psychogenic reaction was a general term, informed by the Freudian school of psychoanalytic psychiatry, used to explain somatic complaints rendered from psychological disturbance. It was later included in the sixth revision of the International Classification of Diseases (ICD-6) in 1948, under the category of 'psychoneurotic disorders'.[44] In these cases, most patients were admitted to the psychiatric department with complaints of headache, dizziness, poor quality of sleep and other physical problems. Most of their 'present illness' all started 'after February 28 Incident'.

For example, a twenty-eight year-old married Taiwanese man, who was a land mortgage broker, visited the psychiatric department because of his suicidal ideation (Suicidversuch). He also had insomnia (Schlafstörung) and angina pectoris (Brustbeklemmung). He was a graduate of Waseda University in Tokyo. Tsung-Yi Lin diagnosed this man with 'psychogenic reaction', a disease directly caused by the February 28 Incident.[45] Another more detailed register shows that a twenty-seven year-old woman visited the psychiatric department because of chest tightness and feelings of distress. She had an elementary school education. In the outpatient department, she complained to the doctor that she felt 'threatened' when other family members were not home. Ten days before her symptoms emerged, she received a telephone call from a certain governmental official, telling her that 'your family has something to do with Lin Rigao (林日高, a legislator, who was arrested after the February 28 Incident)'. Before Lin Rigao was arrested, he often called on her family. Three or four days after the telephone call, she was horrified every time someone knocked on her door. She developed a depressive mood and negative thoughts. Once she had to run away from home because she thought the police were chasing her and, when she returned, she could not recognize her own children. She experienced shallow sleep and terrible thoughts thereafter, such as being chased by people carrying guns. At midnight, when she heard people talking next door, she thought they were bad people; therefore, she kept switching the light on and off. Tsung-Yi Lin diagnosed her as having 'psychogenic reaction' and admitted her to the ward.[46]

However, psychogenic reaction was not the only diagnosis in cases related to the February 28 Incident. A twenty year-old male teacher visited the psychiatric department on 21 April 1947, because of 'Schaflostigkeit' (sleeplessness) and 'Träumreich [sic]' (dream-world). He complained that he had poor sleep quality ever since the February 28 Incident. Apart from insomnia and nightmares, he felt dizzy and had generalized weakness (Allgemeine Kraftlosigkeit) during the day. He was diagnosed as having psychogenic neurasthenische reaktion.[47] Neurasthenia was excluded as a psychiatric disease after the launch of the ICD system. However, as mentioned earlier, during Japanese colonial times, neurasthenia was described as a condition combined with fatigue, anxiety, headache, weakness and other symptoms resulting from nervous exhaustion. In this case, the stress of the February 28 Incident caused the patient's psychogenic reaction and the symptom manifestations resembled those of a case of neurasthenia. 'Neurasthenia' was no longer a privilege of the Japanese people. The colour of colonialism in terms of neurasthenia had gradually faded, becoming a neutral terminology accepted by the Taiwanese people.

On 21 April 1947, a forty-one year-old man visited the psychiatric department because of suicidal ideation. He said he had begun to feel ill since the February 28 Incident. Five days before visiting the hospital, he felt abnormal. During the previous five days, he could not eat and sleep well. During the night, he was terrified by 'ghosts and gods'. His right arm was numb. He was diagnosed as having 'psychogenic depression'. [48]

On 25 July 1949, a twenty-seven year-old elementary school teacher visited the outpatient department. He sought help because the horror experience had severely disturbed his daily life. Since January 1948, he could not stand still. While eating with chopsticks, his hand tremor prevented him from picking up food from the bowl. By August 1948, he began to suffer from slurred speech and a stammer. He rode his bicycle in a serpentine path because of generalized weakness. He said that he had been short-tempered before the February 28 Incident, but was now incapable of getting angry. He was diagnosed as 'Hysterie' with a question mark. This patient called on the doctor one and a half years after the February 28 Incident. The doctor still listed 'February 28 Incident' in the data field under 'aetiology'. This shows the clinician's close attention to, and high regard of, the event and it's prevalence in influencing his diagnoses.[49]

Adjustment Disorders among Chinese Immigrants

In 1949 another epidemic of psychoneurotic disorders began to appear. Newly emerging psychoneurotic cases in Chinese immigrants showed an overturn of power distribution between those diagnosing and the diagnosed, and between the governing and the governed. After the retreat of Chiang Kai Shek's Nationalist Government from Nanjing to Taipei, his troops, followers and those who were driven out by the Communist Party fled to Taiwan. The 2 million new immigrants merged with 6 million other Taiwanese, forming the background constituents of Taiwanese intellectual history. Documents show that beginning in 1946, diagnoses such as psychogenic reaction and neurasthenic reaction in Chinese immigrants increased drastically. As shown in Figure 9.2, the number of patients visiting psychiatric outpatient service increased at a rate of geometric progression from 1949. Figure 9.4 shows that among the numbers of outpatients, there was also an increase among Chinese immigrants. From 1950 to

1953, Chinese immigrants rose from half of the entire outpatient numbers to one third. Most of their complaints matched the general definition of neurasthenia experienced by the Japanese people. Their devastations were not only regarding migration: some personally experienced the Chinese Civil War, some were overwhelmed by the unfamiliar local human and nature conditions and others missed family members who did not move to Taiwan with them.

Diagnoses of these patients varied, although 'psychoneurosis' gradually began to be used because of the introduction of the new disease classification system after 1948. Some diagnoses showed the confusion between psychogenic or nervous disorders. For example, during Japanese colonial times, the term 'neurasthenia' had undergone a transformation phase from physical/organic to psychogenic pathology. A diagnosis such as 'psychogenic neurasthenic reaction' can be found among these immigrant records, emphasizing that the disease was not only a psychological reaction of maladjustment, but also manifested by relatively more severe corporeal symptoms.

For example, in 1946, a twenty-four year-old mainlander woman visited the outpatient department. In the preceding two months she had experienced disorganized speech, irritability and panic. She had graduated from junior high school in China with good grades yet, when Tsung-Yi Lin tested her common sense, she did not know the date of Taiwan's retrocession (*guangfu* 光復). Two months before her visit to the hospital, she was terrified by communist soldiers, particularly when she reported that her body was pressed against one of their Rifle guns. Apart from mental disturbances, she had a good appetite and normal sleep patterns. The doctor diagnosed her as having a psychogenic reaktion (abgerauchen).[50]

A thirty-five year-old soldier came to the hospital because of a 'Kopfschwindel' (headache). Apart from the headache, he also had nightmares and a deteriorating memory. The patient grew tired easily, not only because of the busy administrative work in the military, but also because of poor living quality. He thus visited the psychiatric department for a diagnostic certificate, on which the diagnosis of neurasthenia was given.[51] In another case, a thirty-eight year-old officer of order from the mainland sought psychiatric help. He was a graduate of Xiamen University. In November 1945, he relocated to Taiwan with military troops where, because of his severe homesickness, he experienced 'Heftig Schwindel' (severe vertigo). Once he even abruptly fell in the bathroom. He had a normal appetite and sleep. He was diagnosed as having 'neurasthenische reaction'.[52] In yet another case, a twenty-three year-old politician who worked for the county government sought help from the psychiatric department. He had relocated from Shanghai to Taipei one month before he visited NTUH. His homesickness was so severe that he lost his appetite and his sleep deteriorated from bad to worse. He urinated relatively frequently but defecated only once a day. He was nervous and his memory deteriorated; therefore, he had to quit his work. He was diagnosed as having a neurasthenische reaktion caused by 'excessive nostalgia'.[53]

In 1947, a twenty-two year-old man who worked at the Office of Transportation visited the outpatient department because of 'Kopfschwer Gefühl' (heavy-headed feeling). Before he sought psychiatric help, he was outgoing and had many friends while still in China. He was a college graduate. He had malaria when he was three years old. Before he visited the hospital, he experienced a heavy-headed feeling, loss of appetite, and irregular sleep patterns for six months. Earlier during the war, while still in China, he experienced many difficulties that made him nervous. Now, after his relocation to Taiwan, the nervousness was aggravated by poor communication with local people. In Taiwan, he also developed guilt-ridden thoughts toward his parents. These ideations, however, were not stimulated by the difficult political situation. He missed his family in Shanghai and thought it would be a consolation if he could see them. Tsung-Yi Lin diagnosed him as having psychogenic neurasthenic reaction.[54]

Diasporas, ill adjustment and conflict experiences in Chinese immigrants later became subjects covered by literature, cultural and social studies with the implication of trauma. In a recent study, Aaron William Moore argued that these immigrants, particularly veterans, established a 'language community' to speak of their wartime experiences. They found post-war audiences to be 'either ill-equipped or unwilling to listen' to their private stories. Under this circumstance, their traumatic experiences were not told until much later in unconventional forms of literature, including diaries, testimonials, oral histories, surveys, commercial media and self-published literature.[55] These case notes, instead, directly represent their sufferings in the form of psychoneurosis, providing more concrete sources for scholars to study so-called war trauma of veterans.

Traumatic Neurosis Preceded by Actual Physical Injuries

The term 'trauma' was not classified in the WHO's ICD system or America's DSM system until 1980. In the early post-war period, trauma was applicable only to patients who experienced *bona fide* physical injuries. This is not because mental health professionals ignored the importance of mental deficits caused by non-physical injuries; instead, actual cases of corporeal (particularly head) trauma combined with psychoneurological illness took precedence regarding treatment and research shortly after the war. In these cases, a military surgeon could often tell when a wound had healed successfully, whereas a neuropsychologist or psychiatrist could not be sure that the neurological deficits or mental scars of battle were resolved after medical treatment.[56]

To understand the durable neuropsychological effect caused by head trauma, the Head Injury Advice Bureau of the Department of Health and Social Security (DHSS) commissioned the Neuropsychology Unit at the Radcliffe Infirmary to investigate the psychoneurological defects of servicemen who suffered from real head trauma. Most of these patients initially experienced 'post-traumatic fits' and then developed chronic neurological impairments (hemiplegia, dysphasia, dyslexia, hemianopia and so on).[57] Longitudinal studies have been conducted on the recovery of these injured servicemen. The DHSS study emphasized the test results of their cognition, remaining practiced skills, verbal memory and learning, visual/spatial perceptions, and other basic neurological functions.[58] Despite the research, director Freda Newcombe concluded that these servicemen 'had made remarkably good adjustments, both generally and physically'. In her report to the DHSS, she observed,

> in the interest of the pensioners, I do draw attention to the persistent residual handicaps (of which the men themselves often make light of or which they do not even mention). I do not usually emphasize them in discussion with the pensioners themselves, since this would be of no practical help.[59]

The servicemen or their wives occasionally complained of these so-called persistent residual handicaps during the long-term examinations, for these handicaps were related to depression, changes of mood, and low self-esteem.[60]

Unlike the early separation between psychiatry and neurology in Europe, the two disciplines developed simultaneously in post-war Taiwan. Cases show that during wartime, the surgical department referred patients to the psychiatric department. Psychiatrists also ruled out patients who had actual physical injuries that preceded their mental symptoms. In May 1945, a single Taiwanese man who drove a buffalo wagon for a living was referred to the surgical department of the hospital. While looking for a shed to hide in during the air raid on 16 April, a bombshell penetrated the distal end of his left thigh. The patient developed psychiatric symptoms after the surgical procedures and care. In the afternoon of 7 May, he suddenly hid himself underneath his sickbed and began to shout, 'Air raid!' 'Planes are coming!' 'Flood is coming!' and 'Pigs are coming!'[61] During his agitation, he shattered his cups and bowls. In this case register, hallucination was not recorded and a diagnosis was not given. However, similar cases that were associated with actual physical injuries were diagnosed as 'traumatic neurosis'.

If the onset of injury was determined to be too early to act as a direct cause of the patient's neurosis, the doctor would assume that the disease was not associated with that physical injury and would remove 'trauma' from the diagnosis. However, there was no concrete definition of how long the mental symptoms were to be distanced from the actual trauma.

For example, a twenty-six year-old government official sought help from the psychiatric department. His report indicated that he was admitted a year earlier in Wenjou (溫州) Hospital in China for half a month because of a contusion injury. After discharge, his memory deteriorated and he gradually felt numb. While visiting the psychiatric department, he complained of dizziness, particularly when busy at work. He was diagnosed as having 'Nervosität'.[62] Apparently, the doctor assumed that his symptoms were not caused by the physical injury but by the stress at his recent work.

Medicalizing Common Suffering

While the post-war developing world was facing the rising stimuli of urbanization and industrialization, Taiwan, as part of the Global South, was confronted by the sudden depletion of economics. The epidemics of infectious diseases, inflation, and the shortage of food resources were all new and abruptly emerging external realities that existed as life stressors. Numerous patients suffered because of unexpected, sudden changes in their living standards. When the Chinese civil war reached its peak, hyperinflation affected almost every aspect of living cost in Taiwan, including the price of food resources. Tsung-Yi Lin remembered his father's worry: '[The Chinese Nationalist Government] shipped packs of sugar to Fuzhou and Shanghai. They flocked together and fled to Taiwan, and sold the public goods in order to feed themselves'.[63] Such worry prevailed among the then-native Taiwanese people. For them, the 'recovery' of Taiwan, termed by the new government as '*guangfu*' (光復), was a disaster.

Patient illnesses epitomized the common suffering experience among Taiwanese people. On 15 September 1948, a cake maker sought psychiatric help because of extreme anxiety. He reported to the doctor that because of Taiwan's 'retrocession', he had to close the cake shop because of the inflated price of sugar. He grew weak, and occasionally experienced chest tightness (Brustbeklemmungs-gefühl). His son had also lost his job. Throughout the following days, his son became withdrawn at home. Once he saw his son attempting to burn the Japanese military boots that he kept during the Japanese colonial period, because keeping Japanese daily necessaries was illegal. This made his son suicidal. The cake maker could only sleep two to three hours a day. Described by the patient, 'nerve fire' (神經火) was migrating up and down. He was diagnosed with 'Psychogenic Depression' and was hospitalized for three weeks.[64]

Conclusion

Considerable information can be obtained from analyzing case notes of the Psychiatric Department of National Taiwan University Hospital. In general, they reflect the social and cultural reality at the time of the immediate post-war Taiwan and the social origins of distress among patients and the disease labelling work conducted by clinicians for the purpose of treatment. These patient notes show that rapid social change, immigration, unemployment and other aftermaths of war are important factors facilitating mental disorders. Among patients who were mobilized to use psychiatric services, there are subtle cultural elements such as gender, ethnicity, and language privileges influencing their help-seeking pathways.

Unlike Rosenberg's description of 'epidemic', the surge of these neuropsychotic patients did not create a dramaturgic event in society.[65] In the immediate post-war Taiwan, the medical infrastructure and resources of psychiatric sciences were not sufficient enough for the officials to acknowledge or intervene the increasing help-seeking individuals. The number of case files only represents a handful lot of those who enjoyed accessibility of psychiatric services. These case notes, nevertheless, reveal the actions taken by a young group of medical professionals without governmental support in response to their identity formation, professional ethics and social expectation. In a substantial amount of 'case' studies, examples have been illustrated regarding the contested position of 'cases' between objects of science and the subjective concerns of career scientists. These studies have shown the perpetual contested zones among the state's demand, the professional interests of doctors, the scientific standards of truth and the ideologies of clinicians.[66] Instead of showing the state's social control in other typical 'epidemics', the example in this chapter implies the veiled social criticism among the psychiatric professionals of the origins of social suffering.

This chapter, in addition, contributes to another area in the history of psychiatry. From the perspective of psychiatric classification, the broader picture that emerges from these notes corresponds to the argument of other historical studies on case histories in that they illustrate a picture of patients previously shaded by hazy psychiatric diagnoses. The case records show distinctive disease profiles of each individual. Descriptions of 'present illness' and 'disease history' can also disambiguate flat and rigid disease classifications. The 'impression of disease' and 'aetiology' in the case notes also shows the manners in which doctors attributed psychopathology to the symptoms of patients. NTUH cases not only attest to the emergence of certain psychiatric disorders highly associated with time and space factors, but also imply socio-political meanings behind specific disorders acquired by certain ethnic communities.

From the perspective of language, both continuity and discrepancy of psychiatric theories and languages are evident before and after the Second World War. Although establishment of the Psychiatric Department of NTUH envisaged developing a psychiatric discipline belonging to Chinese, the lack of resources hampered the switch of service languages. The case notes show at least four main written languages: Japanese, German, Chinese and English, each recorded for different purposes. To honestly represent patients, Romanized Taiwanese was employed to record the original complaints expressed in the clinic or at the bedside. Increasing patients either in the outpatient clinic or in the wards not only illustrates the growth of hospital psychiatric services, but also the expansion of medical communities concerning mental health issues in a post-war changing society. Quantitative analysis of service users also indicates the association between the official language of society and service accessibility.

Finally, the problems that psychiatric clinicians faced at NTUH can be considered the prelude of further practices. The discontent of psychiatric classifications resulted in further actions taken by clinicians within the department. Masaaki Matsushita noted that the nosology or classification of disease is closely linked to the medical system, which is subject to the unique sociocultural conditions of a given time and space.[67] Korean psychiatrist Bou-Yong Rhi argued that patterns of classifying mental disorders in each era particularly reflect not only the underlying hypothesis of the pathogenesis of mental disorders at the time, but also the general ideological trends of the era and its concerns on mentally ill patient).[68] Tsung-Yi Lin, as head of the department, was later appointed Medical Officer of the Social Psychiatry Project at the World Health Organization in the 1960s. He was in charge of the process that gave birth to the first internationally acknowledged version of psychiatric disease classification. This sequel requires a topic for future analysis.

10 THE EMERGENCE OF THE PSYCHO-BOOM IN CONTEMPORARY URBAN CHINA

Hsuan-Ying Huang

During the past few years, the vogue enjoyed by psychotherapy in urban China has attracted the attention of Western media.[1] The arrival of this flourishing scene was quick, unanticipated and in sharp contrast to Chinese culture during the Maoist period, when psychology as an academic discipline was first repudiated as 'bourgeois pseudoscience' and then abolished during the Cultural Revolution. The current welcoming of psychotherapy is also a dramatic shift from the earlier post-reform period in which it barely existed in the mental health care system. Although the extent to which psychotherapy has become a common treatment option is uncertain, it is indisputable that counselling or psychotherapy facilities have mushroomed in major cities like Shanghai and Beijing, either as private agencies or as part of public institutions that include hospitals, schools and other government agencies. Additionally, there is a proliferation of short-term courses offered by a growing training industry: many of the courses fill easily as people rush to learn about psychotherapy.

This 'psycho-bloom' (*xinli re* 心理热)[2] is arguably the most salient part of the increasing presence of all things psychological – ideas, views, attitudes, practices and styles – in popular media and everyday life in today's urban China. Local people tend to see it as the natural outcome of three decades of rapid economic growth, often alluding to two intuitively simple and closely related explanations. First, economic development has brought about mounting stress and a number of modern ailments such as anxiety and depression, which must be attended to by a new breed of healers – psychotherapists. Second, as living standards greatly improve, people are paying more attention to their psychological health and are more willing to consume expensive services like talk therapy. It seems that few people question the legitimacy of the psycho-boom given that psychotherapy is known to be an established profession in most developed societies, and that 'the psychological' (*xinli* 心理) has recently become an indispensable dimension of individual and interpersonal experience in urban China.[3]

Does economic prosperity necessarily lead to the popularity of psychotherapy? In what way could an imported cultural artifact prosper in a new social milieu? How does China's psycho-boom differ from the development of psychotherapy in the West and other developing countries? This chapter seeks to challenge the general impressions and the deterministic thinking embraced by many of its participants. The strategy here is neither to provide a comprehensive picture of the psycho-boom nor to construct a detailed history of psychotherapy in the post-reform period. Instead, the intention is to selectively examine the policy context and a number of initiatives endorsed or orchestrated by the state; intriguingly, none of them were issued or carried out by the health authorities. The central argument of this chapter is that the psycho-boom is a popular movement that has emerged, at least partially, as the result of the intended or unintended consequences of these programs. Seeing the craze for psychotherapy training and the rise of a market-oriented training industry as the heart of the movement, this discussion aims to elucidate how these state-related interventions have contributed to the fashioning of psychotherapy training into a commodity targeting the general population, especially the emerging middle class.

The following sections begin with an effort to describe the characteristics of the psycho-boom, then moving to its historical context by examining the time period prior to its advent, including the early post-reform period, when the popular notion of 'psychological counselling' (*xinli zixun* 心理咨询) was invented, and the turn-of-the-century moment, when the foundation for the reform of the mental health care system was laid. The chronicle of the psycho-boom period will subsequently be anchored to a series of undertakings that bear affinities to various state agencies: the Ministry of Labor certification, the television program 'Psychological Interviews' (*xinli fangtan* 心理访谈) and the promotion of psychotherapy in the relief work for survivors of the Wenchuan earthquake. Identifying the movement as the burgeoning of a popular sector alongside the existing mental health care system, discussion will take place as to how these programs created the conditions upon which the psycho-boom has morphed into its current shape and how each of them has made a pivotal contribution. In conclusion, the chapter will return to the local features of the psycho-boom and address the latest state regulation of psychotherapy brought by the Mental Health Law that was enacted in May 2013.

The Psycho-Boom in Urban China

While the boundary between professional psychology and its popular derivatives is not always clear, people are inclined to imagine psychotherapy, or its ideal version, as a specialized treatment attached to a professional community. In the United States and other Western countries where psychological disciplines have developed over many decades, psychotherapy tends to be a subspecialty of, or affiliated with, mental health professions that are regulated by the state through licensure or registration. Typical examples include psychiatry, clinical psychology, counselling psychology and social work. These professions may have basic psychotherapy training in their curricula, but to become a practitioner specializing in psychotherapy, one usually needs to pursue more advanced training. These training programs vary widely depending on the school or orientation to which they belong, but most require an extended period of time and share a similar framework composed of knowledge transmission, supervision of clinical cases and in some instances, personal treatment. The long-term nature of such training processes makes them ideal for ethnographic research on individual therapists and the community at large, as the ethnographies of Tanya Luhrmann and James Davies demonstrate.[4]

The psycho-boom in urban China bears important distinctions from the picture above. Firstly, although many of its leading figures are psychiatrists or academic psychologists, people without professional backgrounds dominate this emerging field. Most of them enter it through the short-term training program for 'psychological counsellors' (*xinli zixun shi* 心理咨询师) established by the Ministry of Labor and Social Security.[5] Secondly, psychotherapy, despite its apparent popularity, has a negligible existence in the training for mental health professionals. As a result, it is not uncommon that psychiatrists, and those who study psychology in universities, lack even the basic understanding of talk therapy. Third, there has been a surge of training courses, but virtually all of these programs are exceedingly short, ranging from a few days to one week at most. Many of them are hosted by private, for-profit agencies and are taught by psychiatrists or psychologists who are employed in the public sector. Fourth, psychoanalysis, the therapeutic school that has been in decline in the West since the rise of psychopharmacology in the 1960s, has gained unmatched popularity in China. While psychoanalysis demands the most lengthy and rigorous training, it is propagated through short-term courses as well. Last, but not least, people engaged in these programs are diverse in terms of their motivations and commitments. A career in psychotherapy practice is but one of many possible outcomes and is, in fact, pursued by a relatively small portion of those who participate in training. Even for the pioneers who venture to become therapists, the career is often a volatile one; as the number of therapists grows rapidly, most do not have enough clients to make ends meet. To some extent therefore, the current psycho-boom seems to be more about the enthusiasm for psychotherapy training than the demand for psychotherapy treatments.[6]

It is not, however, particularly helpful to see the psycho-boom as an emerging occupation whose professionalization is still rudimentary.[7] Instead, it should be conceived more inclusively as a popular movement centered on psychotherapy training. The movement does contain a professional sector that is roughly associated with the pre-existing, formally recognized professions that include psychiatrists, academic psychologists and university counsellors. This professional 'core' has grown substantially but it is still small compared to the broader movement whose momentum is largely encouraged by the surging interest of laypeople. While training agencies and participants typically cite 'training' (*paixun* 培训) as their principle objective, under this stated purpose one can invest in and pursue a wide range of interests. Some participants do consider a new career with various degrees of seriousness, yet some have a self-help or therapeutic agenda; they may seek to solve their own distress, hope to understand themselves more deeply or wish to help their family and friends. Others come to make friends or socialize with people who share similar interests in this tempting, once-forbidden area of knowledge, as the psycho-boom encompasses an abundance of social activities in addition to training events.

The Coining of 'Psychological Counselling'

The reappearance of psychotherapy in the aftermath of the Cultural Revolution occurred at the intersection of academic psychology[8] and psychiatry. These early endeavors were closely related to the coining of the term '*xinli zixun*' (心理咨询), which was, and still is, seen as the literal translation of 'psychological counselling'. It is often used interchangeably with '*xinli zhiliao*' (心理治疗), the term that has denoted 'psychotherapy' since the Republican period, despite a slight difference of meaning that to some extent parallels the distinction in their original context. As in the West, '*xinli zixun*' (psychological counselling) is preferred in non-medical, educational or popular settings; it implies a diluted version of psychotherapy since the term '*zixun*' is a colloquial expression referring to making inquiries, exchanging opinions and seeking advice, all of which have their counterparts in everyday life.[9] However, its first appearance and continued existence in medical settings makes the distinction a very thin one. Eventually, it was adopted by the Ministry of Labor system in the early twenty-first century and has become the dominant term in the psycho-boom since then.

As Dr. Zhao Gengyuan 赵耕源, one of the pioneers of '*xinli zixun*', described in his appraisal of the field's history, the earliest use of this term occurred in a few psychiatric hospitals when the importance of patient education and aftercare began to be acknowledged.[10] '*Xinli zixun*' was considered to be the act of explaining to patients and their families their diagnoses, medication and necessary coping skills. It emerged around 1980 as an innovative intervention to enhance patients' adaptation to life after discharge. Shortly afterward, it was used in a new mode of outpatient clinic in general hospitals, first in Xian in 1982 and then in Guangzhou in 1983.[11] This 'outpatient model' was a walk-in clinic that catered to diverse issues, including psychological symptoms, interpersonal troubles and physical discomforts. Psychosocial aspects were emphasized to some degree, with more time allotted to each visit, but the actual session could involve tasks as varied as psychological testing, physical examination, blood tests and patient education. The objective of such sessions was problem-solving rather than self-exploration; indeed, its pragmatic orientation seemed to have little to do with psychotherapeutic theories or techniques. This model soon earned the endorsement of the professional community. In the early 1990s, it won state support as the Ministry of Health stipulated in the first hospital accreditation standards that all the top-tier, so-called 'Grade Three Class A' (*sanji jiadeng* 三级甲等) hospitals should set up '*xinli zixun*' outpatient clinics. It was also advised that public hospitals above the county level should do so in the long run.

During this period, members of academic psychology – a discipline that had struggled to resurrect itself from the devastation of the Cultural Revolution – established another principal site for the development of psychotherapy. Psychology departments were restored at Peking University, Hangzhou University and at a number of normal or teachers' colleges, but the scale of the discipline remained small. Under such restrictions, its fledgling practical branch advanced along two lines: the establishment of degree programs in counselling or clinical psychology and the inauguration of student counselling centers in colleges. The development of formal training programs was slow whereas college counselling, which also adopted the term '*xinli zixun*', followed a trajectory akin to what was happening in the medical system. As the Hong Kong-based psychologist Seung-Ming Leung and his colleagues indicated, college counselling was boosted by the Ministry of Education's decision to promote 'moral education' (*deyu* 德育) in the early 1990s, as a response to the 1989 student movement.[12] Although college counselling claimed to adopt the new psychological knowledge and practices, to a considerable degree it was derived from the socialist tradition of ideological education or the so-called 'political thought work' (*sixiang zhengzhi gongzuo* 思想政治工作) in higher education. In the 1990s, college counselling facilities were often staffed by former ideological workers, some of whom continue to work and may still have a lingering influence on the field today.

The Turn-of-the-Century Reform

A perception of crisis in mental health and mental health care had begun to emerge in China after a period of rapid economic growth. While the long-term consequences of massive political violence during the Maoist period remain unclear, various mental health issues had surfaced under the drastic transition to market economy. Concurrently, scholars situated between anthropology and psychiatry, led by Arthur Kleinman who pioneered the study of social suffering and Chinese psychiatry in the 1980s, had embarked on exploring these phenomena.[13] Beginning in the mid-1990s, a series of research endeavors revealed notable changes in disease patterns, diagnostic labeling and the mental health care system as a whole. Using newly available official data, Michael Phillips and his colleagues showed that China had one of the highest suicide rates in the world. The data also exposed distinct demographic features: suicide rates were significantly higher in rural areas and among the female population, with rural women being a particularly vulnerable group marked by the frequent use of pesticide ingestion.[14] Sing Lee documented a dramatic shift in the official psychiatric discourse as the once ubiquitous diagnosis of neurasthenia (*shenjing shuairuo* 神经衰弱) languished and was replaced by depression (*yiyuzheng* 抑郁症), a disease category revived in the post-Mao encounter with Western psychiatry.[15] Veronica Pearson and Michael Phillips both presented a grim, almost pre-modern picture in their assessments of China's mental health care system: it had an exclusive orientation toward major psychoses and was highly dependent on institutionalization, yet limited coverage left a substantial proportion of patients untreated.[16] Psychiatric institutions, most of which were public facilities, suffered from shrinking subsidies, and the majority of their personnel lacked formal training. Expectably, the psychosocial needs of patients and their problems outside the psychotic spectrum received scant attention.

Eventually, the turn of the century became a formative period that set the stage for the nation's mental health care reform, which was triggered by its deepening engagement with the international community. In 1993, the World Bank's 'Global Burden of Disease' study brought to light the impacts of psychological and behavioral diseases. In 1996, the World Health Organization (WHO) launched the 'Nations for Mental Health' initiative to promote public recognition and political commitments around the globe. At the WHO/China awareness-raising conference in 1999, the Chinese government designated mental health as an important public health issue and vowed to overhaul the crumbling system. This was a radical change in the position of the state, which had previously denied or downplayed the gravity of these problems. In November 2001, the third National Conference on Mental Health Care was convened in Beijing, during which leading psychiatrists drafted the National Mental Health Plan (2002–10) and the Proposal on Further Strengthening Mental Health Work.[17] The shift in the state's attitude was best exemplified by the dire situation depicted by Vice Minister of Health Yin Dakui at the conference:

> It is estimated that there are sixteen million people suffering from severe mental illnesses in our country. Six million people are afflicted by epilepsy. Each year a quarter million people commit suicide, and suicide attempters could be as many as two million. According to the latest survey, among the 340 million people under the age of seventeen, thirty million are affected by emotional disorders as well as psychologi-

> cal and behavioral problems. Psychiatric diseases among the elderly and the abuse of alcohol and narcotics are increasing, so are the mental illnesses, psychological and behavioral problems in women and the disaster-affected population.[18]

The National Plan, which had the same assessment written into its preamble, and the Proposal identified a number of issues that required urgent attention. These documents became the de facto national policy as the state amplified its investments in public health in the post-SARS period. Mental health care was still dominated by psychiatry, with psychology and education being its auxiliaries, as reflected in the use of '*jingshen weisheng*' (精神卫生) rather than '*xinli weisheng*' (心理卫生) to refer to 'mental health'.[19] The new policy placed capacity building at its forefront; strengthening the professional workforce and expanding treatment coverage were granted top priority status. The emphasis on major psychoses was maintained, but emerging problems such as suicide, depression, dementia and post-disaster conditions appeared in the official discourse for the first time, as did at-risk populations such as children, adolescents and women. The emblematic achievement of this reform was the '686 Project' launched in 2004 and scaled up in 2008. The program, covering more than half of the country's population by the end of 2011, has become the largest treatment and management network for major psychoses in the world.[20]

With much attention focused on severe mental illnesses, minor psychological problems and their treatments occupied an ambiguous position in the reform. The National Plan and the Proposal both used the term 'psychological and behavioral problems' (*xinli xingwei wenti* 心理行为问题) repeatedly, which seemed like an attempt to broaden the scope of mental health concerns. In a few passages, the term 'psychological intervention' (*xinli ganyu* 心理干预) was mentioned without further specification, yet both documents stipulated that the Ministry of Health, in collaboration with the Ministry of Personnel, should set up a certification system for the staff conducing psychological counselling and psychotherapy in hospitals. In 2002, the Ministry of Health added a new kind of 'technician' (*jishi* 技师) – 'psychotherapist' (*xinli zhiliao shi* 心理治疗师) – to its certification for health professionals. However, the new system was restricted to medical personnel and had minimal effects on the upcoming psycho-boom.[21] The Ministry of Health's efforts to make progress within the medical system were immediately eclipsed by another program initiated by the Ministry of Labor and Social Security, which was not even among the six ministries (Ministries of Health, Education, Public Security, Civil Affairs, Justice, and Finance) and one civil organization (Chinese Disabled Persons' Federation) that signed the Proposal.

The Ministry of Labor Certification

In August 2001, the Ministry of Labor and Social Security announced the National Vocational Standards (*guojia zhiye biaozhun* 国家职业标准) for twenty-two occupations, the second round of such stipulations since the publication of the National Occupational Classification in 1999.[22] The inventory included the interim criteria for a new occupation, 'psychological counsellor', which was not among the 1838 kinds of vocations that were already listed in the all-encompassing compendium. Training and certification for this new job were initiated experimentally the following year and then formally launched in 2005. An extensive network of training sites was established in many cities, and the certification test was administered as part of the 'unified national exam' (*quanguo tongkao* 全国统考) conducted each year in May and November. The program was a collaboration between the state department and the China Association for Mental Health (*zhongguo xinli weisheng xiehui* 中国心理卫生协会), the umbrella organization that brought together psychiatry, psychology, education and related social sciences. Since then, several hundred thousand people have attained the certificate, and the system has become the most important medium through which people can gain access to the psycho-boom.[23]

Consistent with China's employment framework, the new occupation had three ranks, but the training and certification for Level One (the most advanced level) was not put into action. The National Vocational Standards stipulated the eligibility, training curriculum and required competencies for the new occupation.[24] Textbooks were published in 2002 and then revised in 2005 with the official inauguration of the program. The ministry saw psychotherapy as an undeveloped field and deliberately set the degree requirements for the program at a lower level to accommodate more candidates. In the beginning, the minimum requirements for Level Three (the entry level) were merely a vocational high school (*zhongzhuan* 中专) degree, which was replaced in 2005 by a college degree without any specification of major. The new requirements for Level Two were raised to a doctoral degree or a master's degree in a related field, or three years of practice after attaining the Level Three certificate. However, these regulations are seldom complied with; it is well acknowledged in the psycho-boom circle that, due to collusion between training agencies and local governments, many people could begin at Level Two without fulfilling these criteria.

The program's mission is ambitious: transforming a person without previous training in medicine, psychology or education into a therapist within an exceedingly short period of time. The curriculum is divided into two parts: essential knowledge and required capabilities. The former includes virtually all the major divisions of the discipline, including 'basic psychology', which refers to biological psychology, social psychology, developmental psychology, abnormal psychology, psychological testing, counselling psychology and related legal matters. The latter is composed of a wide range of practical skills, including diagnosis, counselling or psychotherapy techniques and psychological assessment. The curricula of these two parts are condensed into a two-volume set of textbooks that contain virtually everything one needs to know to excel in the exam. The National Vocational Standards dictates the required training duration: 400 hours for Level Two and 500 hours for Level Three. The course, akin to adult education programs, is held on weekday evenings or during the weekend, and may take four to six months to finish. With the arrival of new technology, the training process has become more flexible in recent years; many agencies now offer online learning so that students can control their own pace. Another popular format is a seven-to-ten-day crash course held immediately preceding the exam. These programs have a remarkably narrow focus on rote learning and exam preparation. In most cases, a field trip to a psychiatric hospital or a counselling center nearby, a few in-class demonstrations or the viewing of popular psychotherapy TV shows would comprise all the 'practicums' of the training.[25]

The certificate is commonly deemed the only 'license' (*zhizhao* 执照) issued at the national level for psychological practitioners. However, this commonsensical understanding may obscure the peculiar effects and origins of this program. Before the Ministry of Labor certification arrived, psychological counselling or psychotherapy only existed in hospitals and college counselling centers. They were considered to be specialized skills without forming the basis of an independent occupation outside these realms. The program is situated between vocational training and adult education; it is far from ideal professional training. Providing a state-sanctioned qualification, the program makes psychological counsellor – which is almost always conflated with psychotherapist – a pursuable vocation, and turns psychotherapy training – which had been reserved for mental health professionals albeit in informal manners – into a purchasable item that can be consumed by the general population.

The program is the convergence of two seemingly irrelevant trajectories: the attempt to create new vocations amid China's labour reform and the efforts of academic psychology to revive a once-suppressed field. The certification was part of the massive National Vocational Qualification (*guojia zhiye zige* 国家职业资格) system, which originated in the labor reform launched during the mid-1990s.[26] Because employment was no longer guaranteed by the state, the Ministry of Labor attempted to transform itself into China's main regulatory body overseeing the training and certification for an entire range of jobs. The system was intended to be all-encompassing, thereby incorporating occupations that were newly emerging or envisioned to be needed when economic development ensued. The training program for psychological counsellors, listed in the 'business and service industry personnel' (*shangye yu fuwu renyuan* 商业

与服务人员) section, was among the state department's earliest undertakings to create new kinds of occupations. Other occupations established in 2001 were anti-erosion worker, automobile repairer, mushroom gardener, tea sampler, restaurant servant and many others. In 2002, these were followed by the announcement of a string of merchandizing jobs such as e-commerce manager, human resources manager and salesman. Most of these efforts failed, as the state had lost much of its command over employment. The system became a redundancy for the nation's gigantic manufacturing and service industry, which usually sought cheap and unskilled labor. It was also unable to compete with degree programs in vocational and higher education, which experienced immense growth in the new century.

Moreover, the Ministry of Labor program was actually a new chapter in the long-term struggle of psychology throughout the history of the People's Republic. Its major proponent was Professor Guo Nianfeng 郭念锋, an eminent scholar at the Institute of Psychology of the Chinese Academy of Sciences and then Vice Chairman of the China Association for Mental Health. Trained in the Soviet-style neuropsychological tradition before the Cultural Revolution, Professor Guo joined the cause to develop psychological counselling in medical institutions in the mid-1980s. Since then, he has been involved in various training projects, including the Institute of Psychology's correspondence school. In an editorial article published on the eve of the launch of the Ministry of Labor certification, Professor Guo saw the late 1950s as the first golden age of Chinese mental health care, during which indigenous modalities such as the Speedy Synthetic Treatment (*kuaisu zonghe liaofa* 快速综合疗法) were developed to combat neurasthenia, the dominant psychosomatic disease of the Maoist period.[27] He cited the presence of psychological counselling services as a major accomplishment since the discipline's rehabilitation in the post-reform period. Yet he cautioned that the largely undertrained workforce was still too small to satisfy the growing demands of society.

> When social demand rapidly rises, all we can do is to resort to non-professionals ... The contradiction [of relying on non-professionals] truly exists, yet from the perspective of development, this is not necessarily distressing. People coming from other backgrounds often have great passion, interest and potential. In some aspects, they are even more qualified than professionals. If we make our continuing education better, the contradiction will absolutely be solved.[28]

The above paragraph summed up the course that the enterprise of psychological counselling had taken during its first decade and a half. The majority of its personnel came from medicine and education; short-term courses focused on knowledge transmission were the only training opportunities available. Shortly afterward, the same model would be applied to the general population as the Ministry of Labor program came into being.

Commoditizing Training

In the beginning, the new occupation did not seem particularly attractive. Among the first group of institutions that were approved to carry out training programs, most were public or semi-official organizations, including the regional branches of the China Association for Mental Health, teaching hospitals and universities.[29] Only a few of them were private agencies. The central government's Bureau of Prisons, the Chinese Youth Development Center of the Communist Youth League and Huaxia Xinli 华夏心理,[30] a pioneering psychotherapy training company, were granted the privilege to establish cross-regional networks of training facilities. This initial framework characterized how the system would proceed in the following years. The penitentiary authorities incorporated psychological counselling into their correctional practices and set up their own training programs. The police and the military soon adopted the same model. In a similar vein, the Communist Youth League, followed by the China Disabled Persons' Federation and the All-China Women's Federation, tried to add the psychological component to their social services. Huaxia Xinli, with its onsite training program in Beijing boasting the most authoritative teaching staff led by Professor Guo Nianfeng, was commissioned to set up a nationwide distance-learning system. It quickly became the largest provider of training for the Ministry of Labor certification; more than 100,000 people have attained their certificates through Huaxia Xinli since 2002. After the system was officially launched in 2005, private companies became the dominant players among course suppliers, turning the enterprise into a for-profit industry. Akin to the alliance between Huaxia Xinli and Professor Guo, training agencies preferred to recruit senior psychiatrists and psychologists working in local hospitals or universities to be their teachers; some of them became their 'star' instructors, business consultants or partners. The training industry produced a powerful discourse that redefined the vocation as a promising career option. A few highly identical paragraphs appeared on tens of thousands of websites related to psychotherapy and were widely circulated during the psycho-boom. For example, the 2006 version of Huaxia Xinli's online advertisement began with an assessment of the nation's mental health that echoed the official discourse of the mental health care reform:

> The number of completed suicides in China has reached 287,000 per year, with an additional two million suicide attempts. There are 25.6 million people suffering from depression; fifteen percent of them have suicidal tendencies, yet only five percent of them receive proper treatment. Dr. Wu Ruihua, a research fellow at the Institute of Psychology, points out that the lack of psychological counseling personnel is a major cause for the relatively high suicide rates in our country. Data show that sixteen million out of our population of 1.3 billion have psychiatric and psychological diseases. It is estimated that 190 million people will need to receive psychological counseling

> in their lifetimes. Also, thirty million out of 150 million adolescents are disturbed by emotional problems or stress.[31]

These descriptions did not specify their sources of information, but the numbers they cited painted the picture of a critical situation that would disquiet every sensible reader. The narrative made an arbitrary assumption that psychological counselling was the solution to these problems before moving on to compare the mental health workforce of the United States and that of China.

> In the United States, every one million people have one thousand psychological counselors, yet in China the number is merely 2.4. In the United States, more than 3000 universities have psychology departments, yet in China there are only sixty or so. What's worse, psychological counseling almost does not exist in our degree programs. The scarce resources are concentrated in a number of universities and research institutions in megacities such as Beijing and Shanghai . . .[32]

The comparison not only exposed China's deficiencies but also implied an exciting message: the deep need for counselling or psychotherapy reflected the enormous potential for this new occupation. While the documents guiding the mental health care reform called for immediate scaling-up of investments by the state, this advertising narrative targeted a different audience; it appealed to those who were interested in this new career option. The vocation that was once juxtaposed with restaurant servant, salesman and other ordinary jobs was refashioned into a prestigious one. A counsellor was no longer an average wage earner or a cog in the mental health care machine, but a distinguished therapist providing luxurious services and charging fairly high hourly fees, as the discourse continued to describe:

> The lucrative incomes make psychological counselors members of the upper-middle class. In the United States, a psychological counselor can earn 150 US dollars per hour. In China, the hourly fee ranges between 100 and 1000 yuan, and the average is around 200 yuan . . . In the Central Business District of Beijing, the charge often reaches 100 US dollors per hour.[33]

A number of practical questions were left unmentioned: Who are the potential customers who could afford such costly services given that almost no insurance plan in China covers psychotherapy conducted in private agencies? Are there enough customers for this novel treatment if the treatment is considered extremely expensive by most of the general population? It seemed to be assumed that the rising middle class, who happened to be the primary patrons of these training programs, would embrace psychotherapy without hesitation and their numbers would soon become robust enough to support this new profession. Nevertheless, Huaxia Xinli's ad proposed that even if the training did not lead to a promising career, it could bring broader significance and reward to one's life, as its last section 'the implications of learning' revealed:

1. In short, [the objectives may include] helping others, helping yourself and self-realization.
2. By learning psychological counseling, you can attain the knowledge and techniques to help people understand themselves and society; to handle various kinds of relationships; to modify thoughts, emotions and reactive styles that are incompatible with the external reality and to master ways to adapt to the outside world.
3. In addition to helping your clients solve their problems and get rid of their troubles, learning psychological counseling can help you master the methods of self-adjustment, by which you can enhance your quality of life, increase your working efficiency, educate your children more successfully and better handle your family relationships. Learning psychological counseling can also amplify your employment and business opportunities, through which you will achieve self-growth and self-development in the end.[34]

During my fieldwork, graduates of the Ministry of Labor program frequently divulged that, except for those who worked in areas where psychological knowledge might be applicable,[35] few of their classmates – typically less than one tenth of the class – went on to become therapists. The reasons listed above accounted for a large part of the participants' motivations.

Televising Psychotherapy

Very few people in China had ever experienced Western-style talk therapy when 'psychological counsellor' suddenly became a career option. The same unfamiliarity applied to not only potential trainees and patients, but also to mental health professionals. The services provided by existing facilities, including 'psychological counselling' clinics in hospitals and college counselling centers, bore limited resemblance to their Western counterparts. Most of the practitioners only had short-term training in which practicums and supervision seldom existed. There were a small number of elite professionals who had direct contact with senior therapists from the West through the legendary Sino-German Course (*zhongde ban* 中德班) and a few other programs.[36] Some of the elite would become influential figures or famous teachers as the training industry emerged in the psycho-boom period, but the influence they had at that moment was nowhere near the celebrity status they achieved later.

A television program that arrived slightly earlier than the official launch of the Ministry of Labor certification in 2005 drastically changed the situation. On December 29, 2004, 'Psychological Interviews', a late-night program featuring 'real', edited psychotherapy sessions, was launched on Channel Twelve 'Society and Law' (*shehui yu fa* 社会与法) of the state-run China Central Television

(CCTV) and broadcast every night from 11:20 to 11:40 pm. The therapy show immediately became the most influential medium through which the general population could gain popular knowledge about everyday psychological problems and their treatments. In the eyes of many participants, the synergy between the Ministry of Labor certification and the CCTV program marked the beginning of the psycho-boom.

The program had a minimalistic setting: the female host, the client (sometimes alone and sometimes accompanied by his or her friends or family members) and the therapist were seated around a table. The absence of a studio audience might strengthen the perception that the spectator was directly peeping into a therapy session. A small group of therapists had made appearances on the show, but two middle-aged male physicians, Drs. Li Zixun Li 李子勋 and Yang Fengchi 杨凤池, who were graduates of the Sino-German Course, were the most welcomed among them and showed up most frequently. The twenty-minute program was intended to simulate a real, though short, one-shot consultation. A typical episode began with a preliminary interview between the host and the client, who always seemed to be a real patient tormented by a real problem. Then, a short film clip helped elucidate the client's personal background in a succinct yet somewhat theatrical manner. What followed was the essential part of the show as the therapist initiated the interview. The conversation between the client and the therapist was often divided into two or three segments, separated by the host's remarks or another short clip. Within the limited time frame, the therapist would perform a succession of masterful techniques: extracting hidden secrets, conducting interesting psychological tests, making penetrating interpretations and providing intelligent advice. Eventually, the trouble would be beautifully solved and the client, who was sometimes on the verge of emotional breakdown in the middle of the session, would be transformed into a much brighter mood.

The program was an immediate success; its impacts could be felt in various aspects of society. First, setting the provision of professional services as its major purpose, the program, akin to a busy psychotherapy clinic, treated hundreds of patients since its inception. Featuring two nationally renowned therapists, it had an incredibly long waiting list of potential clients; numerous volunteers from all over the country signed up, hoping to be treated on the show. The program not only affected those who received consultation sessions but also a much larger population who benefited from seeing how people with similar conditions were treated, as Dr. Yang explained in an interview:

> This is exactly what motivates us to continue showing up on the screen. Since experienced personnel are hard to find in our country, one might not be able to find a 'psychological doctor' (*xinli yishi* 心理医生) even in a pretty large city. When we help one person in an episode, hundreds or thousands of people who have the same

> problem might be helped, too. They do not have the chance to see Dr. Li or me in person, but they feel they have received some assistance when they watch our program.[37]

Second, the show was a theatrical space in which popular psychological knowledge and a myriad of psychological problems were presented in engrossing ways. The viewers became acquainted with a new type of practitioner, the treatment he or she demonstrated and a wide range of issues treatable with such expertise. The powerful image provided by the program shaped the popular perception and understanding of psychotherapy in unprecedented ways; it is widely known that most patients in China sought intense intervention and expected maximum efficacy in the shortest possible time.[38] Third, viewers also learned how to understand a person's mind from a psychological perspective. Josh Krieger, an American psychologist who conducted narrative analyses of the therapist-client interactions in this program, argued that the program educated its viewers to appreciate life and the world from a new perspective informed by psychology, which was quite different from ordinary or traditional standpoints.[39]

Less commonly mentioned were the program's impacts on those who were participating in or were about to join the psycho-boom. The timely arrival of the program not only made Drs. Yang and Li well-known figures in the burgeoning movement, but also produced a paradigmatic image that defined practitioners of the job as it was being made available to the general population: sharp-witted, wise and charming. When I first discovered the psycho-boom phenomena in 2007, a number of web-forums had become public spaces where people convened and discussed various issues related to psychotherapy, including their own experiences of learning or practicing psychotherapy.[40] Most of these participants seemed to be rather new to this enterprise, though occasionally a few well-known figures would show up and interact with their 'fans' (*fensi* 粉丝). 'Psychological Interviews' was always one of the most popular topics on these websites. People would have detailed discussions on each day's show, with a particular emphasis on the therapist's performance. Sometimes they might quarrel over technical issues, but more often idealization was the prevailing mood. To some extent, 'Psychological Interviews' seemed to serve a didactical function in a local world where many people yearned for training opportunities that were not easily obtainable. As mentioned earlier, many training programs would use the show's episodes as tutorials for teaching psychotherapy techniques.

Psychotherapy and the Wenchuan Earthquake

When the devastating earthquake hit the mountainous Wenchuan region in the southwestern province of Sichuan on 12 May 2008, I had been monitoring several psychotherapy web-forums for months. Planning to visit Shanghai and Beijing at the end of June, glancing through these discussion boards every day facilitated an attempt to map out the training agencies and the courses they offered in these two cities. Conducting digital ethnography also provided a form of voyeuristic pleasure; the huge amount of information circulated on these websites was amazing. People were very willing to share all kinds of electronic files, including articles, books and recordings of training courses, with each other. Additionally, many people openly discussed what they experienced in training courses or even what they did or what their patients said in psychotherapy sessions. This reconnaissance period gave the impression that the field was suffused with optimism; painful emotions were dwelled upon but these negative experiences were often surpassed by the exhilaration of understanding the hidden aspects of minds or mastering the therapeutic techniques.

The dominant ethos on these websites immediately changed after the earthquake, as people lamented over the suffering of their compatriots and deliberated about how to help. They talked about certain issues that were seldom touched upon before, including the psychological consequences of natural disasters, post-traumatic stress disorder (PTSD) and the therapy for such conditions. A plethora of information such as research papers and treatment manuals was uploaded to these websites, though it was unclear what insights or capabilities one could gain from the chaotic jumble of materials. It appeared that very few of these people had experience in treating post-traumatic conditions, and that the trauma discourse they were referring to seemed as fresh as the earthquake itself. Surprisingly, the discussions quickly spiraled out of control; in just a few days, these websites were flooded with announcements calling for fellow psychotherapists to travel to Sichuan together as 'volunteers' (*zhiyuanzhe* 志愿者).

This occurance was part of the unprecedented rise of volunteerism in China.[41] The movement had a blatant patriotic undertone and in many aspects harked back to the socialist spirit of making sacrifices for the revolution. After the Wenchuan earthquake, numerous people traveled long distances to the affected region with the intention of providing help; many came on their own rather than with groups organized by governments or semi-official associations. The altruistic spirit was soon extolled and appropriated by the state. A few months later, volunteers came into the national spotlight again at the Beijing Olympics, making 2008 'the year of volunteerism' and a landmark year in the development of civil society in China. However, the people followed on the psychotherapy web-forums were not ordinary volunteers; they assigned a singular mission to themselves: to apply what they had learned in psychotherapy training to console victims of the earthquake. Although much attention was lavished on their goodwill and the psychological modalities they claimed to have mastered, what actually happened in the local world was rarely revealed by the media, possibly due to censorship. Among the several thousand self-proclaimed therapists who arrived in Sichuan, many snatched as many survivors as they could find and persuaded them to receive the unfamiliar treatments. Facing such difficult circumstances, these fledging therapists could only rely on improvisation and experimentation; not infrequently, they invented eccentric therapies that might have produced serious complications. Because of the disruption and trauma they caused, psychotherapists were quickly classified as one of the 'three hazards' in the local area, as exemplified by a popular saying, 'Be watchful of fire, thieves and psychologists' (*fanghuo, fangdao, fang xinli* 防火、防盗、防心理).[42] The messy situation lasted for several months; it was later improved when the state and its affiliated agencies gradually incorporated most of the relief endeavors into areas under their command.[43]

The stories presented to the general public were of a very different kind. The media typically applauded the tremendous efforts of the state-organized relief workers, and the state's growing attention on the psychological consequences of disaster and their remedies was construed as a new and laudable achievement. In fact, the Communist Party had just made some important efforts to weave the once-tabooed psychological vocabulary, including 'psychological harmony' (*xinli hexie* 心理和谐) and 'psychological venting' (*xinli shudao* 心理疏导), into its new ideology of constructing a 'harmonious society'.[44] Immediately after the disaster, one could notice a flooding of psychology-related terms in the state's official discourse, which were simultaneously propagated by the popular media. In the Regulations on the Wenchuan Earthquake Post-Disaster Rehabilitation and Rebuilding issued on 8 June 2008 by the State Council, the term 'psychological aid' (*xinli yuanzhu* 心理援助) was mentioned twice.[45] Psychology made a more potent presence in the General Planning on the Wenchuan Earthquake Post-Disaster Rehabilitation and Rebuilding, which was published three months later.[46] More than half of the 'spiritual home' (*xinling jiayuan* 心灵家园) section was dedicated to related issues, and a number of psychological concepts, including 'psychological rehabilitation' (*xinli kangfu* 心理康复), 'psychological intervention' (*xinli ganyu* 心理干预) and 'psychological trauma' (*xinli chuangshang* 心理创伤) were elicited.

All these terms that saturated the public arena in the aftermath of the earthquake were naturally associated with, if not equated to, psychotherapy or psychological counselling, the terms that the general population had most often heard in regards to psychology in general since the inception of the psycho-boom. Television channels rushed to feature psychotherapists in various programs covering the earthquake. While the psychological dimensions of trauma received substantial attention, psychotherapy was imagined as the sole solution and one with magical efficacy. Following is one example that illustrates the exaltation and mystification of psychotherapy in the post-earthquake relief work. On 29 May 2008, CCTV's 'Psychological Interviews' launched a special series, 'Rebuilding the Psychological Home' (*chongjian xinling jiayuan* 重建心

灵家园). The first episode of the series featured Dr. Liu Jin from China's Center for Disease Control, a self-labeled psychologist from Shandong, and Professor Zhang Kan 张侃, President of the Chinese Psychological Society and Director of the Institute of Psychology of the Chinese Academy of Sciences. During the interview, Professor Zhang, who was a leading expert in engineering psychology rather than clinical psychology, said that there were more than 2,000 people providing psychological assistance in the affected region, but this was still seriously inadequate. In a passionate yet weary tone, he continued:

> The earthquake affected more than six million people. Even if we set the incidence rate (of PTSD) at as low as one per cent, there will be 60,000 patients who need psychological treatments, and all the work has to be done on a one-on-one basis.

The female host repeated the last phrase 'one-on-one', and Professor Zhang stressed that for such difficult patients, this was the only cure.

The Post-earthquake Boom

The psycho-boom was already quite visible around 2005–6. In addition to the Ministry of Labour program that served as the primary channel through which most people entered or encountered the psycho-boom, short-term training courses and workshops on various psychotherapy schools or topics quickly emerged, targeting those who aspired to learn more or something else. After the Wenchuan earthquake in 2008, the field entered a new phase of accelerated growth. A number of prominent therapists toured the vast country, giving various kinds of workshops and courses to a rapidly expanding audience; among the most successful ones were several 'masters' who graduated from the legendary Sino-German course. Therapists from Hong Kong, Taiwan, Japan, Europe and North America also arrived to explore the market of psychotherapy training. Together they offered opportunities ranging from the most elite-oriented – such as the direct candidate program administered by the International Psychoanalytical Association[47] and the Internet-based psychoanalytic psychotherapy training run by the China-American Psychoanalytic Alliance,[48] both of which were non-profit endeavors aiming to provide highly rigorous training to the future leaders of the profession– to those having an explicit self-help or self-exploration agenda, some of which were even laced with New Age or spiritual flavors. With thriving and diverse training endeavors, participants could select from an abundance of training opportunities and assemble unique pathways for themselves.

Media and the state response to disasters continue to advance Chinese public awareness and interest in psychotherapy. While 'Psychological Interviews' maintains its unique niche by showing 'real' therapy to the audience, programs featuring celebrity psychologists have multiplied. This new generation of 'psychological programs' (*xinli jiemu* 心理节目) are more entertainment-oriented; they tend to adopt a talk-show format in which the psychologist is one of the distinguished guests.[49] At the end of my fieldwork in mid-2011, most TV channels offered at least one such kind of program. After the Wenchuan earthquake, state-orchestrated relief work that gives prominence to its psychological component has become the reflex response to any major natural or artificial disaster. Psychotherapy gained massive attention through catastrophes like the Yushu earthquake (2010), Zhouqu landslide (2010), Wenzhou train crash (2011) and numerous less severe incidents. The immense publicity was accompanied by the inflation of the value of psychotherapy, which had been depicted as a luxurious service since the psycho-boom appeared. During 2009–10, psychotherapy fees in Beijing rose more than fifty per cent in one year, which paralleled the steep escalation of real estate prices amid the state's ambitious stimulus plan.[50]

In the past several years, the psycho-boom has developed into a massive social world composed of a diverse array of persons, networks, institutions and events. On the one hand, this social world is comparable to the early stages of professionalization in many other countries, when healers, dilettantes and charlatans co-inhabit the landscape of healing practices.[51] On the other hand, it bears structural resemblance to what David Palmer describes as the '*qigong* milieu' in his ethnography on *qigong* – the re-invented healing tradition that swept through the country in the 1980s and 1990s – namely, 'a nebula of networks and associations' in which 'many types of popular activities and networks flourished'.[52] Similarly, people from various backgrounds come together and form intricate networks in the psycho-boom. In addition to a multitude of training activities, the psycho-boom also includes a profusion of social activities. Its members often dine together, visit each other's offices or collaborate on business plans. A large proportion of participants are women aged between twenty-five and forty-five and who come from the relatively well-off strata of the urban population. On the contrary, most of the 'masters' are men in their forties or early fifties.

Local people often divide this enormous social world into three broad categories based on a person's primary job affiliation. The first is psychiatry and medicine. Most of the well-known therapists are psychiatrists or physicians by training, and many psychiatric and general hospitals have departments bearing names such as 'psychological counselling', 'clinical psychology' (*linchuang xinlixue* 临床心理学) or simply 'psychology'. In most cases, physicians but not psychologists staff these units, and the kinds of treatments provided in these facilities vary greatly. The second is the education system, which used to consist of only academic psychology and college counselling. Recently, student counselling has blossomed in primary and secondary education, too. These two categories are often lumped in a more inclusive category, 'the system' (*tizhi* 体制), as both of them mainly belong to the public sector.

These two sectors, namely, psychiatry/medicine and academic psychology/school counselling saw a significant growth during the past decade. However, the recent boom is marked by the rapid expansion of the third category, the so-called 'social sector' (*shehui shang de* 社会上的) that refers to the vast majority of psycho-boom members who are not employed by 'the system'. Included in this category are the so-called 'hobbyists' (*aihaozhe* 爱好者), for whom coming to psychotherapy courses has become a cherished pastime, as well as therapists who are involved in practice. The boundary between 'hobbyist' and therapist is thin, as most of these therapists have exceedingly low caseloads and work on a part-time basis in private counselling centers or psychotherapy clinics. Since licensure for psychotherapy does not exist, these agencies can attain only an ambiguous status by registering as education or consulting companies at the business bureaus of local governments. People may begin their practice on a whim, only to find it difficult to make a living. This sector is therefore highly versatile and unstable: some of its members quickly drop out of the field, and some try to find a foothold in various businesses triggered by the psycho-boom, including employment assistance programs (EAPs) and the sale of psychological paraphernalia.[53] However, quite a few participants carry on with the training or practice of psychotherapy, seeing it as a hobby, a career or a self-exploratory journey; they tend to be wealthier and do not have to worry about their livelihoods.

Conclusion

This chapter examines the recent psycho-boom in urban China from the perspective of policy and state-related interventions. Before the movement emerged in the early 2000s, psychotherapy was an unfamiliar treatment claimed to exist on the fringes of psychiatry and psychology. When the state's health authorities embarked on the mental health care reform at the turn of the century, the psychological enterprise received limited attention, and the eruption of the psycho-boom was almost inconceivable. Nevertheless, the actions and strategies taken by various state agencies, psychological professionals and private ventures have transformed psychotherapy training into an alluring object to which the general population has access. Numerous people join these training programs for various reasons and constitute a huge social world in which middle-class women dominate.

The present is a particularly interesting moment for the psycho-boom. To begin with, the Mental Health Law that was enacted in May 2013 may intervene in the development of the psycho-boom through the medicalization of psychotherapy.[54] In stark contrast to the fluidity and flexibility that the past decade enjoyed, the law makes a clear distinction between psychotherapy and psychological counselling, which have been conflated since the latter was invented in the early 1980s. Psychotherapy is now defined as a medical treatment that shall be conducted by medical personnel in medical settings. The law also stipulates that psychiatric facilities should have specialized personnel providing psychotherapy, but leaves the training and certification for such professionals undefined. Recently, it has been heard that the Ministry of Labor certification will include significant changes in 2014: On the one hand the training and certification will become more rigorous. On the other hand psychological counselling, now defined as non-medical in nature, will be seen as a health-promoting procedure rather than a treatment modality.

Second, psychological technologies are quickly being incorporated into the practices of various public agencies. Historically, hospitals and schools had been the primary sites at which psychotherapy or psychological counselling developed, and the Ministry of Labor program had been used for training the psychological personnel in the police, prisons and military since its outset. In recent years the public agencies responsible for social and community services have followed in those footsteps and increasingly adopted psychological knowledge and techniques in the management of marginalized or disadvantaged populations, as anthropologist Jie Yang reported in her case studies.[55] In many cases, these public agencies assign their personnel to the Ministry of Labor program for training. It is thus unclear to what extent these services have been psychologized since the training tends to be short and superficial.

Given the role that the state-related interventions described in this article played in the psycho-boom, the latest mental health legislation and the permeation of psychology into public services may again have profound intended or unintended consequences on its development. Will the psycho-boom, particularly its 'social sector' composed of laypeople, continue to thrive? If yes, in what way will it maintain its momentum? How will diverse actors in the popular movement respond to the new policies? Will the enormous interest in psychotherapy extend from training to treatment and be able to support a new mental health profession? Will a certain part of the movement undergo an adequate professionalization process, and will the fledging professional community be able to transform the imported therapeutics to fit local needs? These questions will have great implications not only for the psycho-boom but also for China's mental health care system and the psychological well-being of its vast population.

Acknowledgements

My deepest gratitude goes to the psychotherapists I encountered in the social world of the psycho-boom. I am indebted to Drs. Yu Xin, Xiao Zeping and Qiu Jianyin for arranging the institutional support at the Institute of Mental Health at Peking University and Shanghai Mental Health Center during my fieldwork. Throughout my research, I benefited greatly from discussions with my friends who are psychiatrists in Taiwan: Shan Yu, Wang Sheng-Chang, Chien Yi-Ling, Liu Shu-Tsen, Yang Ming-Min, Chen Jia-Shin, Chou Jen-Yu and Wang Hao-Wei. I also thank Arthur Kleinman, Byron Good and Benjamin Penny for their valuable suggestions and critiques on previous drafts.

11 AFTERWORD: REFRAMING PSYCHIATRY IN CHINA

Nancy N. Chen

Psychiatry in contemporary China has multiple influences or genealogies reflecting distinct institutional frameworks of knowledge, practice and care. Whether from imperial medical doctors, Western missionary physicians, mental hygiene programs, international classification categories, or Big Pharma drugs, the formations of contemporary Chinese psychiatry are deeply shaped by foundational practices of psychiatry from earlier periods. Scholars of medicine and madness have long considered psychiatry as a key site to examine cultural beliefs and societal values. This afterword addresses the places, practices and people that animated Chinese psychiatry, as well as specific themes and tensions that emerge in this volume. Through imperial case histories, mental illness categories and institutional histories, the authors focus on notions of selfhood, professional knowledge and confinement that reflect particular notions of governance and care. Rather than argue that contemporary psychiatry in China is merely a continuation of earlier formations, the authors collectively unpack such spaces of containment to reframe categories of emotion and ongoing family state relations.

The volume advances in chronological formation beginning with Imperial China and early formations of wellbeing. In her examination of dreams and nightmares of late Ming China, Vance shows how dreams were intimately linked to emotions and the body revealing potential energetic blockages that could lead to illness or disease. Unlike concepts of Cartesian dualism which contended that mind and body were quite separate spheres, medical treatises of the era extensively addressed proscriptions for proper sleep habits, recognizing that bodily practices could impact mental wellbeing. Dreams were not simply individual experiences but were related to broader social and political contexts. While Vance's topic may initially seem quite distinct from the following chapters, which focus more specifically on the growing institutionalization of Chinese psychiatry, the chapter serves as an important site to consider folk or traditional notions of medicalization and mental hygiene. Even in twenty-first century China, it is still not uncommon to find patients who raise deep concerns and seek mental health care for restless sleep or nightmares in their clinical narratives.

Throughout the volume, authors keenly engage with the critical nexus between narrative and case history. Case histories, especially in Chinese medicine, are richly textured documents of affective social landscapes. The analysis of such documents offers scholars a vivid lens onto social relations, embodiment and psychological categories. Case studies offer textured accounts of personal turmoil and familial encounters with insanity as many authors address in their chapters. In Chapter Three's discussion of the imperial period, Simonis critically examines cases of *dian* and *kuang* to question these categories of pathology. Moreover, he eschews the term 'mental illness' since it was rarely used by Chinese. Simonis prefers instead to use the term 'psycho-behavioral' to encompass the range of emotional distress and other behaviors. While, earlier conceptions of *dian* and *kuang* were not necessarily tied to emotion, mental instability gradually came to be linked through humoral theories of emotions and their influence on the mind and body such as excessive inner heat. Emetics and other forms of treatment focused on organic means of addressing disruptive symptoms in a patient rather than transforming troubling social relations. Simonis notes that case files emerged in late imperial times as a preferred method to record different instances or trajectories of illness over a lifetime. By the 19th century, this format offered doctors the professional basis for comparative etiology, diagnosis and therapeutic strategy.

Chen's discussion of case histories in Chapter Two reflects on the lesser known practice of counter therapy in which talk cures and emotional manipulation were utilized in the treatment of mental disorders. Chen raises a key question of why emotional therapy did not become the main form of treatment. Then, as perhaps even in the present, it seemed that physicians' preferred method was drug therapy. Narrative relies on clear communication between a patient, family members and the doctor. Moreover, while ordinary communication is already influenced by differences in status, gender and age, incidents of emotional disturbances that run the gamut of agitation, anxiety, suspicion, anger, fright, etc. can further complicate therapeutic engagement. Emotional therapy not only required extensive knowledge on the part of the physician but also time. Chen suggests that the labor-intensive element of such therapy rather than the somatization of emotional disturbances led to the preference of drug therapy.

The role of Western missionary physicians and, by extension, psychiatric hospitals in early-twentieth-century China is a key narrative that several chapters in this volume address – notably Chapters Four, Five and Seven. This period of psychiatry in China is a moment of dramatic encounters not just between Chinese and Westerners but also of transformations for family systems. The construction of asylums devoted specifically to psychiatric patients rendered confinement visible such that mentally ill persons were no longer locked away at homes. Such institutions were dramatic new spaces that enabled families to care for members whose behaviors or symptoms were no longer manageable at home. In Chapter Four, Szto offers one of the most concise and thorough discussions of the architecture and design philosophies that shaped European and American hospitals for the insane and the eventual transfer to building the Kerr Refuge for Insane in southern China. Dr. Kerr's efforts to utilize vernacular architecture principles and local materials for an inviting atmosphere in addition to moving his own family into the space completed the mission of creating a psychiatric space that embodied familial care.

While Szto addresses the spatial elements of missionary asylums, Ma and Shapiro engage with the impact of institutionalization for society, especially families. Beginning with contemporary examples of domestic confinement, where mentally ill relatives are locked away sometimes for decades by family members, in Chapter Five Ma contends that the burden of legal responsibility for mentally ill has continued to be on family members throughout the long twentieth century into the present. Ma examines the category of Chinese families suggesting that this social unit was also a key site of transformation with the introduction of missionary psychiatry. Asylums were transforming intimate forms of social relations through shaping family entities, not just asylum patients, as biopolitical subjects. Rather than being confined to foreign spatial and temporal settings, missionary medical discourse contended that psychiatric patients were being liberated from oppressive incarceration in family compounds. The alliance of local elites and police further shaped the psychiatric ward as an extension of familial engagement – one that focused on care rather than suffering or constraints. In spite of this dichotomy, family members were actively engaged in care of patients through the provision of food, medicines and visitations at the Kerr Refuge. Such material forms of engagement are still present today in Chinese psychiatric hospitals where family members attend visiting hours to speak with physicians about recovery or medications. By claiming that patients were emancipated subjects, Ma contends that such governance in the psychiatric context was a particular form of colonial dialectic to proclaim missionary enlightenment. She suggests that contemporary proclamations of emancipation can easily extend this mode of civilizing subjects through mental health cases.

As the profession of psychiatry began to expand in the Republican era with more specialized hospitals, new categories of pathology emerged to encompass different subjects of disorderly behavior, such as women and foreigners. Decades after the establishment of the Kerr Refuge and other wards across China, Shapiro examines, in Chapter Seven, the near inescapable pathology of women in a marriage system under the strains of vast economic and social change. Case histories of this period showed that some female patients sought refuge as patients, preferring to be admitted into the asylums rather than remain with in laws or in a polygamous arrangement. Domestic conflict during 1920s and1930s China was attributed to women's discord with the confines of a patriarchal marriage system.

It was not only Chinese who faced psychological maladies in the midst of vast shifts in family and marriage systems of the early twentieth century. Many foreigner expatriates who resided in China then also experienced forms of malaise referred as 'Oriental nerves' or tropical neuroses. The cases of neurasthenia discussed by Wang in Chapter Six predates Arthur Kleinman's later ethnographic study of neurasthenia in 1980s China by six decades.[1] Those susceptible to the nervous disorder in these two periods could not be more different in terms of racial and class backgrounds – white missionaries or Chinese intellectuals and workers. However, the focus on organic causes and constitutional weakness of sufferers in the context of challenging work environments suggest similar approaches to explanatory models. Initial blame on the weak internal constitutions of foreigners who could not handle the moral deterioration of life in the Far East later turned to heat and excessive sunlight for Western soldiers. Wang's analysis of the American psychiatrist McCartney and his evolving theories about neurasthenia opens up the perplexing category further, demonstrating how a category can be porous, contradictory and, above all, inherently culture bound.

It is tempting to assume that since psychiatry was introduced by foreign doctors, that the practice simply entailed Western ideals inserted into Chinese medical practice. Instead, the chapter by Blowers and Wang, Chapter Eight, as well as that of Wu, Chapter Nine, turn this notion over to address instead how psychiatry in China came to be firmly rooted in modern medical practice and knowledge making through its practitioners and their visions of academic medicine. Blowers and Wang trace the brief flourishing of psychotherapy and psychology during the 1930–60s, a critical period when Chinese physicians engaged in debates about mental hygiene and therapy. Their analysis of *West Wind*, a leading journal of this time, offers insight into the emerging professional world for practitioners which included training students, counseling patients and intellectual exchanges. Like earlier chapters, which focused on the role of Western missionary doctors, this chapter offers fascinating insight onto leading Chinese psychiatrists and psychotherapists who forged new paths for treatment with hybrid knowledge. There remains a lacunae of information about the promotion of mental hygiene during the socialist era of 1950–70s. However, through the life trajectories of the Chinese doctors whose lives and professional careers underwent dramatic shifts, Blowers and Wang bring to life the world of Chinese psychotherapy before its initial closure in the tumultuous 1960s.

Across the straits, Wu offers a parallel view onto the world of Chinese psychiatry in post-WWII Taiwan. Through case histories and the professional histories of key practitioners, we see a different professional context in which new formations of institutionalization addressed large numbers of psychological traumas in a diverse society that included Japanese, mainland Chinese and ethnic Taiwanese as well as indigenous people and other Chinese ethnic groups. The earlier influence of Japanese-German medicine continued in this period as seen through markers of race and illness categories used in case histories. Wu queries how psychiatrists in this context rendered invisible certain forms of trauma while others were given extensive description and carefully documented in statistics.

As the respective opening and ending chapters, Vance and Huang demonstrate a key theme of the volume which addresses the role of emotion in therapy. In the present context, the resource of time remains a critical issue in the treatment of psychiatric subjects. However, emotional therapy continues as a popular treatment available to all citizens which Huang addresses in Chapter Ten, discussing the phenomenal growth of psychotherapy in contemporary China. Rather than simply link what he refers to as the psycho-boom to economic prosperity, Huang argues that extensive popular interest in psychology in the early economic reform period led to the phenomenal growth of psychotherapy in China today. Talk shows, news articles and the rapid growth of training schools for therapists led to the counselling industry as a new cultural entity. The legacy of historic turmoil during the twentieth century is less emphasized than the recent 2008 Wenchuan earthquake which drew official recognition of such practitioners through licensing. Huang raises a key point of how the different disciplines of psychology, psychotherapy and psychiatry have been mostly conflated in the public view which the 2013 Mental Health Law seeks to redress. Another contribution of this volume has been the careful analysis of each of these subdisciplines during distinct periods of knowledge and psychiatric practice.

A key question for this volume is how did Chinese physicians engage with global psychiatry? During the late twentieth century, Chinese psychiatrists adopted international diagnostic categories and classifications such as the Diagnostic and Statistical Manual of Mental Disorders of the American Psychiatric Association and the International Classification of Diseases (ICD-9) of the World Health Organization. The Chinese professional community has also engaged in active translation of the latest Western psychiatric articles and international classification categories into Chinese, categories in the Chinese Classification of Mental Disorders (CCDM) being crucial sites of cultural translation.[2] Parallel to psychiatry in Western, post-industrial nations, there is an increased usage of psychopharmacology. During the mid to late 1990s, the pharmaceutical industry introduced new drugs to the Chinese market and multinational as well as local firms have been active in making psychotropic drugs available and an integral part of consumer life. Such practices raise key questions about the dark side of globalization, which enable swift introduction of material goods and symbolic meanings that undermine local and alternative healing systems. In recent years other means for families to seek advice and help outside of the psychiatric unit, with regard to mental health, have arisen. One noteworthy trend has been hotlines, which people can call anonymously for help, whilst the Chinese popular press and magazines have, in recent years, taken on stories that deal with social issues such as mental illness. Besides seeking a range of clinical practitioners, such as Traditional Chinese Medicine or biomedical, family members can write to newspapers or journals seeking advice and a number of private mental health clinics have opened. In addition, outreach education programs in mental health have been introduced to the school curriculum.

The rural-urban difference in access to medical care, especially psychiatric care, which continues in the present era is not addressed in the volume. Larger research hospitals and the majority of professionals are mainly located in cities. It is important to note however that, by contrast to the early twentieth century when psychiatric hospitals were private, mental health wards are now public and state owned. The number of beds for mentally ill clients has also increased. In 1948 there were only 1,100 beds for 500 million people (a ratio of 0.22 beds per 10,000 people), with 50 to 70 trained physicians and even fewer nurses. By 1995 the number of beds significantly increased to 120,000–130,000 beds or about 1.1 beds per 10,000 people. In larger psychiatric hospitals with several hundred inpatients, 80 to 90 percent of the patient population consisted of chronic schizophrenic patients for whom family care was no longer viable. While the majority of patients were schizophrenic, there were also clinical cases of depression, neurological disorders, neurasthenia and psychosomatic disorders. Regional differences in hospital stays between rural patients and urban patients also persist, due to health insurance in mainly urban regions. Moreover, in terms of percentage there are more severe cases among mentally ill patients due to relatively late diagnosis in rural regions.[3] The number of beds is still quite low in comparison to other countries with smaller populations and there is a heavy reliance on family and community managed care, especially for outpatient beds.

May 2013 was notable for two major events in psychiatry which will shape the profession in decades to come. The fifth edition of the Diagnostic and Statistical Manual (DSM–V) was released after a decade of discussions in panels, conferences and forums. The standardization of global diagnostic categories, yet inclusion of culturally specific forms of mental illness, reflects ongoing development of the profession as a practice that spans public policy, social debates and cultural norms. At the same time, China's new mental health law, which was passed earlier in 2012, came into effect.[4] The impact of this legislation will continue to unfold throughout the decade, however, its emergence reflects the prioritization of mental health in twenty-first-century China. The state focus reflects a widespread social interest that began two decades earlier, when psychology literature became popular forms of self-care and improvement accompanying economic transformations in China. Public awareness of mental health needs significantly increased with the much publicized recovery efforts of the 2008 Sichuan earthquake. The new mental health law of 2013 seeks to shift the majority of care from specialized psychiatric hospitals to more general hospitals and community health clinics with the capacity of reaching out to a wider population. In an era of de-institutionalization and managed care, which characterizes psychiatric care in most post-industrial nations, sustainable alternative forms of mental health care are of great significance.

In sum, the contributors of this volume offer keen insights onto the formations of Chinese psychiatry as it evolved in different periods to address specific behaviors and social relations. Rather than solely link the grand narrative of psychiatry in China to economic or political transformation, the authors reveal the cultural frameworks that give shape to categories of behavior as well as the affective landscapes of emotional distress and suffering in each era. In doing so, the volume expands prior scholarship on psychiatry and mental illness in China in significant ways.

NOTES

Chiang, 'Historicizing Chinese Psychiatry'

1. This book would not have been conceivable without the pioneering scholarship of, among others, J. J. Kao, *Three Millennia of Chinese Psychiatry* (New York: Institute for Advanced Research in Asian Science and Medicine, 1979); A. Kleinman, *Patients and Healers in the Context of Culture: An Exploration of the Borderland between Anthropology, Medicine and Psychiatry* (Berkeley, CA: University of California Press, 1980); H. Agren, 'The Conceptual History of Psychiatric Terms in Traditional Chinese Medicine', in *Explorations in the History of Science and Technology in China*, eds Li Guohao et al. (Shanghai: Shanghai Chinese Classics, 1982), pp. 573–81; M. Li Chiu, *Mind, Body and Illness in a Chinese Medical Tradition* (PhD Dissertation, Harvard University, 1986); R. S. Chin and Ai Li S. Chin, *Psychological Research in Communist China: 1949–1966* (Boston, MA: MIT Press, 1987); V. W. Ng, *Madness in Late Imperial China: From Illness to Deviance* (Norman, OK: University of Oklahoma Press, 1990); V. Pearson, 'The Development of Modern Psychiatric Services in China, 1891–1949', *History of Psychiatry* 2:6 (1991), pp. 133–47; Ming Li, 'Psychology in China: A Brief Historical Review', *Journal of Psychology*, 128:3 (1994), pp. 281–7; H. Shapiro, 'The View From A Chinese Asylum: Defining Madness in 1930s Peking' (PhD Dissertation, Harvard University, 1995); and N. Chen, *Breathing Spaces: Qigong, Psychiatry and Healing in China* (New York: Columbia University Press, 2003).
2. For an erudite study of the history of concepts and practices of hygiene in relation to the modernizing Chinese body politic from late Qing to the Republican period, see R. Rogaski, *Hygienic Modernity: Meanings of Health and Disease in Treaty-Port China* (Berkeley, CA: University of California Press, 2004).
3. This quote originally appeared in André Tridon's 'Introduction' to S. Freud, *Dream Psychology: Psychoanalysis for Beginners* (New York: James A. McCann, 1920).
4. M. F. Reiser, 'The Dream in Contemporary Psychiatry', *American Journal of Psychiatry*, 158:3 (2001), pp. 351–9.
5. On the introduction of psychoanalysis to China, see Jingyuan Zhang, *Psychoanalysis in China: Literary Transformations, 1919–1949* (Ithaca, NY: Cornell University Press, 1992); Tao Jiang and P. J. Ivanhoe (eds), *The Reception and Rendition of Freud in China: China's Freudian Slip* (New York: Routledge, 2013).
6. As quoted in Chapter One, p. 17.
7. As quoted in Chapter Two, p. 39.
8. As quoted in Chapter Four, p. 82.

9. For an in-depth discussion of Selden's involvement in the Kerr Refuge, see Pearson, 'The Development of Modern Psychiatric Services in China', pp. 133–47
10. See Figures 5.2 and 5.3 in Chapter Five, p. 103.
11. W. Anderson, R. C. Keller and D. Jenson (eds), *Unconscious Dominions: Psychoanalysis, Colonial Trauma and Global Sovereignties* (Durham, NC: Duke University Press, 2011).
12. W. Anderson, 'The Trespass Speaks: White Masculinity and Colonial Breakdown', *American Historical Review* 102:5 (1997), pp. 1343–70; W. Anderson, *Colonial Pathologies: American Tropical Medicine, Race and Hygiene in the Philippines* (Durham, NC: Duke University Press, 2006), pp. 130–57.
13. As quoted in Chapter Six, p. 124.
14. V. Schwarcz, *The Chinese Enlightenment: Intellectuals and the Legacy of the May Fourth Movement of 1919* (Berkeley, CA: University of California Press, 1990).
15. J. Gregory Lutz, *China and the Christian Colleges, 1850–1950* (Ithaca, NY: Cornell University Press, 1971); P. Bailey, *Reform the People: Changing Attitudes Towards Popular Education in Early Twentieth Century China* (Edinburgh: Edinburgh University Press, 1990); Zheng Wang, *Women in the Chinese Enlightenment: Oral and Textual Histories* (Berkeley, CA: University of California Press, 1999); D. Ko, *Cinderella's Sisters: A Revisionist History of Footbinding* (Berkeley, CA: University of California Press, 2005); D. Ko and Zheng Wang (eds), *Translating Feminisms in China* (London: Wiley-Blackwell, 2007).
16. See, for example, S. Glosser, *Chinese Visions of Family and the State, 1915–1953* (Berkeley, CA: University of California Press, 2003).
17. Tze-lan Deborah Sang, *The Emerging Lesbian: Female Same-Sex Desire in Modern China* (Chicago, IL: University of Chicago Press, 2003); Haiyan Lee, *Revolution of the Heart: A Genealogy of Love in China, 1900–1950* (Stanford, CA: Stanford University Press, 2006); W. Larson, *From Ah Q to Lei Feng: Freud and Revolutionary Spirit in 20th Century China* (Stanford, CA: Stanford University Press, 2008); H. Chiang, 'Epistemic Modernity and the Emergence of Homosexuality in China', *Gender and History*, 22:3 (2010), pp. 629–57.
18. M. Bullock, *An American Transplant: The Rockefeller Foundation and Peking Union Medical College* (Berkeley, CA: University of California Press, 1980). On the development of Western medicine in modern China, see also B. Andrews, *The Making of Modern Chinese Medicine, 1850–1960* (Vancouver: University of British Columbia Press, 2014); and H. Chiang (ed.), *Historical Epistemology and the Making of Modern Chinese Medicine* (Manchester: Manchester University Press, 2015).
19. C. Furth, *A Flourishing Yin: Gender in China's Medical History, 960–1665* (Berkeley, CA: University of California Press, 1999); F. Simonis, 'Mad Acts, Mad Speech and Mad People in Late Imperial Chinese Law and Medicine' (PhD dissertation, Princeton University, 2010); Hsiu-fen Chen, 'Medicine, Society and the Making of Madness in Imperial China' (PhD dissertation, University of London, 2003).
20. Wen-Ji Wang, '*West Wind Monthly* and the Popular Mental Hygiene Discourse in Republican China', *Taiwanese Journal for Studies of Science, Technology and Medicine*, 13 (2011), pp. 15–88.
21. On the mental hygiene movement in postwar Taiwan, see Hans Tao-Ming Huang, *Queer Politics and Sexual Modernity in Taiwan* (Hong Kong: Hong Kong University Press, 2011), pp. 31–52.
22. See, for example, Hsien Rin 林憲, *Wenhua jingshen yixue de zengwu: Cong Taiwan dao Riben* 文化精神醫學的贈物: 從台灣到日本 [The Gift of Cultural Psychiatry: From

Taiwan to Japan] (Taipei: Xinling gongfang, 2007); Wen-Shing Tseng 曾文星, *Yige rensheng, sanzhong wenhua: Zhongguo、Riben、Meiguo wenhua dui renge xingcheng de ziwo fenxi* 一個人生，三種文化：中國、日本、美國文化對人格形成的自我分析 [One Life, Three Cultures: The Self-Analysis on Personality Shaped by China, Japan, and America] (Taipei: Psychology, 2010).

23. For the English translation of the law, see H. H. Chen et al., 'Mental Health Law of the People's Republic of China (English Translation with Annotations)', *Shanghai Archives of Psychiatry* 24:6 (2012), pp. 305–21.
24. Sing Lee, 'From Diversity to Unity: The Classification of Mental Disorders in 21st-Century China', *Psychiatric Clinics of North America*, 24: 3 (2001), pp. 421–31.
25. A. Kleinman, Yunxiang Yan, Jing Jun, Sing Lee, Everett Zhang, Pan Tianshu, Wu Fei and Jinhua Guo, *Deep China: The Moral Life of the Person* (Berkeley, CA: University of California Press, 2011).
26. See, for example, M. Vaughan, *Curing Their Ills: Colonial Power and African Illness* (Cambridge: Polity, 1991); W. Ernst, *Mad Tales from the Raj: European Insane in British India, 1800–58* (New York: Routledge, 1991); J. McGulloch, *Colonial Psychiatry and the 'African Mind'* (Cambridge: Cambridge University Press, 1995); J. Sadowsky, *Imperial Bedlam: Institutions of Madness in Colonial Southwest Nigeria* (Berkeley, CA: University of California Press, 1999); C. Hartnack, *Psychoanalysis in Colonial India* (Oxford: Oxford University Press, 2001); D. Bhugra and R. Littlewood (eds), *Colonialism and Psychiatry* (Oxford: Oxford University Press, 2001); S. Mahone, 'The Psychology of Rebellion: Colonial Medical Responses to Dissent in British East Africa', *Journal of African History*, 47:2 (2006), pp. 241–58; H. Pols, 'The Development of Psychiatry in Indonesia: From Colonial to Modern Times', *International Review of Psychiatry* 18:4 (2006), pp. 363–70; R. Keller, *Colonial Madness: Psychiatry in French North Africa* (Chicago, IL: University of Chicago Press, 2007); S. Mahone and M. Vaughan (eds), *Psychiatry and Empire* (Basingstoke: Palgrave Macmillan, 2007); W. Ernst and T. Muller (eds), *Transnational Psychiatries: Social and Cultural Histories of Psychiatry in Comparative Perspectives, c. 1800–2000* (Newcastle: Cambridge Scholars Publishing, 2010); W. Anderson, R. C. Keller and D. Jenson (eds), *Unconscious Dominions: Psychoanalysis, Colonial Trauma and Global Sovereignties* (Durham, NC: Duke University Press, 2011); J. Saha, 'Madness and the Making of Colonial Order in Burma', *Modern Asian Studies*, 47:2 (2013), pp. 406–35; M. Heaton, *Black Skins, White Coats: Nigerian Psychiatrists, Decolonization and the Globalization of Psychiatry* (Athens, OH: Ohio University Press, 2013); and W. Ernst, *Colonialism and Transnational Psychiatry: The Development of an Indian Mental Hospital in British India, c. 1925–1940* (London: Anthem Press, 2013).
27. The themes of colonialism are also relatively less pertinent to the history of psychiatry in Japan. The parallels to China suggest that further comparative work would be desirable. See, for example, Shigehisa Kuriyama, 'The Historical Origins of 'Katakori'', *Japan Review* 9 (1997), pp. 127–49; Akihito Suzuki, 'Family, the State and the Insane in Japan, 1900–1945', in R. Porter and D. Wright (eds), *Psychiatric Confinement in International Perspective* (Cambridge: Cambridge University Press, 2003), pp. 193–225; Akihito Suzuki, 'A Brain Hospital in Tokyo and Its Private and Public Patients, 1926–1945', *History of Psychiatry* 14 (2003), pp. 337–60; Akihito Suzuki, 'Between Two Psychiatric Regimes: Migration and Psychiatry in Early Twentieth-Century Japan', in A. McCarthy and C. Colebourne eds, *Migration, Ethnicity and Mental Health: International Perspectives, 1840–2010* (London: Routledge, 2012), pp. 141–51; and Junko Kitanaka,

Depression in Japan: Psychiatric Cures for a Society in Disease (Princeton, NJ: Princeton University Press, 2011).

28. R. Munro, Human Rights Watch and Geneva Initiative on Psychiatry, *Dangerous Minds: Political Psychiatry in China Today and Its Origins in the Maoist Era* (New York: Human Rights Watch, 2002); R. Munro, *China's Psychiatric Inquisition: Dissent, Psychiatry and the Law in Post-1949 China* (London: Wildy Simmonds and Hill, 2006).

1 Vance, 'Exorcising Dreams and Nightmares in Late Ming China'

1. For more on Ge Hong, see R. F. Campany, *To Live as Long as Heaven and Earth: A Translation and Study of Ge Hong's Traditions of Divine Transcendents* (Berkeley, CA: University of California Press, 2002).
2. Shang Wei addressed the question of readership and approach to reading in late imperial China, arguing that *Jin Ping Mei*, with its complicated multi-layered format, conveyed a new vision of the world that called for new strategies of reading and comprehension, requiring readers to depart from methods of reading intensely, character by character. See Shang Wei, "Jin Ping Mei' and Late Ming Print Culture', in J. T. Zeitlin, L. H. Liu and E. Widmer (eds), *Writing and Materiality in China: Essays in Honor of Patrick Hanan* (Cambridge, MA: Harvard University Asia Center, 2003), pp. 187–238.
3. *Concise Oxford Dictionary*, ed. by Catherine Soanes, 11th edition (Oxford: Oxford University Press, 2008), s. v. 'Dream'.
4. Ling Shaowen 凌紹雯 et al. (eds), *Kangxi zi dian* 康熙字典 [Kangxi dictionary] (Shanghai: Hong bao zhai, 1890), under '*meng* 夢".
5. He Dongru 何棟如, *Meng lin xuan jie* 夢林玄解 [An Explication of the Profundities in the Forest of Dreams], from a photographic reprint of the Ming Chongzhen edition (1628–44) housed in the Shanghai Lexicographical Library. This photographic reprint is published in *Xuxiu siku quan shu* 續修四庫全書 [Continuation to the Complete Four Treasuries Library] *zi bu* 子部 *shu shu lei* 術數類, vols 1063–4 (Shanghai: Shanghai Guji chubanshe, 2002), p. 602. This edition is widely available in major universities, libraries and archives. Because of its availability, I cite this copy. I have located fifteen extant 1636 copies of *Forest of Dreams* (one in the United States, three in Japan, three in Taiwan and eight in the People's Republic of China) and confirmed that the first page of each of the the first fascicles was printed from the same woodblock. I have also confirmed that the section entitled 'Dream Exorcism' is identical in each of the aforementioned extant fifteen copies, so I do not discuss other textual differences in this chapter. Unless otherwise noted, all translations are my own.
6. He Dongru, *Forest of Dreams*, vol. 1063, p. 605.
7. Several examples of '*rang* 禳' suggest that disaster may be averted by means of virtuous behaviour or conduct. One example reads: 'the king said it would be possible to avert disaster by behaving virtuously'. Kong Yingda 孔穎達 (ed.), *Chongkan song ben shisanjing zhushu fujiao kanji* 重刊宋本十三經注疏附校勘記 [Song Commentary on the Thirteen Classics], no. 4, pp. 113–2, available online through *Zhongyang Yanjiuyuan Hanji dianzi wenxian ziliao ku* 中央研究院漢籍電子文獻資料庫 [Academia Sinica Scripta Sinica Database] at http://hanji.sinica.edu.tw/, [accessed December 2011]. A second example reads: 'if the ruler cultivates virtue in order to avert disaster, then perhaps it is possible to attain foodstuffs, though there are no foodstuffs'. *Tiao ri fa* 調日法 [Methods of Adjusting the Day], *Luli qi ming tian li yi* 律曆七明天曆一 [Calendrical Laws 7, Daily Calendar 1], *Di qishisi zhi di ershiqi* 第七十四志第二十七 [Record Num-

ber 74, Number 27], in *Song shi* 宋史 [Song Histories], 1686, available online through *Zhongyang Yanjiuyuan Hanji dianzi wenxian* 中央漢籍電子文獻 [Academia Sinica Scripta Sinica Database] at http://hanji.sinica.edu.tw/, [accessed December 2011].

8. U. Englehardt, 'Longevity Techniques and Chinese Medicine', in L. Kohn (ed.), *Daoism Handbook*, vol. 2. (Leiden: Brill, 2000), pp. 74–108. See also Chen Hsiu-fen 陳秀芬, *Yangsheng yu xiushen: wan ming wenren de shenti shuxie yu shesheng jishu* 養生與修身：晚明文人的身體書寫與攝生技術 [Nourishing Life and Cultivating the Body: Writing the Literati's Body and Techniques for Preserving Health in the Late Ming] (Taipei: Daoxiang chubanshe, 2009).
9. Englehardt, 'Longevity Techniques and Chinese Medicine', pp. 74–108.
10. He Dongru, *Forest of Dreams*, vol. 1064, p. 302.
11. Ibid.
12. Ibid., pp. 302–3. The quoted passage echoes proscriptions in Gao Lian's (1573–1620) work on prolonging life, which was first published between 1591 and 1620. See Gao Lian 高濂, *Zun sheng ba jian* 《遵生八箋》 [Eight Essays on Cherishing Life] (Chengdu: Bashu shu she, 1992), pp. 370–2.
13. He Dongru, *Forest of Dreams*, vol. 1064, p. 312.
14. The Chinese sexagenary cycle is a system for recording hours, days, months and years. Recorded usage dates to the Shang dynasty. Each set of terms in the sexagenary cycle comprises two Chinese characters, the first representing a term from the ten heavenly stems (*tiangan* 天干) and the second from the twelve earthly branches (*dizhi* 地支). The term combines the first heavenly stem with the first earthly branch; the second term combines the second heavenly stem with the first earthly branch. The cycle continues, generating a total of sixty distinct terms. After sixty, the cycle repeats itself. The ten heavenly stems and twelve earthly branches (collectively known as ganzhi 干支) are elements of a cyclic character numeral system and used in the calculation and division of time. The ten heavenly stems are: *Jia* (甲), *Yi* (乙), *Bing* (丙), *Ding* (丁), *Wu* (戊), *Ji* (己), *Geng* (庚), *Xin* (辛), *Ren* (壬) and *Gui* (癸). The twelve earthly branches are: *Zi* (子), *Chou* (丑), *Yin* (寅), *Mao* (卯), *Chen* (辰), *Si* (巳), *Wu* (午), *Wei* (未), *Shen* (申), *You* (酉), *Xu* (戌) and *Hai* (亥). The heavenly stems are associated with the concepts of yin, yang and the Five Phases. The earthly branches also identify the twelve months of the year, twelve zodiac animals (the twelve zodiac animals are also used as mnemonics), directions, seasons, months and the hour of the day in the form of double-hours.
15. Specific reasons for the choice of tiger time are not given in the encyclopedia. Perhaps it is because tiger (*yin*) represents wood according to five phases theory; since the pillow was to be made of wood, it might have been important to match the qualities of the pillow with the correct time (matching wood with wood). Nathan Sivin detailed the ways in which early alchemists depended upon numerological correlations, correspondences and resonances in order to manipulate and control time. In their quest to attain elixirs of immortality, Daoist adepts carefully timed alchemical processes. See N. Sivin, 'Chinese Alchemy and the Manipulation of Time', *Isis*, 67:239 (1967), pp. 516–26.
16. He Dongru. 何棟如, *Meng lin xuan jie* 夢林玄解 [An Explication of the Profundities in the Forest of Dreams], Ming Chongzhen edn (1628–44), Chinese Collection, Harvard Yenching Library Rare Book Collection.
17. See M. E. Lewis, *Writing and Authority in Early China* (Albany, NY: State University of New York Press, 1999).
18. C. Despeux, 'Women in Daoism', in *Daoism Handbook*, p. 499.
19. Ibid., p. 528.

20. I. L. Legeza, *Tao Magic: The Secret Language of Diagrams and Calligraphy* (London: Thames and Hudson, 1975).
21. Here, Laozi's method is not equivalent to the exorcism of nightmares. The term used (*bi* 避) implies avoidance, evasion, or escape. It appears together with such terms as 'the world' (*shi* 世), 'rain' (*yü* 雨), 'summer heat' (*shu* 暑) and 'difficulties' (*nan* 難).
22. He Dongru, *Forest of Dreams*, vol. 1064, p. 303.
23. Ibid.
24. The term also carried connotations of submission or eliminating discomfort or pain. The goal of this technique of suppression was to benefit oneself and avoid or deflect disaster in the future. See Luo Zhufeng 罗竹风 (ed.), *Hanyu da cidian* 漢語大詞典, [Comprehensive Chinese Word Dictionary], 12 vols (Shanghai: Shanghai Cishu chubanshe, 1986), under 'yansheng 厭勝 ' .
25. He Dongru, *Forest of Dreams*, vol. 1064, p. 306.
26. Ibid.
27. Ibid., p. 310.
28. At least in contemporary Daoist rituals, talismans themselves are not actually swallowed. Sometimes the talisman is placed in a vessel filled with liquid. The power of the talisman transfers to the liquid, which is then imbibed. Some talismans are burned and the ashes placed in water, which is then consumed. The methodology is not explicitly stated in *Forest of Dreams*; however, it seems likely that one of the aforementioned procedures was adopted. Another option might have involved the substitution of paper for peach wood.
29. He Dongru, *Forest of Dreams*, vol. 1064, p. 283.
30. Ibid., p. 282.
31. Ibid., p. 281.

2 Chen, 'Emotional Therapy and Talking Cures in Late Imperial China'

1. In this study, 'late Imperial China' roughly refers to the period during the twelfth and the nineteen centuries.
2. Wu Kun 吳昆, *Yifang kao* 醫方考 [Research on Medical Formulas], (1586; Jiangsu: Jiangsu kexue jishu chubanshe, 1985), fascicle 3, ch. 27, p. 201.
3. Zhang Congzheng 張從正, 'Rumen shiqin 儒門事親' [The Scholar Serving His Kin], *Zihe yiji* 子和醫集 [The Medical Collection of Zhang Zihe] (Beijing: Renmin weisheng chubanshe, 1994/6), fascicle 3, p. 109; Xu Yongcheng 徐用誠 and Liu Chun 劉純, 'Yuji weiyi 玉機微義' [Esoteric Meanings of the Jade Secrets], *Liu chun yixue quanshu* 劉純醫學全書 [The Complete Medical Works of Liu Chun] (Beijing: Zhongguo zhongyiyao chubanshe, 1999), fascicle 16, p. 245; Xu Chunfu 徐春甫, *Gujin yitong daquan* 古今醫統大全 [Collection of Medical Traditions in the Past and Present] (1556; Beijing: Renmin weisheng chubanshe, 1991), fascicle 41, p. 1187; Zhang Zhicong 張志聰, *Huangdi neijing suwen jizhu* 黃帝內經素問集註 [The Inner Canon of the Yellow Emperor: Annotation on Basic Questions] (1670; Hangzhou: Zhejiang guji chubanshe, 2002), fascicle 2A, ch. 5, p. 42.
4. N. Sivin, 'Emotional counter-therapy', in *Medicine, Philosophy and Religion in Ancient China* (Hampshire: Variorium, 1995), part 2, pp. 1–19; F. Simonis, 'Mad Acts, Mad Speech and Mad People in Late Imperial Chinese Law and Medicine' (PhD dissertation, Princeton University, 2010), p.88.

5. I capitalize the names of these visceral organs since they are not fully identical with the anatomical entities of modern bio-medicine. These organs in Chinese medicine have more functional and complicated interrelationship, according to the theory of systematic correspondence. N. Sivin, *Traditional Medicine in Contemporary China* (Ann Arbor, MI: The University of Michigan, 1997), pp. 124–33.
6. Wang Bing 王冰, *Huangdi neijing suwen* 黃帝內經素問 [The Inner Canon of the Yellow Emperor: Basic Questions] (762; Beijing: Renmin weisheng chubanshe, 1996), fascicle 2, ch. 5, pp. 37–42. Similar but slightly different descriptions of these paragraphs can be found in ibid., fascicle 6, ch. 19, pp. 124–5; fascicle 19, ch. 67, pp. 374–85.
7. Ibid., fascicle 2, ch. 5, p. 34; fascicle 6, ch. 19, pp. 124–5; fascicle 11, ch. 39, pp. 221–2.
8. Zhang Zhicong, *The Inner Canon of the Yellow Emperor: Annotation on Basic Questions*, fascicle 2a, ch. 5, pp. 43–4.
9. Shigehisa Kuriyama, *The Expressiveness of the Body and the Divergence of Greek and Chinese Medicine* (New York: Zone Book, 1999), p. 103.
10. Chao Yuanfang 巢元方, *Zhu bing yuan hou lun* 諸病源候論 [The Treatise on Causes and Symptoms of Medical Disorders] (762; Beijing: Renmin weisheng chubanshe, 1991/1996 [610]), fascicle 13, pp. 400–1.
11. Chen Yan 陳言, *San yin ji yi bing zheng fang lun* 三因極一病證方論 [The Treatise on the Three Causes Unified: Diseases, Symptoms and Recipes] (1174; Beijing: Remin weisheng chubanshe, 1963), fascicle 2, p. 19; Yan Yonghe 嚴用和, *Jisheng fang* 濟生方 [Recipes for Aiding Life] (1253; Beijing: Renmin weisheng chubanshe, 1956), vol. 2, fascicle 5–6, pp. 153–206.
12. See, for example, Fei Boxiung 費伯雄, *Yi chun sheng yi* 醫醇賸義 [The Supplementary Meanings of Medical Essence], in Cao Bingzhang 曹炳章 (ed.), *Zhongguo yixue dacheng xuji* 中國醫學大成續集 [The Great Collection of Chinese Medical Works: Supplementary Volumes] (Shanghai: Shanghai kexue jishu chubanshe, 2000), vol. 29, fascicle 2, pp. 195–6.
13. Wu Kun, *Research on Medical Formulas*, fascicle 3, ch. 27, pp. 201–4.
14. Zhang Jiebin, *Lei jing* 類經 [The Classified Canon], 1624 edn, National Library, Taipei, fascicle 31, pp. 31a–37a.
15. Chen Menglei 陳夢雷 et al. (eds), 'qingzhi men' 情志門 [Category of Emotions] in *Gujin tushu jicheng yibu quanlu* 古今圖書集成 [Past and Present Synthesis of Books and Illustrations] (Taipei: Xinwenfeng chuban gongsi, 1979 [1723]), fascicle 321, pp. 2368–73.
16. Zhang Zhicong, *Huangdi neijing lingshu jizhu* 黃帝內經靈樞集註 [The Inner Canon of the Yellow Emperor: Annotation on The Divine Pivot] (1670; Hangzhou: Zhejiang guji chubanshe, 2002), fascicle 4, p. 228; Guo Aicun 郭靄春 (ed.), *Huangdi neijing lingshu jiaozhu yuyi* 黃帝內經靈樞校注語譯 [The Inner Canon of the Yellow Emperor: Annotation and Translation of The Divine Pivot] (Tianjin: Tianjin kexue jishu chubanshe, 1989), ch. 29, p. 256.
17. Zhang Congzheng, *The Scholar Serving His Kin* , fascicle 3, pp. 106, 109–10.
18. Ibid., p. 110.
19. Ibid.
20. Ibid., p. 111.
21. See, for example, Wang Ji 汪機 and Chen Jue 陳桷 (eds), 'Shishan yian' 石山醫案 [Stone Mountain Medical Case Histories], *Wang Shishan yixue quanshu* 汪石山醫學全書 [The Complete Medical Works of Wang Ji] (Beijing: Zhongguo zhongyiyao chubanshe, 1999), fascicle 2, pp. 97–8; Yang Jizhou 楊繼洲, *Zhenjiu dacheng* 針灸大成

[The Great Achievements of Acupuncture and Moxibustion] (1601; Beijing: Renmin weisheng chubanshe, 1997), fascicle 9, pp. 373–4.

22. Zhang Jiebin, *The Classified Canon*, fascicle 12, pp. 39a–39b.
23. Wu Jutong 吳鞠通, *Yi yi bing shu* 醫醫病書 [Curing The Ills of Medicine] (1798; Jiangsu: Jiangsu kexue jishu chubanshe, 1985), p. 16. My interpretation of Wu's passage mainly follows Fabien Simonis's translation. Please see Chapter Three in this book, especially pp. 68–9.
24. Lin Peiqin 林佩琴, *Lei zheng zhi cai* 類證治裁 [Categories of Symptoms and Treatments], 1884 edn (1851; Beijing: Zhongguo zhongyiyao chubanshe, 1999), fascicle 3, p. 197.
25. Chen Hsiu-fen 陳秀芬, 'Dang bingren jian dao gui: shilun mingqing yizhe duiyu xiesui de taidu 當病人見到鬼：試論明清醫者對於「邪祟」的態度' [When Patients met Ghosts: A Preliminary Survey of Scholarly Doctors' Attitudes towards 'Demonic Affliction' in Ming-Qing China] in Lin Fushi 林富士 (ed.), *Zongjiao yu yiliao* 宗教與醫療 [Religions and Medicine] (Taipei: Lianjing chuban shiye gufen youxian gongsi, 2011), pp. 356–62.
26. Zhang Congzheng, *The Scholar Serving His Kin* , fascicle 7, p. 206.
27. Ibid., pp. 202–3.
28. Ibid., p. 207.
29. Ibid. Also see: Sun Yikui 孫一奎, 'Chi sui xuan zhu 赤水玄珠' [Red Water and Black Pearl], in *Sun Yikui yixue quanshu* 孫一奎醫學全書 [The Complete Medical Works of Sun Yikui] (Beijing: Zhongguo zhongyiyao chubanshe, 1999), fascicle 14, p. 330.
30. Zhang Congzheng, *The Scholar Serving His Kin* , fascicle 7, pp. 207–8; Wei Zhixiu 魏之琇 (ed.), *Xu mingyi leian* 續名醫類案 [Supplements to Famous Physicians' Classified Medical Cases] (1770; Taipei: Hongye chubanshe, 1971), fascicle 21, p. 517.
31. They can be found in Xu Yongcheng and Liu Chun, *Esoteric Meanings of the Jade Secrets*, fascicle 16, pp. 243–5; Sun Yikui, *Red Water and Black Pearl*, fascicle 9, pp. 206–7; Wang Kentang 王肯堂, 'Zhengzhi zhunsheng zabing 證治準繩雜病' [Standard for Diagnosis and Treatment: Miscellaneous Disorders], in *Wang kentang yixue quanshu* 王肯堂醫學全書 [The Complete Medical Works of Wang Kentang] (Beijing: Zhongguo zhongyiyao chubanshe, 1999), vol. 2, pp. 60–1.
32. Zhang Congzheng, *The Scholar Serving His Kin* , fascicle 3, p. 111. Also see: Wang Ji, *Stone Mountain Medical Case Histories*, fascicle 2, p. 97.
33. Zhang Congzheng, *The Scholar Serving His Kin* , fascicle 3, p. 111.
34. Zhu Zhenheng 朱震亨, 'Mai yin zheng zhi 脈因證治' [Pulses, Causes, Symptoms and Therapy], in *Danxi yiji* 丹溪醫集 [Medical Collection of Zhu Danxi] (Beijing: Renmin weisheng chubanshe, 1993/5), fascicle 2, pp. 839–40.
35. Zhu Zhenheng, *Danxi xinfa* 丹溪心法 [Zhu Danxi's Heart Method] (1481/1601; Beijing: Renmin weisheng chubanshe, 1993/5), fascicle 5, p. 483.
36. Chen Menglei et al. (eds), *Past and Present Synthesis of Books and Illustrations*, fascicle 295, p. 260.
37. Jiang Guan 江瓘 and Jiang Yingsu 江應宿 (eds), *Mingyi lei'an* 名醫類案 [Famous Physicians' Classified Medical Cases] (1591; Taipei: Hongye shuju, 1971/1994), fascicle 2, p. 74; Wu Kun, *Research on Medical Formulas*, fascicle 27, pp. 202–3.
38. Yu Zhen 俞震 (ed.), *Gujin yian an* 古今醫案按 [Comments on Medical Cases, Past and Present] (1778; Beijing: Renmin weisheng chubanshe, 2010), fascicle 5, p. 168.

39. Wan Quan 萬全, 'Yangsheng siyao 養生四要' [The Four Essentials of Nourishing Life], in *Wan mizhai yixue quanshu* 萬密齋醫學全書 [The Complete Medical Works of Wan Mizhai] (Beijing: Zhongguo zhongyiyao chubanshe, 1999), fascicle 2, p. 14.
40. Zhang Jiebin, *jingyue quanshu* 景岳全書 [The Complete Works of Zhang Jingyue] (1624; Beijing: Renmin weisheng chubanshe, 1997), fascicle 19, p. 442.
41. Wang Ji, *Stone Mountain Medical Case Histories*, fascicle 2, p. 98. According to Wu Kun, this noble man was a Minister Han 韓 and the physician was Zuo Youxin 左友信.; see Wu Kun, *Research on Medical Formulas*, p. 202.
42. Wang Ji, *Stone Mountain Medical Case Histories*, fascicle 2, p. 98. Wu Kun's *Research on Medical Formulas* notes that this physician was Dai Nianren 戴念仁; see p. 203.
43. Yu Zhen (ed.), *Comments on Medical Cases, Past and Present*, fascicle 6, p. 221.
44. Wang Ji, *Stone Mountain Medical Case Histories*, fascicle 2, p.98. According to Chen Jue, the compiler of *Stone Mountain*, the physician in this medical case should be Wang Ji. But the later medical works mentioned that the physician had actually been Han Shiliang 韓世良. Wu Kun, *Research on Medical Formulas*, fascicle 27, pp. 203–4; Zhang Jiebin, *The Classified Canon*, fascicle 12, pp. 39b–40a; Wei Zhixiu, *Supplements to Famous Physicians' Classified Medical Cases*, fascicle 10, p. 232.
45. J. Grant, *A Chinese Physician: Wang Ji and the Stone Mountain Medical Case Histories* (London: RoutledgeCurzon, 2003), pp. 98–9.
46. Lu Yitian 陸以湉, *Jingjiao lenglu yihua* 精校冷廬醫話 [Medical Discourses at the Studio of Lenglu] (1857; Taipei: Guoli zhongguo yiyao yanjiusuo, 1966), fascicle 2, p. 61.
47. Wu Jingzi 吳敬梓., *Rulin waishi* 儒林外史 [The Scholars] (Taipei: Lianjing chuban shiye gongsi, 1985 [1749?]), ch. 3, pp. 30–3.
48. Wei Zhixiu (ed.), *Supplements to Famous Physicians' Classified Medical Cases*, fascicle 21, p. 528; Chen Shanggu 陳尚古, 'Zanyunlou zasuo 簪雲樓雜說' [Miscellaneous Talks at the Zanyun Building], in *Biji xiaosuo daguan* 筆記小說大觀 [Great Spectacle of Jotting Books] (Taipei: Xinxing shuju, 1974), series 3, vol. 10, p. 6435b.
49. Qing Chengzi 青城子, Ziyi xubian 志異續編 [Supplementary Compilation to Strange Records], in Great Spectacle of Jotting Books, vol.22, fascicle 4, pp.5780a-5781b.
50. Zhang Congzheng, *The Scholar Serving His Kin*, fascicle 3, p. 83; fascicle 6, p. 173; fascicle 7, pp. 212–13.
51. Sivin, 'Emotional counter-therapy', p. 17.
52. Zhang Congzheng *The Scholar Serving His Kin* , fascicle 3, p. 112.
53. H. Chen, 'Between Passion and Repression: Medical Views of Demon Dreams, Demonic Fetuses and Female Sexual Madness in Late Imperial China', *Late Imperial China*, 32:1 (2011), p. 63.
54. Xu Yongcheng and Liu Chun, *Esoteric Meanings of the Jade Secrets*, fascicle 16, p. 245.
55. Yang Jizhou, *The Great Achievements of Acupuncture and Moxibustion*, fascicle 9, p. 375.
56. Wang Kentang, *Standard for Diagnosis and Treatment: Miscellaneous Disorders*, vol. 2, pp. 61–2.
57. Sivin, 'Emotional counter-therapy', p. 17.

3 Simonis, 'Medicaments and Persuasion: Medical Therapies for Madness in Nineteenth-Century China'

1. The case of Mr. Bao appears in the 'Insanity' 癲狂 section of Wu Tang's case collection: *Wu Jutong yian* 吳鞠通醫案 [Wu Jutong's Medical Case Files], in Li Liukun 李劉坤 (chief ed.), *Wu Jutong yixue quanshu* 吳鞠通醫學全書 [The Complete Medical Books of Wu Jutong] (Beijing: Zhongguo Zhongyiyao chubanshe, 1999), fascicle 2, p. 257. The case is undated, but the structure of the book suggests that it took place sometime between 1809 and 1827 (inclusively).
2. See F. Simonis, 'Mad Acts, Mad Speech and Mad People in Late Imperial Chinese Law and Medicine' (PhD dissertation, Princeton University, 2010), ch. 3–9, pp. 26–406.
3. I have analysed thirteen different terms by which a man's insanity was referred to in a criminal report dated 1736. See Simonis, 'Mad Acts', pp. 518–20.
4. A partial facsimile of the original Mawangdui manuscripts that appears on p. 194 (fourth line from the right) of D. Harper, *Early Chinese Medical Literature* (London: Royal Asiatic Society, 1998), clearly shows the compound *dianji* 瘨疾. Modern editions use the conventional modern characters *dianji* 癲疾 instead of the more authentic form. The character *dian* 瘨 also appears in the *Classic of Poetry*, where it refers to a generic 'malady'.
5. Luo Mei 羅美, 'Dian kuang xian zheng' 癲狂癇證 [The Symptoms of *Dian*, *Kuang* and *Xian*], *Gujin mingyi huicui* 古今名醫匯粹 [Florilegium from Illustrious Physicians Past and Present], fascicle 6, (Beijing: Zhongyi guji chubanshe, 1999), p. 206.
6. See Simonis, 'Mad Acts', pp. 418–19.
7. For more on 'trials of the insane', see P. Katz, *Divine Justice: Religion and the Development of Chinese Legal Culture* (London and New York: Routledge, 2009), pp. 105–9.
8. See K. C. Wong, 'A short history of psychiatry and mental hygiene in China', *Chinese Medical Journal*, 68 (1950), pp. 44–8; I. Veith, 'Psychiatric Thought in Chinese Medicine', *Journal of the History of Medicine and Allied Sciences*, 10 (1955), pp. 261–8; Shou Meilong 壽梅隆, 'Zuguo yixue zhong jingshenbingxue de fazhan yu chengjiu' 祖國醫學中精神病學的發展和成就 [Psychiatric Developments and Achievements in the Medicine of the Fatherland], *Xin Zhongyiyao* 新中醫藥 [New Chinese Medicine], 8:6 (1957), pp. 3–9; Xue Meng 薛盟, 'Zuguo yixue dui jingshenbing de renshi he zhiliao' 祖國醫學對精神病的認識和治療 [Knowledge and Treatment of Mental Illness in the Medicine of the Fatherland], *Zhejiang zhongyi zazhi* 浙江中醫雜誌 [Zhejiang Chinese Medicine Journal], 10 (1959), pp. 17–20; J. C. C. Cheng, 'Psychiatry in Traditional Chinese Medicine', *Canadian Psychiatric Association Journal*, 15 (August 1970), pp. 399–401; Tseng Wen-shing, 'The Development of Psychiatric Concepts in Traditional Chinese Medicine', *Archives of General Psychiatry*, 29 (1973), pp. 569–75; J. J. Kao, *Three Millennia of Chinese Psychiatry* (New York: The Institute for Advanced Research in Asian Science and Medicine, 1979); Liu Xiehe, 'Psychiatry in Traditional Chinese Medicine', *British Journal of Psychiatry*, 138 (1981), pp. 429–33; Fong Wing Loi 方永來 and Lee Cheng-yu 李政育, *Zhongguo chuantong yixue zhi jingshenbinglixue* 中國傳統醫學之精神病理學 [Psychopathology in Chinese Traditional Medicine] (Taipei: Qiye shuju, 1981–5); H. Ågren, 'The Conceptual History of Psychiatric Terms in Traditional Chinese Medicine', in Li Guohao, Zhang Mengwen and Cao Tianqin (eds), *Explorations in the History of Science and Technology in China* (Shanghai: Chinese Classics Publishing House, 1982), pp. 575–81; T'ien Ju-k'ang, 'Traditional Chinese Beliefs and Attitudes towards Mental Illness', in W. S. Tseng and D. Wu (eds), *Chinese Culture*

and Mental Health (New York: Academic Press, 1985), pp. 67–82; He Yumin 何裕民, *Zhongguo chuantong jingshenbinglixue* 中國傳統精神病理學 [Traditional Chinese Psychopathology] (Shanghai: Shanghai kexue puji chubanshe, 1995); and Liao Yuqun, 'The history of psychiatric diagnosis in traditional Chinese medicine', in Yosio Kawakita, Shizu Sakai and Yasuo Otsuka (eds), *History of Psychiatric Diagnoses* (Tokyo: Ishigaku Euro-America, Inc., 1997), pp. 239–51.

9. The expression 'grand titration' is from J. Needham, *The Grand Titration: Science and Society in East and West* (Cambridge: Cambridge University Press, 1969).
10. In addition to the titles cited in note 8, see Huang Jian 黃健, 'Zhubing yuanhou lun dui Zhongguo gudai jingshenbingxue de gongxian' 《諸病源候論》對中國古代精神病學發展的貢獻 [The Contributions of the *Treatise on the Origins and Symptoms of the Illnesses* to the Development of Ancient Chinese Psychiatry], *Zhonghua yishi zazhi* 中華醫史雜誌 [Chinese Journal of Medical History], 24:4 (1994), pp. 207–10; Huang Jian 黃健, 'Zhu Danxi yu woguo gudai de jingshenbingxue' 朱丹溪與我國古代的精神病學 [Zhu Danxi and Ancient Chinese Psychiatry], *Zhejiang Zhongyi zazhi* 浙江中醫雜誌 [Zhejiang Journal of Traditional Chinese Medicine], 30:8 (1995), pp. 365–6; and Huang Jian 黃健 and Guo Liwa 郭麗娃, 'Zhang Jingyue Zhongyi jingshenbingxue chutan' 張景岳中醫精神病學思想初探 [Preliminary Explorations on Zhang Jiebin's Thinking on TCM Psychiatry], *Zhonghua yishi zazhi* 中華醫史雜誌 [Chinese Journal of Medical History], 26:4 (1996), pp. 245–7.
11. These compilations are Hua Beiling 華蓓苓, Zhou Changfa 周長發 and Zhu Xinghai 朱興海, *Dian Kuang Xian* 癲狂癇 [*Dian*, *Kuang* and *Xian*] (Beijing: Zhongyi guji chubanshe, 1990); Shi Yuguang 史宇廣 and Shan Shujian 單書建 (eds), *Dangdai mingyi linzheng jinghua: dian kuang xian zhuanji* 當代名醫臨證精華–癲狂癇專輯 [The Best Therapies of Famous Contemporary Physicians: Dian-Kuang-Xian Volume] (Beijing: Zhongyi guji chubanshe, 1997); and Shan Shujian 單書健 and Chen Zihua 陳子華 (eds), *Gujin mingyi linzheng jinjian: dian kuang xian juan* 古今名醫臨證金鑒–癲狂癇卷 [The Golden Mirror of the Therapies of Famous Physicians Past and Present: Dian-Kuang-Xian Volume] (Beijing: Zhongguo Zhongyiyao chubanshe, 1999). Hans Ågren speaks of *dian*, *kuang* and *xian* as 'the three main madnesses' and 'the core triad of behavioural disorders in China'; Ågren 'The Conceptual History of Psychiatric Terms', p. 575. Nancy Chen claims that madness was 'differentiated into the three main categories of *dian*, *kuang* and *xian*'; N. Chen, 'Translating Psychiatry and Mental Health in Twentieth-Century China' in L. Liu (ed.), *Tokens of Exchange: The Problem of Translation in Global Circulations* (Durham, NC: Duke University Press, 1999), pp. 305–27, on p. 307. Chen Hsiu-fen calls them 'three major types of madness'; Chen Hsiu-fen 'Medicine, Society and the Making of Madness in Imperial China' (PhD dissertation, School of Oriental and African Studies, University of London, 2003), p. 78. Angelika Messner considers them as 'significant concepts for madness [*Irresein*] in late imperial times'; A. Messner, *Medizinische Diskurse zu Irresein in China (1600–1930)* (Stuttgart: Franz Steiner Verlag, 2000), p. 85.
12. For a more sustained critique of the *dian-kuang-xian* approach to insanity in Chinese medical history, see Simonis, 'Mad Acts', pp. 5–6, 43.
13. *Kuang* had been paired with *dian* since at least the first century BC, when *dian* was mostly understood as a disorder characterized by seizures. For more on the semantic evolution of *dian* and its relation to *kuang*, see Simonis, 'Mad Acts', pp. 47–53, 232–7, 298–304.
14. The expression 'behavioural dislocations' is from G. E. Berrios, 'Obsessional disorders during the nineteenth century: terminological and classificatory issues', in W. F. Bynum,

R. Porter and M. Sheperd (eds), *The Anatomy of Madness*, vol. 1: *People and Ideas* (London and New York: Tavistock, 1985), pp. 166–87, on p. 166.

15. See J. Kim, *Supervenience and Mind: Selected Philosophical Essays* (Cambridge: Cambridge University Press, 1993); and E. Savellos and U. Yalcin (eds), *Supervenience: New Essays* (Cambridge: Cambridge University Press, 1995).
16. I explain this transformation of the etiology of insanity in more detail in F. Simonis, 'Ghosts or mucus? Medicine for madness: new doctrines, therapies and rivalries', in J. Lagerwey (ed.), *Modern Chinese Religion*, Part 1: *Song, Liao, Jin and Yuan* (960–1368) (Leiden: Brill, forthcoming).
17. For more on this issue, see Ch'en Hsiu-fen 陳秀芬, 'Dang bingren jiandao gui: shilun Ming Qing dui "xiesui" de taidu' 當病人見到鬼: 試論明清醫者對「邪祟」的態度 [When Patients Saw Ghosts: A Preliminary Survey of the Attitudes of Ming and Qing Doctors toward Spectral Affliction], *Guoli zhengzhi daxue lishi xuebao* 國立政治大學歷史學報 [The Journal of History of National Chengchi University], 30 (2008), pp. 43–86; and Simonis, 'Mad Acts', chapter 8, pp. 326–66.
18. See respectively *Huainan zi* 淮南子 (late 2nd century BC), 'Jingshen xun' 精神訓 [Quintessential Spirit]; and Wang Qiyuan's 王啟源 preface to Luo Denggao's 駱登高 *Yilin yizhi* 醫林一致 [Unity in the Forest of Medicine] (1703).
19. Nathan Sivin makes similar points in N. Sivin, 'Emotional Counter-therapy', in *Medicine, Philosophy and Religion in Ancient China* (Aldershot, England: Ashgate, 1995), part 2, pp. 1–3.
20. *Zhangshi yitong* 張氏醫通 [Mr. Zhang's Comprehensive Medicine] fascicle 14, last entry of the section on *kuang* (狂門); in Zhang Minqing 張民慶, Wang Xinghua 王興華 and Liu Huadong 劉華東 (eds), *Zhang Lu yixue quanshu* 張璐醫學全書 [The Complete Medical Books of Zhang Lu] (Beijing: Zhongguo Zhongyiyao chubanshe, 1999), p. 467B.
21. The earliest and latest dated cases in Wu's case collection are from 1793 and 1833 respectively.
22. For more on Warm illnesses, see M. Hanson, *Speaking of Epidemics in Chinese Medicine: Disease and the Geographic Imagination in Late Imperial China* (London and New York: Routledge, 2011).
23. I discuss the rising dominance of this notion of illness and its effect on textual forms in F. Simonis, 'Illness, Texts and "Schools" in Danxi Medicine: A New Look at Chinese Medical History from 1320 to 1800', in B. Elman (ed.), *Antiquarianism, Language and Medical Philology: From Early Modern to Modern Sino-Japanese Medical Classics* (Leiden: Brill, forthcoming).
24. For more on the case form in Chinese medicine, see C. Cullen, 'Yi'an: The Origin of a Genre of Chinese Medical Literature', in E. Hsü (ed.), *Innovation in Chinese Medicine* (Cambridge: Cambridge University Press, 2001), pp. 292–323; and the relevant articles in C. Furth, J. Zeitlin and Hsiung Ping-chen (eds), *Thinking with Cases: Specialist Knowledge in Chinese Cultural History* (Honolulu, HI: University of Hawai'i Press, 2007).
25. 'Diankuang' 癲狂, *Wu Jutong's Medical Case Files*, in *The Complete Medical Books of Wu Jutong*, fascicle 2, ppp. 257A–B. The chronological arrangement of the dated cases in this section and the rest of the collection suggests that the undated cases were also chronologically arrayed.
26. For more on Wang's edition of the *Inner Canon*, see Qian Chaochen 錢超塵 (chief ed.), 'Huangdi neijing wenxian ji yuyan wenzi yanjiu' 《黃帝內經》文獻及語言文字研

究 [Research on the Documentation, Language and Written Style of the *Yellow Emperor's Inner Canon*] in Wang Hongtu 王洪图 (chief ed.), *Huangdi neijing yanjiu dacheng* 黃帝內經研究大成 [Complete Research on the *Yellow Emperor's Inner Canon*] (Beijing: Beijing chubanshe, 1997), pp. 15–107; and P. Unschuld, *Huang Di Nei Jing Su Wen: Nature, Knowledge, Imagery in an Ancient Chinese Medical Text* (Berkeley and Los Angeles, CA: University of California Press, 2003), pp. 39–58.

27. Basic Questions 11.6b, in chapter 40; in Zhang Dengben 張登本 and Sun Lijun 孫理軍 **(eds),** *Wang Bing yixue quanshu* 王冰醫學全書 [The Complete Medical Books of Wang Bing] (Beijing: Zhongguo Zhongyiyao chubanshe, 2006), p. 190A. *Dian* 瘨 in the passage that Wang was glossing should have read *ju* 疽 ('furuncles'). The sentence 'mineral drugs: eruption of furuncles; herbal drugs: manic fits' [石藥發疽 芳草發狂] appears in Huangfu Mi's 皇甫謐 *Zhenjiu jiayi jing* 針灸甲乙經 [AB Canon of Acumoxa], fascicle 11, part 5,'Wuqi yifa, xieke, huangdan 五氣溢發消渴黃癉' [Overflow of the Five Qi, Diabetes and Jaundice].
28. For more details on this shift in the meaning of *dian* outside medicine, see Simonis, 'Mad Acts', pp. 49–53.
29. In Song Naiguang 宋乃光 (chief ed.), *Liu Wansu yixue quanshu* 劉完素醫學全書 [The Complete Medical Books of Liu Wansu] (Beijing: Zhongguo Zhongyiyao chubanshe, 2006), p. 98B.
30. For more on the historical importance of Zhu Zhenheng's approach to medical learning, refer to Simonis, 'Illness, Texts and 'Schools' in Danxi Medicine'.
31. For more on counter-affect therapy, refer to Sivin, 'Emotional Counter-Therapy', pp. 1–19; Simonis, 'Mad Acts', pp. 88–94; and Ch'en Hsiu-fen's article in this volume. Modern Chinese scholars usually call this form of treatment the 'psychological healing method' (*xinli liaofa* 心理療法). See Xiao Guogang 蕭國鋼, *Rumen shiqin yanjiu* 儒門事親研究 [Research on The Scholar Serving his Kin] (Beijing: Zhongyi guji chubanshe, 1998), p. 16; and editorial comments in Deng Tietao 鄧鐵濤 (chief ed.), *Zihe yiji* 子和醫集 [Collected Medical Works of Zhang Congzheng] (Beijing: Renmin weisheng chubanshe, 1994), p. 404. The primary sources usually spoke of the 'overcoming of emotions' (*qing sheng* 情勝) or a variant thereof, in which 'overcoming' alluded to the 'mutual conquest' or 'mutual overcoming' (*xiangsheng* 相勝) cycle of the Five Agents (*wuxing* 五行).
32. See Yu Tuan 虞摶, 'Dian kuang xian zheng' 癲狂癇證 [*Dian*, *kuang* and *xian* disorders], and 'Lun' 論 [Discussion] in *Yixue zhengchuan* 醫學證傳 [The Correct Transmission of Medical Learning], 1515 edn (Beijing: Zhongyi guji chubanshe, 2002), fascicle 5, p. 309: 'Many people with lofty aspirations but who cannot fulfil their purpose have it [*dian*]' (多為求望高遠不得志者有之); and Sun Yikui 孫一奎, 'Dian kuang xian bian' 癲狂癇辨 [Distinctions between *dian, kuang* and *xian*], *Yizhi xuyu* 醫旨緒餘 [Residual (Discussions) on the Purport of Medicine], in Han Xuejie 韓學傑 and Zhang Yinsheng 張印生 (eds), *Sun Yikui yixue quanshu* 孫一奎醫學全書 [The Complete Medical Books of Sun Yikui], 1584 edn (Beijing: Zhongguo Zhongyiyao chubanshe, 1999), fascicle 1, p. 674: 'Many people with high ambitions but [whose achievements] do not follow their desires have it [*dian*]' (此志願高大而不遂所欲者多有之).
33. See Simonis, 'Mad Acts', chapters 5 and 6, pp. 136–263.
34. For information on the high number of doctors who could see the same patient when complicated illnesses arose, see Jiang Zhushan 蔣竹山, 'Qi Zhongmin gong riji zhong de yibing guanxi shiliao daodu' 《祁忠敏公日記》中的醫病關係史料導讀 [Guided Reading of Historical Sources on Doctor–Patient Relations in *Diary*

of Sire Qi Zhongmin] 2006, at www2.scu.edu.tw/history/PDF.report2006Jiang.pdf [accessed 15 November 2011]; and Zhu Pingyi 祝平一, '"Yao yi bu si bing, Fo du you yuan ren": Ming Qing de yiliao shichang, yixue zhishi yu yibing guanxi' 藥醫不死病，佛度有緣人：明、清的醫療市場、醫學知識與醫病關係 ['Drugs Cure Non-Mortal Illnesses; The Buddha Saves Those Who are so Destined': The Medical Market, Medical Knowledge and Doctor–Patient Relations in the Ming-Qing Period], *Zhongyang yanjiuyuan jindaishi yanjiusuo jikan* 中央研究院近代史研究所集刊 [Bulletin of the Institute of Modern History, Academia Sinica], 68 (2010), pp. 1–50.

35. J. Goldstein, *Console and Classify: The French Psychiatric Profession in the Nineteenth Century*, 1987 edn (Chicago, IL: University of Chicago Press, 2001), p. 383.
36. In Simonis, 'Mad Acts', chapter 13, pp. 509–43, I provide abundant evidence that ordinary Chinese people, by contrast, commonly traced madness (either their own or that of others) to various social stresses and failures.
37. Deng Tietao 鄧鐵濤 and Qiu Shijun 邱仕君, 'Wenbing xueshuo de fazhan he yufang baojian' 溫病學說的發展和預防保健 [The Development of the Warm-Illness Theory and its Prophylactic Health Practices]健, in Li Jingwei 李經緯 and Lin Zhaogeng 林昭庚 (chief eds), 'Zhongguo yixue tongshi' 中國醫學通史 [General History of Chinese Medicine] *Gudai juan* 古代卷 [Ancient Times] (Beijing: Renmin weisheng chubanshe, 2000), pp. 577–82, on p. 580.
38. This paste of Wu's invention, which was taken in the form of pellets, contained dozens of ingredients, some quite expensive. Wu typically used it at the end of his treatments of Warm-factor disorders to replenish Yin and balance Yang. The recipe appears in *Wenbing tiaobian* 溫病條辨 [Systematic Distinctions on Warm-Factor Illnesses], '*Qiuzao*' 秋燥; [Autumnal Dryness], in *The Complete Medical Books of Wu Jutong*, fascicle 3, p. 100A, and (with slight differences) in 'Yeshi' 噎食 [Dysphagia], *Wu Jutong yian* 吳鞠通醫案 [Wu Jutong's Medical Case Files], in *The Complete Medical Books of Wu Jutong*, fascicle 3, p. 291B.
39. Emplotment (*mise en intrigue*), a concept coined by literary theorist Paul Ricœur, refers to ways of presenting facts or claims in a narrative fashion. In H. White, *Tropics of Discourse: Essays in Cultural Criticism* (Baltimore: Johns Hopkins University Press, 1978), H. White, *The Content of the Form: Narrative Discourse and Historical Representation* (Baltimore: Johns Hopkins University Press, 1987) and other works, Hayden White argues that all historical texts, even non-narrative ones, are emplotted in ways that impart narrative meaning to facts despite their author's intention. Emplotment can of course be used purposely, as Wu Tang did in his medical case files.
40. *Tongmen xu zhi* 童門須知 [What Needs to be Known About Children], cited in W. T. Rowe, *Saving the World: Chen Hongmou and the Elite Consciousness in Eighteenth-Century China* (Stanford, CA: Stanford University Press, 2001), p. 417.
41. The citation is from C. Bell, *Ritual: Perspectives and Dimensions* (Oxford and New York: Oxford University Press, 1997), p. 117.
42. See A. Kleinman, *Rethinking Psychiatry: From Cultural Category to Personal Experience* (New York: The Free Press, 1988), pp. 108–41.
43. Many issues discussed in T. J. Csordas, 'The Affliction of Martin: Religious, Clinical and Phenomenological Meaning in a Case of Demonic Oppression', in A. Gaines (ed.), *Ethnopsychiatry: The Cultural Construction of Professional and Folk Psychiatries* (Albany, NY: State University of New York Press, 1992), pp. 125–70, apply very well to the case of Mr. Bao.

44. 'Interactive' and 'indifferent' kinds: I. Hacking, *The Social Construction of What?* (Cambridge, MA: Harvard University Press, 1999), pp. 115–17. Other citation: D. Holland, W. Lachicotte Jr., D. Skinner and C. Cain, *Identity and Agency in Cultural Worlds* (Cambridge, MA and London: Harvard University Press, 1998), p. 8. For another take on how some therapeutic processes allow patients to re-symbolize their experience in beneficial ways, see E. Corin, 'Facts and Meaning in Psychiatry: An Anthropological Approach to the Lifeworld of Schizophrenics', *Culture, Medicine and Psychiatry*, 14 (1990), pp. 153–88.
45. *Yi yi bing shu* 醫醫病書 [Curing the Ills of Medicine], in *The Complete Medical Books of Wu Jutong*, p. 150A.
46. For more on inner harm in Li Gao's writings, see Simonis, 'Mad Acts', pp. 99–103.
47. In the mapping of the Five Agents (*wuxing* 五行) on internal organs, Wood was paired with the Liver and Earth with the Stomach. 'Wood-riding-on-Earth' referred to a process by which excessive Liver Wind (or more rarely excessive Qi from the Gallbladder, which was the Yang counterpart of the Liver and thus also associated with Wood) encroached on the functions of the Stomach or the Spleen (the two Earth viscera). Depending on which scenario unfolded, the symptoms of 'Wood-riding-on-Earth' included vomiting and stomach pains or abdominal distension and coldness of the limbs. For a mention of 'Wood-riding-on-Earth' in Wu Tang's own works, see 'Yeshi' 噎食 [Dysphagia], *Curing the Ills of Medicine*, in *The Complete Medical Books of Wu Jutong*, p. 158B.
48. 'Zhi neishang xu zhuyou lun' 治內傷須祝由論 [On the Necessity of Invoking the Cause When Treating Inner Harm], *Curing the Ills of Medicine*, in *The Complete Medical Books of Wu Jutong*, p. 150.
49. 'Zhong zhang' 腫脹 [Swellings and bloats], *Wu Jutong's Medical Case Files*, in *The Complete Medical Books of Wu Jutong*, fascicle 2, p. 270.
50. Elsewhere in *Curing the Ills of Medicine*, Wu claimed that dysphagia often arose from anger long pent-up [其得病之由　多由怒鬱日久]; 'Yeshi' 噎食 [Dysphagia], *Curing the Ills of Medicine*, in *The Complete Medical Books of Wu Jutong*, p. 158A. See also the reference cited in the previous note.
51. The phrase is from Holland et al., *Identity and Agency in Cultural Worlds*, p. 3.
52. The citation is from H. Fabrega, Jr., 'The Position of Psychiatry in the Understanding of Human Disease', *Archives of General Psychiatry*, 32 (1975), pp. 1500–12, on p. 1500.

4 Szto, 'Psychiatric Space and Design Antecedents: The John G. Kerr Refuge for the Insane'

1. C. Selden, *Work Among the Chinese Insane And Some of its Results, 1901–1903* (Canton, China: The China Baptist Publication, Guangzhou Psychiatric Hospital Archives, 1903).
2. N. Diamant, 'China's 'Great Confinement': Missionaries, Municipal Elites and Police in the Establishment of Chinese Mental Hospitals', *Republican China*, 19:1 (1993), pp. 3–50; E. Goffman, *Asylums: Essays on the Social Situation of Mental Patients and Other Inmates* (New York: Anchor Books, 1959); J. J. Kao, *Three Millennia of Chinese Psychiatry* (New York: The Institute for Advanced Research in Asian Science and Medicine, 1979); V. Pearson, 'The Development of Modern Psychiatric Services in China, 1891–1949', *History of Psychiatry* 2:6 (1991), pp. 133–47; L. Topp, J. Moran and J. Andrews (eds), *Madness, Architecture and the Built Environment: Psychiatric Spaces in Historical*

Context (London: Routledge, 2007); C. Yanni, *The Architecture of Madness: Insane Asylums in the United States* (Minneapolis, MN: University of Minnesota Press, 2007).

3. B. Edginton, 'The Well-Ordered Body: The Quest for Sanity through Asylum Architecture', *Canadian Bulletin of Medical History*, 11:2 (1994), pp. 375–86; R. Porter and D. Wright (eds), *The Confinement of the Insane: International Perspectives, 1800–1965* (New York: Cambridge University Press, 2003); R. Porter, W. F. Bynum and M. Shepherd (eds), *The Anatomy of Madness: Essays in the History of Psychiatry* (London: Routledge, 1988); Topp, Moran and Andrews (eds), *Madness, Architecture and the Built Environment.*
4. *The John G. Kerr Refuge for Insane* is the original name of the hospital. Scientific nomenclature influenced its name change so that 'Insane Asylum' replaced 'Refuge' in 1901 and 'Asylum' was changed to 'Hospital' in 1904. The People's Republic of China (PRC) changed the name to *The Guangzhou Psychiatric Hospital* in 1949. Today, the hospital is called the *Guangzhou Brain Hospital.* In this study the terms 'refuge', 'institution', 'insane asylum' and 'asylum care' are used interchangeably.
5. C. Selden, 'The John G. Kerr Refuge for Insane', *The China Medical Journal*, 22:2 (March 1908), pp. 84.
6. Guangzhou and Canton refer to the same city. *Guangzhou* is the historic name of the ancient port city and provincial capital of Guangdong. It is the name of the city today. *Canton* is a mispronunciation, in a British accent, of Guangdong. Throughout the nineteenth century and for most of the twentieth century the descriptor Canton was used.
7. Porter and Wright (eds), *The Confinement of the Insane.*
8. A. Scull, *Museums of Madness: The Social Organization of insanity in Nineteenth Century England* (New York: St. Martin's Press 1979); Yanni, *The Architecture of Madness,* pp. 1–15; Topp, Moran and Andrews (eds), *Madness, Architecture and the Built Environment.*
9. P. Szto, 'Cultural context and social technology transfer: the case of Canton, China', *International Journal of Social Welfare* 16:1 (2007), pp. 55–64, on p. 56.
10. Szto, 'Cultural context and social technology transfer', p. 56.
11. Y. Tsu, *The Spirit of Chinese Philanthropy: A Study in Mutual Aid* (New York: AMS Press, 1912), p. 70.
12. V. W. Ng, *Madness in Late Imperial China: From Illness to Deviance* (Norman, OK: University of Oklahoma Press, 1990)
13. D. Y. F. Ho, 'On the concept of face', *American Journal of Sociology*, 81:4 (1976), pp. 867–84; D. Ho, 'The concept of 'face' in Chinese-American interaction', in W. C. Hu and C. L. Grove (eds), *Encountering the Chinese: A guide for Americans* (Yarmouth, ME: Intercultural Press, 1991), pp. 111–24.
14. M. H. Bond (ed.), *The Psychology of the Chinese People* (Hong Kong: Oxford University Press, 1986), p. 243.
15. S. Naquin and E. S. Rawski, *Chinese Society in the Eighteenth Century* (New Haven, CT: Yale University Press, 1987).
16. K. Frampton, *Studies in Tectonic Culture: The Poetics of Construction in Nineteenth and Twentieth Century Architecture*, ed. J. Cava (Cambridge, MA: The MIT Press, 1995), p. 8.
17. M. J. Dear and S. M. Taylor, *Not on Our Street: Community Attitudes to Mental Health Care* (London: Pion Limited, 1982); C. Philo, *A Geographical History of Institutional Provision for the Insane from Medieval Times to the 1860s in England and Wales: The Space Reserved for Insanity* (Lewiston, NY: Edward Mellen Press, 2004).

18. Robert Morrison (1782–1834) was the first Protestant missionary to China who arrived in 1804 under the sponsorship of the London Missionary Society.
19. A. Scull, *Madhouses, Mad-Doctors and Madmen: The Social History of Psychiatry in the Victorian Era* (Philadelphia, PA: University of Pennsylvania Press, 1983), p. 10.
20. M. Kerr, 'Presbyterian Board of Foreign Missions action' (Philadelphia, PA: Presbyterian Historical Archives, n.d.).
21. A. Deutsch, *The Mentally Ill in America: A history of Their Care and Treatment from Colonial Times* (New York: Doubleday, Doran & Company, Inc., 1937); N. Tomes, *The Art of Asylum-Keeping: Thomas Story Kirkbride and the Origins of American Psychiatry* (Philadelphia, PA: University of Pennsylvania Press, 1984); Yanni, *The Architecture of Madness*, pp. 24–9.
22. In the Sermon on the Mount Jesus said, 'You are the light of the world. A city on a hill cannot be hidden' (Matthew 5:14).
23. N. Pevsner, *A History of Building Types* (Princeton, NJ: Princeton University Press, 1976), p. 139.
24. Ibid.
25. Ibid., p. 141.
26. Ibid., p. 147.
27. Ibid.
28. P. Day, *A New History of Social Welfare* (New Jersey: Prentice Hall, 1989).
29. Pevsner, *A History of Building Types*, p. 150.
30. Ibid., p. 139.
31. The transfer of psychiatric space also took hold in India, Africa and Southeast Asia as a function of colonialization. The focus here is on the transfer to China.
32. C. Rosenberg, *The Care of Strangers: The Rise of America's Hospital System* (New York: Basic Books, 1987).
33. T. A. Markus, *Buildings and Power: Freedom and Control in the Origin of Modern Building Types* (London: Routledge, 1993); C. Stevenson, *Medicine and Magnificence: British Hospital and Asylum Architecture, 1660–1815* (New Haven, CT: Paul Mellon Centre for Studies in British Art and Yale University Press, 2000).
34. Tomes, *The Art of Asylum-Keeping*, p. 131.
35. Ibid., p. 5.
36. Deutsch, *The Mentally Ill in America*, p. 77.
37. Tomes, *The Art of Asylum-Keeping*, p. 4.
38. G. Grob, *The Mad Among Us: The History of the Care of America's Mentally Ill* (New York: Free Press, 1994), p. 29.
39. *An Account of the Events Surrounding the Origins of Friends Hospital & A Brief Description of the Early Years of Friends Asylum, 1817–1820* (Philadelphia, PA: Winchell Company, 1988), p. 9.
40. P. F. Clement, 'The Philadelphia Welfare Crisis of the 1820s', *The Pennsylvania Magazine of History and Biography*, 105:2 (April 1981), p. 59.
41. *An Account of the Events*, p. 16.
42. Grob, *The Mad Among Us*, p. 64.
43. The Pennsylvania Hospital for the Insane is called today The Institute of Pennsylvania Hospital.
44. Tomes, *The Art of Asylum-Keeping*, p. 139.
45. Ibid.
46. Yanni, *The Architecture of Madness*, p. 38.

47. J. G. Kerr, *Medical Missions.* (Canton, China: Presbyterian Board of Publication and Sabbath-School Work, 1895), p. 21.
48. *Jefferson Alumni Bulletin* (Philadelphia, PA: Jefferson Hospital Library Archives, August 1963).
49. Canton Medical Hospital Annual Report, *Medical Missionary Society* (Philadelphia, PA: Presbyterian Historical Archives, 1872), pp. 17–18.
50. Selden, 'The John G. Kerr Refuge for Insane', p. 83.
51. J. G. Kerr, 'The 'Refuge for the Insane', Canton', *The China Medical Missionary Journal,* 12: 4 (December, 1898), p. 178.
52. J. G. Kerr, *A Guide to the City and Suburbs of Canton* (Shanghai-Singapore-Yokohama: Kelly & Walsch, Ltd, 1918), p. 11.
53. Selden, *Work Among the Chinese Insane And Some of its Results, 1901–1903.*
54. C .C. Selden, 'Work Among the Chinese Insane and Some of its Results', *The China Medical Missionary Journal,* 19:1 (January 1905), Guangzhou Psychiatric Hospital Archives, p. 8.
55. W. Cadbury and M. Jones, *At the Point of a Lancet: One Hundred Years of the Canton Hospital, 1835–1935* (Hong Kong and Singapore: Kelly and Walsh, Limited, 1935); B. C. Henry, *The Cross and the Dragon or Light in the Broad East* (New York: Anson D. F. Randolph and Company, 1885).
56. Henry, *The Cross and the Dragon*, p. 51.
57. J. D. Thompson and G. Goldin, *The Hospital: A Social and Architectural History* (New Haven: Yale University Press, 1975), p. 79.
58. *Report for the years 1907 and 1908* (Canton, China: China Baptist Publication Society, 1909), inside cover.
59. H. Noyes, *China Born: Adventures of a Maverick Bookman* (San Francisco, CA: China Books & Periodicals, Inc., 1989), p. 14.
60. Kerr, 'The 'Refuge for the Insane', Canton', p. 178.
61. Selden, 'Work Among the Chinese Insane', p. 1.
62. C. C. Selden, 'The Need of More Hospitals for Insane in China', *The China Medical Journal,* 24 (1910), p. 326.
63. Kerr, 'The 'Refuge for the Insane', Canton', p. 178.
64. Selden, 'The Need of More Hospitals for Insane in China', p. 328.
65. In a personal interview in 1994 with *Mo Gan Ming*, the hospital's superintendent between 1945 and 1988, shared with the author that during the Japanese occupation of Canton (1938 to 1945) three French Catholic nuns managed the hospital. He reported the hospital treated between 600–700 patients and that the mortality rate was extremely high due to malnutrition. He estimated approximately 300 patients died annually.
66. Selden, *Work Among the Chinese Insane And Some of its Results, 1901–1903*, p. 6.
67. D. Brady, 'Review of *Hospital and Asylum Architecture in England 1840–1914: Building for Health Care* (London: Mansell Publishing, 1991) by Jeremy Taylor', *Medical History,* 38:2 (1994), pp. 219–20.

5 Ma, 'An Iron Cage of Civilization? Missionary Psychiatry, the Chinese Family and a Colonial Dialectic of Enlightenment'

1. S. LaFraniere, 'Neglect and Abuse: Life in Shadows for Mentally Ill in China', *New York Times,* 10 November 2010 at http://www.nytimes.com/2010/11/11/world/asia/11psych.html?scp=1&sq=mentally%20ill%20china&st=cse [accessed 25 February 2012].
2. For example, see http://roll.sohu.com/20120221/n335385091.shtml, [accessed 2 June 2013].
3. C. Selden, 'The John G. Kerr Refuge for Insane', *The China Medical Journal*, 22:2 (March 1908), pp. 82–91.
4. J. Harris, 'Pinel Delivering the Insane', *Archives of General Psychiatry,* 60:6 (2003), p. 552.
5. For example, A. H. Woods, 'The Nervous Diseases of the Chinese', *Archives of Neurology and Psychiatry* (1929), pp. 542–70, on p. 569.
6. See, for example, Jie Li, 'The First Psychiatric Hospital in China', *The British Journal of Psychiatry,* 197 (2010), p. 440. Lulu Zhang & Yuping Ning, 'Guangzhou Psychiatric Hospital: the Oldest Psychiatric Hospital in China', *Psychiatry*, 7 (2010), pp. 53–4., on p. 53.
7. J. J. Kao, *Three Millennia of Chinese Psychiatry* (New York: The Institute for Advanced Research in Asian Science and Medicine, 1979), p. 18. See also P. Szto, *The Accommodation of Insanity in Canton, China: 1857–1935* (Doctoral dissertation, University of Pennsylvania, 2002).
8. Nianqun Yang, *Zaizao Bingren: Zhong Xi Yi Chongtu Xia De Kongjian Zhengzhi (1832–1985)* [Remaking 'Patients': Politics of Space in the Conflicts between Traditional Chinese Medicine and Western Medicine (1832–1985)] (Beijing: China Renmin University Press, 2006).
9. See Yang, Remaking 'Patients', p. 8 for a similar critique of the impact-response framework in historical studies of Western medicine in China. But his own analysis perceives the Kerr Refuge as 'basically a transplantation and copy of the York retreat in Britain' and it also takes the missionaries' description of the constraining Chinese family at face value.
10. J. Comaroff, *Body of Power, Spirit of Resistance: The Culture and History of a South African People* (Chicago, IL:: University of Chicago Press, 1985). In particular, Comaroff's work has pointed out to me the dialectics in 'the historical articulation of systems dominant and subordinate' and the 'reciprocal determination' between the colonizers' and the colonized people's understandings of themselves and each other (p. 252). Also see R. Rogaski, *Hygienic Modernity: Meanings of Health and Disease in Treaty-Port China* (Berkeley, CA: University of California Press, 2004).
11. M. Weber, *Economy and Society*, trans G. Roth & C. Wittich (Berkeley, CA: University of California Press, 1978), p. 25.
12. Ibid. Instrumental rationality is also called means-end rationality.
13. M. Weber, *The Protestant Ethic and the Spirit of* Capitalism, trans. T. Parsons (New York: Scribner, 1976); M. Weber, *Weber: Political Writings (Cambridge Texts in the History of Political Thought)*, trans. Ronald Speirs (Cambridge: Cambridge University Press, 1994).
14. T. Barlow, 'Colonialism's Career in Postwar China Studies', *Positions* (1993), pp. 224–67. D. Chakrabarty, *Provincializing Europe: Postcolonial Thought and Historical Difference* (Princeton, NJ: Princeton University Press, 2000); G. Spivak, 'Can the Subaltern Speak?' in Cary Nelson & Lawrence Grossberg (eds), *Marxism and the Interpretation of Culture* (Urbana, IL: University of Illinois Press, 1998), pp. 271–313.

15. V. Schwarcz, *The Chinese Enlightenment: Intellectuals and the Legacy of the May Fourth Movement of 1919* (Berkeley, CA: University of California Press, 1990).
16. S. Glosser, *Chinese Visions of Family and the State, 1915–1953* (Berkeley, CA: University of California Press, 2003); J. Stacey, *Patriarchy and Socialist Revolution* (Berkeley, CA: University of California Press, 1983).
17. M. Horkheimer and T. Adorno, *Dialectic of Enlightenment: Philosophical Fragments*, trans. Edmund Jephcott (Stanford, CA: Stanford University Press, 1947), p. 2.
18. Ibid., p. 9.
19. Other scholars who have deconstructed the notion of universal patriarchy include M. Rosaldo, 'The Use and Abuse of Anthropology: Reflections on feminism and cross-cultural understanding', *Signs*, 5:3 (1980), pp. 389–417. Also see Chakrabarty, *Provincializing Europe*, pp. 214–36.
20. Barlow, 'Colonialism's Career in Postwar China Studies', p. 229.
21. A. L. Stoler, *Carnal Knowledge and Imperial Power: Race and the Intimate in Colonial Rule* (Berkeley, CA: University of California Press, 2002).
22. Barlow, 'Colonialism's Career in Postwar China Studies', p. 254.
23. Ibid.
24. Tong Lam, *A Passion for Facts: Social Surveys and the Construction of the Chinese Nation-State, 1900–1949* (Berkeley, CA: University of California Press, 2010).
25. For studies on the biologized and desiring individual, see for instance H. Chiang, 'Epistemic Modernity and the Emergence of Homosexuality in China', *Gender and History*, 22:3 (2010), pp. 629–57. For studies on the biopolitics of population, see for instance Lam, *A Passion for Facts*, pp. 50–74. Rogaski, *Hygienic Modernity*, pp. 1–21 and S. Lei, 'Moral Community of *Weisheng*: Contesting Hygiene in Republican China', *East Asian Science, Technology and Society: an International Journal* 3 (2009) pp. 475–504 both focus on individual-population dynamics in the hygienic projects.
26. M. Thompson, 'Foucault, Fields of Governability and the Population-Family-Economy Nexus in China', *History and Theory*, 51 (2012), pp. 42–62.
27. M. Foucault, 'Nietzsche, Genealogy, History' in Paul Rabinow (ed.), *The Foucault Reader* (New York: Pantheon, 1977), p. 78.
28. In fact, some scholars have pointed out that Foucault's scattered discussions of the family constitute a genealogy, a decisive shift 'from an axiomatic of alliance to an axiomatic of sexuality' in Europe and America in the eighteenth and nineteenth centuries'; Thompson, 'Foucault, Fields of Governability and the Population-Family-Economy Nexus in China', p. 44. See also C. Taylor, 'Foucault and Familial Power', *Hypatia*, 27:1 (2012), pp. 201–18. While benefiting from their insights on genealogies of the family, I nevertheless do not take the Euro-American notions of domesticity in Foucault's work for granted.
29. M.-R. Trouillot, *Silencing the Past: Power and the Production of History* (Boston, MA: Beacon Press, 1995).
30. C. Wenyon, 'Letter to the Editor', *China Medical Missionary Journal*, 6 (1892), p. 6.
31. R. Porter, 'Diseases of Civilization', in W. F. Bynum and R. Porter (eds), *Companion Encyclopedia of the History of Medicine* (London: Routledge, 1993), pp. 585–600.
32. See Chapter Four, pp. 71–90.
33. J. Harvey, 'The Insane in China', in *The China Medical Journal* (1920), pp. 104–5, on p. 104.
34. Selden, 'The John Kerr Refuge for the Insane', pp. 82–91. Similar general discussions could also be found in, for example, C. C. Selden, 'II. Treatment of the Insane', *The China Medical Journal* (1909), pp. 221–32.

35. Chakrabarty, *Provincializing Europe*, pp. 121–2.
36. Ibid., p. 119.
37. J. Allen Hofmann, 'A Report of the Patients Discharged from the John G. Kerr Hospital for Insane During 1912' *The China Medical Journal* (1913), pp. 369–79, on p. 370.
38. C. C. Selden, 'A Work for the Insane in China: The John G. Kerr Refuge for Insane, Fong Tsuen, Canton', *The Chinese Recorder*, XL (May 1909), pp. 262–7.
39. J. G. Kerr, 'The 'Refuge for the Insane', Canton', *The China Medical Missionary Journal*, 12: 4 (December, 1898), p. 177–8. Italics added.
40. Chakrabarty, *Provincializing Europe*, pp. 118.
41. F. Simonis, 'Mad Acts, Mad Speech and Mad People in Late Imperial Chinese Law and Medicine' (PhD dissertation, Princeton University, 2010), pp. 780–1.
42. V. W. Ng, *Madness in Late Imperial China: From Illness to Deviance* (Norman, OK: University of Oklahoma Press, 1990).
43. de Certeau distinguishes spatial strategy and tactics. While official strategies divide and police urban space, people in their everyday life often engage in tactics that negotiate and resist these official spatial boundaries and claim meanings of space on their own terms. See M. de Certeau, *The Practice of Everyday Life* (Berkeley, CA: University of California Press, 1984).
44. C. C. Selden, 'The Need of More Hospitals for Insane in China', *The China Medical Journal*, 24 (1910), p. 325–30.
45. Selden, 'The John G. Kerr Refuge for the Insane', p. 83.
46. The other half was transferred from the Government Lunatic Asylum in Hong Kong. See Selden, 'II. Treatment of the Insane', p. 231.
47. The John G. Kerr Refuge for the Insane, Report for 1909 (Canton, China: The China Baptist Publication Society, 1909), p. 4. Missionaries themselves used the word 'belief'.
48. Selden, 'A Work for the Insane in China', pp. 262–7.
49. For example, see Woods, 'The Nervous Diseases of the Chinese', p. 569.
50. Selden 'II. Treatment of the Insane', p. 228.
51. Ibid.
52. Kerr, 'The 'Refuge for the Insane', Canton', pp. 177–8.
53. N. Diamant, 'China's 'Great Confinement': Missionaries, Municipal Elites and Police in the Establishment of Chinese Mental Hospitals', *Republican China*, 19:1 (1993), pp. 3–50
54. Simonis, 'Mad Acts', pp. 326–66.
55. J. L. McCartney, 'Neuropsychiatry in China; A Preliminary Observation', *China Medical Journal* (1926), pp. 617–26, on p. 621.
56. Horkheimer & Adorno, *Dialectic of Enlightenment*, p. 9.
57. The idea of materialization of the body through reiteration of a norm comes from J. Butler, *Bodies That Matter: On the discursive limits of 'sex'* (New York: Routledge, 1993).
58. R. Ross, 'The Treatment of the Insane', *The China Medical Journal* (1920), pp. 580–1.
59. Ibid., p.581.
60. D. Haraway, 'Situated Knowledges: The Science Question in Feminism and the Privilege of Partial Perspective', *Simians, Cyborgs and Women: The reinvention of nature* (New York: Routledge, 1991), pp. 183–201. Haraway argues that with the use of a prosthesis, our body reaches outward and perceives reality through mingling with other bodies, which are never just distant objects.
61. Hoffmann, 'A Report of the Patients Discharged', pp. 369–79, on p. 379.

62. For the rise of the eugenic subject and its accompanying moral discourse in the U.S., see W. Kline, *Building a Better Race: Gender, Sexuality and Eugenics from the Turn of the Century to the Baby Boom* (Berkeley, CA: University of California, 1995).
63. Harvey, 'The Insane in China', p. 104.
64. R. M. Ross, 'Mental Hygiene', *The China Medical Journal* (1926), pp. 8–13, on p. 10.
65. Yumin He, *Chinese Traditional Psychopathology* (Shanghai, China: Shanghai Popular Science Press, 1995).
66. For example, The John G. Kerr Hospital for the Insane, Report for the Years 1922 and 1923 (Canton, China: The China Baptist Publication Society, 1923).
67. Foucault also analyzes the modern family as a disciplinary power that is plugged into medical control, a space in which parents become doctor-figures, closely monitoring and correcting children's behavior and psychological status. See M. Foucault, *Abnormal: Lectures at the Collège de France, 1974–1975* (New York: Picador, 2003).
68. Ross, 'Mental Hygiene', p.13.
69. Ibid., p.10.
70. D. Kevles, *In the Name of Eugenics: Genetics and the Uses of Human Heredity* (Cambridge, MA: Harvard University Press, 1985), p. 107.
71. Ross, 'Mental Hygiene', p. 10.
72. Ibid., p. 11.
73. Woods, 'The Nervous Diseases of the Chinese', p. 565.
74. McCartney, 'Neuropsychiatry in China', p. 836.
75. Woods, 'The Nervous Diseases of the Chinese', p. 566. Italics added.
76. McCartney, 'Neuropsychiatry in China', p. 837.
77. A. H. Woods, 'Removal of the Cause', *The China Medical Journal* (1928), pp. 366–8, on p. 367.
78. Pan Guangdan, *Feng Xiaoqing: Yijian Yinglian zhi Yanjiu* [Feng Xiaoqing: A Study of Narcissism] 1929 edn reprinted in Pan Naimu & Pan Naihe (eds), *Pan Guangdan Wenji* [Collection of Pan Guangdan's Work], vol. 1. (Beijing: Peking University Press, 2002), vol. 1, pp. 1–66.
79. Haiyan Lee, *Revolution of the Heart: A Genealogy of Love in China, 1900–1950* (Stanford, CA: Stanford University Press, 2006) pp. 191, 216.
80. G. Blowers, 'Bingham Dai, Adolf Storfer and the Tentative Beginnings of Psychoanalytic Culture in China: 1935–1941', *Psychoanalysis and History,* 6:1 (2004), pp. 93–105.
81. Bingham Dai, 'Personality Problems in Chinese Culture', *American Sociological Review,* 4:5(1941), pp. 688–96.
82. A. H. Woods, 'A Memorandum to Chinese Medical Students on the Medicolegal Aspects of Insanity', *National Medical Journal of China,* 9 (1923), pp. 203–12, on p. 204.
83. The Commission on Extraterritoriality, *The Provisional Criminal Code of the Republic of China Embodying Presidential Mandates, the Provisional Criminal Code Amendment Act, the Revised Draft of the Law on Offences Relating to Morphine, Revised Regulations Governing Military Criminal Cases, Regulations Governing Naval Criminal Cases* (1923).
84. Chakrabarty, *Provincializing Europe*, pp. 97–113.
85. Barlow argues in her study on cultural colonialism's influences on Cold War China studies that 'when you erase a mark what you have is an erasure. The displaced knowledge is never fully replaced by what succeeds it. That is the reason why I argue throughout this essay that occluding one thing [colonialism as a category, semicolonialism in China] enabled another thing [Cold War China studies]'. Barlow, 'Colonialism's Career in Postwar China Studies', p. 225. The logic applies here.

6 Wang, 'Tropical Neurasthenia or Oriental Nerves? White Breakdowns in China'

1. G. B. Price, 'Discussion on the Causes of Invaliding from the Tropics', *British Medical Journal* (15 November 1913), pp. 1290–3, on p. 1291.
2. 'The Health of Missionaries', *China Medical Journal*, 29:5 (1915), pp. 331–5.
3. F. Oldt, 'Nervous Disorders of Sexual Origin', *China Medical Journal*, 33:5 (1919), pp. 446–53.
4. W. Lennox, *The Health of Missionary Families in China: A Statistical Study* (Denver, CO: University of Denver, 1920), pp. 92f, 118.
5. F. Sargent II, 'Tropical Neurasthenia: Giant or Windmill?', *Environmental Physiology and Psychology in Arid Conditions* (Geneva: UNESCO, 1963), pp. 273–314; D. Kennedy, 'Diagnosing the Colonial Dilemma: Tropical Neurasthenia and the Alienated Briton', in D. Ghosh and D. Kennedy (eds), *Decentring Empire* (Hyderabad, India: Orient Longman, 2006), pp. 157–81.
6. Sir R. Havelock Charles, 'Neurasthenia and its Bearing on the Decay of Northern Peoples in India', *Transactions of the Royal Society of Tropical Medicine and Hygiene*, 7:1 (1913), pp. 2–31, on p. 11.
7. G. T. Trewartha, 'Recent Thought on the Problem of White Acclimatization in the Wet Tropics', *Geographical Review*, 16:3 (1926), pp. 467–78, on p. 476.
8. C. J. Singapore, 'Mental Irritability and Breakdown in the Tropics', *British Medical Journal* (13 March 1926), pp. 503–4.
9. M. Jackson, 'Mental Irritability and Breakdown in the Tropics', *British Medical Journal* (22 May 1926), p. 884; J. W. Linsay, 'Mental Irritability and Breakdown in the Tropics', *British Medical Journal* (29 May 1926), p. 920; H. M. Hanschell, 'Mental Irritability and Breakdown in the Tropics', *British Medical Journal* (10 April 1926), p. 676; R. van Someren, 'Mental Irritability and Breakdown in the Tropics', *British Medical Journal* (27 March 1926), p. 596; M. Iles, 'Mental Irritability and Breakdown in the Tropics', *British Medical Journal* (10 April 1926), p. 676; E. R. Hunt, 'Mental Irritability and Breakdown in the Tropics', *British Medical Journal* (10 April 1926), pp. 676–7; L. D. Parson, 'Mental Irritability and Breakdown in the Tropics', *British Medical Journal* (22 May 1926), p. 884; R. M. Barrow, 'Mental Irritability and Breakdown in the Tropics', *British Medical Journal* (4 April 1926), p. 634; 'Neurosis in the Tropics', *British Medical Journal* (17 March 1928), pp. 445–52.
10. W. E. Masters, *Essentials of Tropical Medicine* (London: John Bale, Sons & Danielsson, 1920), p.26; Ch. Joyeux, *Précis de Médecine Coloniale* (Paris: Masson et Cie, 1927), pp. 251–2; L. Rogers and J. W. D. Megaw, *Tropical Medicine* (London: J. & A. Churchill, 1930), pp. 481–3.
11. P. H. Manson-Bahr, *Manson's Tropical Diseases*, 10th edn (London: Cassell & Co., Ltd, 1935), p. 604.
12. D. Kennedy, 'The Perils of the Midday Sun: Climatic Anxieties in the Colonial Tropics', in J. M. MacKenzie (ed.), *Imperialism and the Natural World* (Manchester: Manchester University Press, 1990), pp. 118–40.
13. Kennedy, 'Diagnosing the Colonial Dilemma', pp. 157–81.
14. W. Anderson, 'The Trespass Speaks: White Masculinity and Colonial Breakdown', *American Historical Review* 102:5 (1997), pp. 1343–70; W. Anderson, *Colonial Pathologies: American Tropical Medicine, Race and Hygiene in the Philippines* (Durham, NC: Duke University Press, 2006), pp. 130–57. A similar argument recently has been made

in a wider colonial context. See S. Maß, 'Welcome to the Jungle: Imperial Men, 'Inner Africa' and Mental Disorder in Colonial Context', in M. Reinkowski and G. Thum (eds), *Helpless Imperialists: Imperial Failure, Fear and Radicalization* (Göttingen: Vandenhoeck & Ruprecht, 2013), pp. 92–116.

15. A. Crozier, 'What Was Tropical about Tropical Neurasthenia? The Utility of the Diagnosis in the Management of British East Africa', *Journal of the History of Medicine and Allied Sciences*, 64:4 (2009), pp. 518–48.
16. S. Mahone, 'The Psychology of Rebellion: Colonial Medical Responses to Dissent in British East Africa', *Journal of African History*, 47:2 (2006), pp. 241–58. For another interesting analysis on the use of neurasthenia in constructing the identity of the colonized population in the history of European psychiatry, see I. L. Christensen and S. Rud, 'Arctic Neurasthenia: The Case of Greenlandic Kayak Fear 1864–1940', *Social History of Medicine* 26:3 (2013), pp. 489–509.
17. Yu-Chuan Wu and Huei-Wen Teng 巫毓荃，鄧惠文, 'Re, shenjing shuairuo yu zaitai riren: Zhimin wanqi taiwan de jingshen yixue lunshu 熱、神經衰弱與在台日人: 殖民晚期台灣的精神醫學論述' [Neurasthenia and the Japanese Colonizers: The Psychiatric Discourses in the Late Colonial Taiwan], *Taiwan: A Radical Quarterly in Social Study*, 54 (2004), pp. 61–103.
18. Yu-Chuan Wu巫毓荃, 'Sixiang bing yu 'xing zhenghouqun': Rizhi wanqi taiwan ri tai ren nanxing de xinqizheng 思鄉病與「性症候群」：日治晚期台灣日台人男性的心氣症' [Nostalgia and 'Sexual Syndrome': Hypochondriasis and Masculinity in Late Colonial Taiwan], *Journal of Women's and Gender Studies*, 21 (2006), pp. 1–46.
19. D. N. Livingstone, 'Tropical Climate and Moral Hygiene: The Anatomy of a Victorian Debate', *British Journal for the History of Science*, 32 (1999), pp. 93–110.
20. W. Anderson, 'Biomedicine in Chinese East Asia: From Semicolonial to Postcolonial?' in A. Ki Che Leung and C. Furth (eds), *Health and Hygiene in Chinese East Asia: Politics and Publics in the Long Twentieth Century* (Durham, NC: Duke University Press, 2010), pp. 273–8.
21. W. Flynt and G. W. Berkle, *Taking Christianity to China: Alabama Missionaries in the Middle Kingdom, 1850–1950* (Tuscaloosa, AL: The University of Alabama Press, 1997), pp. 118–21; J. G. Lutz, 'Attrition among Protestant Missionaries in China, 1807–1890', *International Bulletin of Missionary Research* 36:1 (2012), pp. 22–7.
22. Annual reports of the Army Medical Department only provided statistic data on 'the diseases of the nervous system', without further explanation on their etiology or regional variations. See *Army Medical Department Report for the Year 1890*, vol. 32 (London: Harrison and Sons, 1892), p. 114; *Army Medical Department Report for the Year 1891*, vol. 33 (London: Harrison and Sons, 1893), p. 117; *Army Medical Department Report for the Year 1896*, vol. 38 (London: Harrison and Sons, 1897), p. 126; *Army Medical Department Report for the Year 1897*, vol. 39 (London: Harrison and Sons, 1898), p. 50.
23. M. Duncan, *The Missionary Mail to Faithful Friends and Candid Critics* (London: Elliot Stock, 1900), pp. 44–5; P. S. Grant, *Observations in Asia* (New York: Brentano's, 1908), pp. 134–5; H. B. Taylor, 'A Plea for the Wider Use of Psycho–Therapy, with Report of Cases', *China Medical Journal*, 24:2 (1910), pp. 104–9; The Missionaries in the Field, *White unto Harvest* (Minneapolis, MN: The Board of Foreign Missions, 1919), p. 52.
24. J. Speicher, *The Conquest of Cross in China* (London: Fleming H. Revell Company, 1907), p. 211; T. Richard, *Forty-Five Years in China: Reminiscences by Timothy Richard* (New York: Frederick A. Stokes Company, 1916), p. 60; S. Grypma, *Healing Henan: Canadian Nurses at the North China Mission, 1888–1947* (Vancouver: UBC Press,

2008), p. 14; E. L. Blumhofer et al. (eds), *Pentecostal Currents in American Protestantism* (Urbaba and Chicago, IL: University of Illinois Press, 1999), pp. 33–4.

25. 'Lottie Moon Letter, P'ingtu, December 13, 1886', *Foreign Mission Journal* 18.8:2 (1887), p. 12.
26. D. D. Main, 'Hang-Chow Medical Mission', *Medical Mission Quarterly* 8 (1894), pp. 19–22, on p. 21.
27. A. Crombie, 'Maladies of European Children in Hot Climates', *British Medical Journal* (14 September 1901), pp. 694–9, on. p. 698.
28. 'The Inter-Provincial Conference, January 1920', in *The Challenge of China: Being the Report of a Deputation Sent out to Visit the China Mission Fields of the BMS 1919 1920* (London: The Carey Press, 1920), pp. 24–43, on p. 26.
29. For instance, cases of 'nervous prostration and debility' and neurasthenia were rarely recorded in the medical reports of the Imperial Maritime Customs during the period from 1890 to 1900. See 'Dr J. H. Lowry's Report on the Health of Wenchow', *Medical Reports of the Imperial Maritime Customs of China*, 42 (1891), pp. 19–20; 'Dr W. H. Park's Report on the Health of Soochow', *Medical Reports of the Imperial Maritime Customs of China*, 53 (1897), pp. 19–20; 'Dr Alfred Hogg's Report on the Health of Wenchow', *Medical Reports of the Imperial Maritime Customs of China*, 54 (1897), pp. 43–4.
30. N. MacLeod, 'The Bromide Sleep: A New Departure in the Treatment of Acute Mania', *British Medical Journal* (20 January 1900), pp. 134–6. See also Howard Chiang, 'An Early Hope of Psychopharmacology: Bromide Treatment in the Turn-of-the-Twentieth-Century Psychiatry', *Historia Mediciae*, 1:1 (2009), pp. 1–7.
31. 'In the Court of Consuls', *North-China Herald* (24 July 1909), pp. 216–21, pp. 241–3; 'A Vancouver Tragedy', *North-China Herald* (11 December 1909), p. 631.
32. 'The Story of a Mother in China', *North-China Herald* (12 December 1910), p. 561; 'Of Interest to Ailing Wives', *North-China Herald* (29 April 1911), pp. 315–16. For the use of the Pink Pills in British Malaya, see M. K. Cody, 'A Paler Shade of White', in L. van der Putten and M. K. Cody (eds), *Lost Times and Untold Tales from the Malay World* (Singapore: NUS Press, 2009), pp. 82–96.
33. 'Health of Missionaries', *China Medical Journal*, 39:8 (1925), pp. 714–17.
34. Sir R. Havelock Charles, 'On Special Factors Influencing the Suitability of Europeans for Life in the Tropics', *British Medical Journal* (24 September 1910), pp. 869–74, on p. 872.
35. A. H. Smith, *The Uplift of China* (New York: Missionary Education Movement of the United States and Canada, 1912), pp. 9–10.
36. Price, 'Discussion on the Causes of Invaliding from the Tropics', p. 1291, 1293.
37. 'The Health of Missionaries', *China Medical Journal*, 29:5 (1915), pp. 331–5.
38. A. H. Smith, *A Manual for Young Missionaries to China* (Shanghai: The Christian Literature Publishing House, 1918), pp. 6–7.
39. Price, 'Discussion on the Causes of Invaliding from the Tropics', pp. 1291, 1293. J. Hudson Taylor, 'The Missionary: His Qualifications, Introduction to His Work and Mode of Life', *Records of the General Conference of the Protestant Missionaries of China* (Shanghai: American Presbyterian Mission Press, 1890), pp. 145–52, on pp. 148–9; W. H. Boone, *Health Hints for Missionaries to China* (Shanghai: Medical Missionary Association of China, 1907); F. K. Sanders, *The Fourth Report of the Board of Missionary Preparation (For North America)* (New York: The Board of Missionary Preparation, 1914); R. A. Semple, *Missionary Women: Gender, Professionalism and the Victorian Idea of Christian Mission* (Rochester, NY: Boydell, 2003), pp. 30–1.

40. 'Notes and Comments', *China Medical Journal*, 29:5 (1915), p. 358.
41. 'The Health of Missionaries', *China Medical Journal*, 29:5 (1915), pp. 331–5; ''Accidie' and Summer Vacations', *China Medical Journal*, 31:5 (1917), pp. 408–11; 'Health of Missionaries', *China Medical Journal*, 39:8 (1925), pp. 714–17, on p. 716; W. W. Cadbury, 'An Analysis of the Health of a Missionary Community in South China during a Period of Thirteen Years', *China Medical Journal*, 39:8 (1925), pp. 723–44, on p. 743.
42. Ibid., p. 731.
43. T. E. Egerton Shore, 'Salaries, Furloughs, etc.', *Fifteenth Conference of the Foreign Missions Boards in the United States and Canada* (New York: Foreign Missions Library, 1908), pp. 121–32; J. W. Wood, 'Furloughs and their Use', *Foreign Missions Conference of North America* (New York: Foreign Missions Library, 1912), pp. 179–91; W. D. Mackenzie, 'Board of Missionary Preparation Report', *Foreign Missions Conference of North America* (New York: Foreign Missions Conference, 1914), pp. 80–100, on pp. 93–4.
44. W. B. Billinghurst, 'Mental Irritability and Breakdown in the Tropics', *British Medical Journal* (27 March 1926), pp. 846–7.
45. A. S. McNeil, 'Mental Irritability and Breakdown in the Tropics', *British Medical Journal* (8 and 25 May 1926), pp. 595–6.
46. Ibid. For tropical clothing and colonial identity, see R. Johnson, 'European Cloth and 'Tropical' Skin: Clothing Material and British Ideas of Health and Hygiene in Tropical Climates', *Bulletin of the History of Medicine*, 83:3 (2009), pp. 530–60.
47. M. Gijswijt-Hofstra and R. Porter (eds), *Cultures of Neurasthenia from Beard to the First World War* (Amsterdam: Rodopi, 2001).
48. W. Anderson, 'Immunities of Empire: Race, Disease and the New Tropical Medicine, 1900–1920', *Bulletin of the History of Medicine*, 70:1 (1996), pp. 94–118.
49. M. Harrison, *Public Health in British India: Anglo-Indian Preventive Medicine 1859–1914* (Cambridge: Cambridge University Press, 1994), pp. 36–59; M. Harrison, *Climates and Constitutions: Health, Race, Environment and British Imperialism in India, 1600–1850* (Oxford: Oxford University Press, 1999).
50. K. L. MacPherson, *A Wilderness of Marshes: The Origins of Public Health in Shanghai, 1843–1893* (Lanham, MD: Lexington Books, 2002); Shang-Jen Li 李尚仁, *Diguo de yishi: Wanbade yu yingguo redai yixue de chuangjian* 帝國的醫生：萬巴德與英國熱帶醫學的創建 [The Imperial Doctor: Patrick Manson and the Creation of the British Tropical Medicine] (Taipei: Asian Culture Press, 2012), pp. 59–72.
51. J. Oppenheim, *'Shattered Nerves': Doctors, Patients and Depression in Victorian England* (Oxford: Oxford University Press, 1991).
52. J. L. Hevia, 'Leaving a Brand on China: Missionary Discourse in the Wake of the Boxer Movement', in T. E. Barlow (ed.), *Formations of Colonial Modernity in East Asia* (Durham, NC: Duke University Press, 1997), pp. 112–39, on p. 131.
53. For a nineteenth-century example of the role British medical practitioners in China played in the imperial medical network at large, see Shang-Jen Li, 'Eating Well in China: Diet and Hygiene in Nineteenth-Century Treaty Ports', in Angela Ki Che Leung and C. Furth (eds), *Health and Hygiene in Chinese East Asia: Politics and Publics in the Long Twentieth Century* (Durham, NC: Duke University Press, 2010), pp. 109–31.
54. Sanders, *The Fourth Report of the Board of Missionary Preparation (For North America)*, pp. 31, 88, 118, 216, 228.
55. In Frederick Sargent's extremely exhaustive review of the medical literature on tropical neurasthenia published from 1900 to 1959, 'political situation' was not singled out by

the contemporary sources as one of the socio-economic characteristics of the tropical milieu. See Sargent II, 'Tropical Neurasthenia', pp. 295–6.

56. This is not to suggest that there was no medical missionary involvement in the treatment of mental illness during the same period. See Chapters Four and Five in this volume, pp. 71–90 and 91–110 and N. Diamant, 'China's 'Great Confinement'?: Missionaries, Municipal Elites and Police in the Establishment of Chinese Mental Hospitals', *Republican China*, 19:1 (1993), pp. 3–50.
57. Kennedy, 'The Perils of the Midday Sun', p. 123.
58. Rogers and Megaw, *Tropical Medicine*, pp. 481–2; A. C. Reed, 'Tropical Neurasthenia', *American Journal of Tropical Medicine* 22:2 (1942), pp. 127–30; Sargent II, 'Tropical Neurasthenia', pp. 273–314.
59. See for instance M. Prince et al., *Psychotherapeutics: A Symposium* (Boston, MA: Richard G. Badger, 1919).
60. 'Review of *Collected Papers of Analytic Psychology*, by C. G. Jung', *China Medical Journal*, 30:5 (1916), pp. 381–3; 'Review of *Handbook of Suggestive Therapeutics, Applied Hypnotism and Psychic Science*, by Henry S. Munro', *China Medical Journal*, 31:4 (1917), pp. 358–60; 'Review of *Advanced Suggestion (Neuro-Induction)*, by Haydn Brown', *China Medical Journal*, 33:2 (1919), p. 196; 'Review of *A Manual of Neurasthenia (Nervous Exhaustion)*, by Ivo Geikie Cobb', *China Medical Journal* 34:4 (1920), p. 457; 'Review of *Treatment of the Neuroses*, by Ernest Jones', *China Medical Journal* 34:4 (1920), pp. 457–8.
61. J. C. Cormack, 'Unconscious Therapeutics', *China Medical Journal*, 38:6 (1924), pp. 505–18.
62. E. M. Merrins, 'The Emmanuel Movement in China', *China Medical Journal*, 24:1 (1910), pp. 28–34.
63. Taylor, 'A Plea for the Wider Use of Psycho-Therapy', pp. 104–9.
64. 'Tropics and Nerves', *The North-China Herald* (22 September 1923), pp. 813–14. The article to which the news report was referring is T. S. Rippon, 'The Effect of Tropical Climate on Physical and Mental Efficiency', *Proceedings of the Royal Society of Medicine*, 16 (1923), pp. 45–54.
65. 'Tropics and Nerves', pp. 813–14.
66. For one of the latest studies on the development of psychoanalysis in the colonial context, see W. Anderson, R. C. Keller and D. Jenson (eds), *Unconscious Dominions: Psychoanalysis, Colonial Trauma and Global Sovereignties* (Durham, NC: Duke University Press, 2011).
67. Oldt, 'Nervous Disorders of Sexual Origin', p. 448.
68. Ibid., p. 452.
69. M. Culpin, 'An Autobiography', *Occupational Psychology*, 23 (1949), pp. 139–52; M. d'Eimar de Jabrun, 'Culpin, Millais (1874–1952)', *Australian Dictionary of Biography* (National Centre of Biography, Australian National University), http://adb.anu.edu.au/biography/culpin-millais-12872/text23247 [accessed 12 July 2013].
70. M. Culpin, 'An Examination of Tropical Neurasthenia', *Proceedings of the Royal Society of Medicine*, 26:7 (1933), pp. 911–22; M. Culpin, 'Neurasthenia in the Tropics', *Practitioner*, 85 (1935), pp. 146–54.
71. 'Neuroses in the Tropics', *British Medical Journal* (17 March 1928), pp. 448–9, on p.449; H. B. Day, 'Discussion on Neuroses in the Tropics', *Proceedings of the Royal Society of Medicine*, 21:9 (1928), pp. 1667–76, on p. 1676.

72. J. L. McCartney, 'Overt Transference', *Journal of Sex Research*, 2:3 (1966), pp. 227–37, on p. 223.
73. J. L. McCartney, 'Neuropsychiatry in China; A Preliminary Observation', *China Medical Journal*, 40:7 (1926), pp. 617–26; J. L. McCartney, 'Neuropsychiatry in China', *Archives of Neurology and Psychiatry*, 18:7 (1927), pp. 87–95.
74. J. L. McCartney, 'Oriental Nerves', *China Journal of Science and Art*, 4:2 (1926), pp. 84–91, on p. 89.
75. Ibid., p. 87.
76. J. C. Thompson, 'Tropical Neurasthenia: A Deprivation Psychoneurosis', *Military Surgeon*, 54 (1924), pp. 319–27.
77. McCartney, 'Oriental Nerves', p. 90.
78. Ibid.
79. Ibid., pp. 90–1.
80. For the concept of relocation costs, see P. D. Curtin, *Death by Migration: Europe's Encounter with the Tropical World in the Nineteenth Century* (Cambridge: Cambridge University Press, 1989).
81. J. L. McCartney, 'Chinese Military Medicine', *U. S. Naval Medical Bulletin*, 25:4 (1927), pp. 783–816.
82. J. L. McCartney, 'Headaches: With Special Reference to those of Psychogenic Origin', *China Medical Journal*, 39:1 (1925), pp. 32–40.
83. J. L. McCartney, 'Psychogenic Headaches, With the Treatment of a Case', *National Medical Journal of China*, 12:5 (1926), pp. 358–71.
84. J. L. McCartney, 'The Call to Foreign Missions: Its Effect on Unstable Personalities', *Mental Hygiene*, 12 (1928), pp. 521–9, on p. 525. The same opinion was recorded on a 1928 *Time* report on McCartney's speech at the National Institute of Mental Hygiene. See 'Morbid Missionaries', *Time Magazine*, 12:4 (1928), p. 20.
85. McCartney, 'The Call to Foreign Missions', p. 524.
86. Ibid., p. 529.
87. Anderson, *Colonial Pathologies*, p. 155.
88. It is important to note that 'neurasthenia' as a diagnosis itself declined during the same period. See E. Shorter, *From Paralysis to Fatigue: A History of Psychosomatic Illness in the Modern Era* (New York: Free Press, 1992); M. Micale, *Approaching Hysteria: Disease and its Interpretation* (Princeton, NJ: Princeton University Press, 1995); R. E. Taylor, 'Death of Neurasthenia and its Psychological Reincarnation', *British Journal of Psychiatry*, 179 (2001), pp. 550–7. For the climactic and physiological models, see P. E. Turner, *A Tropical Medical Manual Specially Prepared for the Use of Salvation Army Officers*. 3rd edn (London: International Headquarters, 1942), p. 61.
89. W. R. Logan, 'Psychical Illness among the Services in Singapore', *Journal of Mental Science*, 87 (1941), pp. 241–55; F. G. Crandall, 'Observations of a Medical Officer in the South Pacific Area', *California and Western Medicine*, 59:6 (1943), pp. 319–22; T. Rowland Hill, 'Tropical Neurasthenia', *Lancet* (13 March 1943), pp. 332–3; H. B. Craigie, 'Two Years of Military Psychiatry in the Middle East', *British Medical Journal* (22 July 1944), pp. 105–9; H. J. Trenchard, 'Inability to Work in a Tropical Climate', *British Medical Journal* (21 September 1946), pp. 416–18.
90. See for instance W. Ernst, 'Idioms of Madness and Colonial Boundaries: The Case of the European and 'Native' Mentally Ill in Early Nineteenth-Century British India', *Comparative Studies in Society and History*, 39:1 (1997), pp.153–81.
91. Culpin, 'An Examination of Tropical Neurasthenia', pp. 920–1.

92. Ibid., p. 921.
93. McCartney's own knowledge of the Orient can be found in a novel he composed in 1953 about missionary lives in West China. See J. L. McCartney, *Frustrated Martyr: A Novel of a Medical Missionary in West China* (New York: Exposition Press, 1953).
94. For the case of the Japanese ruled Manchuria, see J. Matsumura, 'Eugenics, Environment and Acclimatizing to Manchukuo: Psychiatric Studies of Japanese Colonists', *Niho Ishigaku Zasshi*, 56:3 (2010), pp. 329–50.
95. T. E. Barlow, 'Introduction: On 'Colonial Modernity'', in T. E. Barlow (ed.), *Formations of Colonial Modernity in East Asia* (Durham, NC: Duke University Press, 1997), pp. 1–20, on p. 5; B. Goodman, 'Improvisations on a Semicolonial Theme, or, How to Read a Celebration of Transnational Urban Community', *Journal of Asian Studies* 59:4 (2000), pp. 889–926; R. Rogaski, *Hygienic Modernity: Meanings of Health and Disease in Treaty-Port China* (Berkeley, CA: University of California Press, 2002), pp. 10–15.
96. 'The Health of Missionaries', *China Medical Journal*, 29:5 (1915), p. 331.
97. Lutz, 'Attrition among Protestant Missionaries in China, 1807–1890'; M. Jennings, ''This Mysterious and Intangible Enemy': Health and Disease amongst the Early UMCA Missionaries', *Social History of Medicine* 15:1 (2002), pp. 65–87; C. M. Good Jr., *The Steamer Parish: The Rise and Fall of Missionary Medicine on an African Frontier* (Chicago, IL:: University of Chicago Press, 2004), pp. 266–7.
98. M. Vaughan, 'Healing and Curing: Issues in the Social History and Anthropology of Medicine in Africa', *Social History of Medicine* 7:2 (1994), pp. 283–95.
99. Jennings, ''This Mysterious and Intangible Enemy'', p. 67.
100. W. Anderson, 'Postcolonial Technoscience', *Social Studies of Science*, 32:5/6 (2002), pp. 643–58; J. Secord, 'Knowledge in Transit', *Isis*, 95:4 (2004), pp. 654–72; K. Raj, 'Beyond Postcolonialism ... and Postpositivism: Circulation and the Global History of Science', *Isis*, 104:2 (2013), pp. 337–47.
101. For the relation between the London School and colonial policy, see M. Worboys, 'Manson, Ross and Colonial Medical Policy: Tropical Medicine in London and Liverpool, 1899–1914', in R. MacLeod and M. Lewis (eds), *Disease, Medicine and Empire: Perspectives on Western Medicine and the Experience of European Experience* (London: Routledge, 1988), pp. 21–37.
102. Culpin, 'Neurasthenia in the Tropics', p. 154. For Culpin's research project in connection with the scientific study of work-related issues, see R. S. F. Schilling, 'Industrial Health Research: The Work of the Industrial Health Research Board, 1918–1944', *British Journal of Industrial Medicine* 1:3 (1944), pp. 145–52.
103. It seems that the earlier derogatory reference to an unstable and even morbid personality was no longer appropriate for those who fought bravely for the country. J. L. McCartney, 'Tropical Neuropsychiatry', *War Medicine*, 4 (1943), pp. 351–66; 'Blonds Crack in Tropics', *Science News Letter* (22 May 1943), p. 324.
104. For the breakdown of colonial boundaries in history of medicine, see also Anderson, *Colonial Pathologies*, pp. 227–33; R. Bivins, 'Coming 'Home' to (post)Colonial Medicine: Treating Tropical Bodies in Post-War Britain', *Social History of Medicine*, 26:1 (2012), pp. 1–20.
105. McCartney observed that psychiatrists at the Peking Union Medical College ascribed the mental unbalance of Western sojourners to the influence of 'food, climate, economic readjustments'. See 'Morbid Missionaries', p. 20. For the development of dynamic psychiatry in Republican China, see Wen-Ji Wang 王文基, '''Dangxia weiren zhi daren': Dai Bingham de suren jingshen fenxi 「當下為人之大任」：戴秉衡的俗人精神

分析' ['This All-Important Job of Being Human at the Present': Bingham Dai's Lay Psychoanalysis], *New History*, 17:1 (2006), pp. 91–142.

106. See Chapters Four and Five in this volume, pp. 71–90 and 91–110.
107. Shixie Liu, 'Neurasthenia in China: Modern and Traditional Criteria for its Diagnosis', *Culture, Medicine and Psychiatry*, 13:2 (1989), pp. 163–86; on p. 166.

7 Shapiro, 'Pathologizing Marriage: Neuropsychiatry and the Escape of Women in Early Twentieth-Century China'

1. On *tan* (mucus), see F. Simonis, 'Mad Acts, Mad Speech and Mad People in Late Imperial Chinese Law and Medicine' (PhD dissertation, Princeton University, 2010), pp. 73–135. Simonis's work also reveals the relative paucity of medical records on the 'madness' of women during the late imperial period.
2. 'Poverty' and 'disease' were the leading causes of suicide for men. S. Gamble, assisted by J. S. Burgess, *Peking: A Social Survey* (New York: George H. Doran Company, 1921), p. 418.
3. R. S. Watson, 'Girls' Houses and Working Women: Expressive Culture in the Pearl Delta, 1900–41', in M. Jaschok and S. Miers (eds), *Women and Chinese Patriarchy: Submission, Servitude and Escape* (Hong Kong: Hong Kong University Press, 1994); p. 33.
4. Ibid., pp. 31, 35–6; M. Jaschok, 'On the Lives of Women Unwed by Choice in Pre-Communist China', *Republican China*, 10:1a (Nov 1981); J. Stockard, *Daughters of the Canton Delta: Marriage Patterns and Economic Strategies in South China, 1860–1930* (Stanford, CA: Stanford University Press, 1992).
5. M. Jaschok, *Concubines and Bondservants: The Social History of a Chinese* Custom (Hong Kong: Oxford University Press, 1988); J. M. Carroll, 'A National Custom: Debating Female Servitude in Late Nineteenth-Century Hong Kong', *Modern Asian Studies*, 43:6 (2009), pp. 1463–93.
6. M. Topley, 'Marriage Resistance in Rural Kwangtung', in M. Wolf and R. Witke (eds), *Women in Chinese Society* (Stanford, CA: Stanford University Press, 1975), pp. 67–88.
7. 'Taonü Ke Dashen 逃女柯大詵' [Runaway Girl Ke Dashen], *Chahar shen zhengfu gongbao* 察哈尔省政府公报 [Chahar Provincial Government Gazette], 894 (1935), p. 3.
8. From 1928 to 1949, Beijing was named 'Beiping' 北平 'Northern Peace', when the Nationalist (KMT, GMD) government established its capital in Nanjing.
9. J. Chen, *Guilty of Indigence: The Urban Poor in China, 1900–1953* (Princeton, NJ: Princeton University Press, 2012).
10. I. Pruitt, *A Daughter of Han, the Autobiography of a Chinese Working Woman* (Stanford, CA: Stanford University Press 1967), pp. 31–4.
11. M. Elvin, 'Tales of *Shen* and *Xin*: Body-Person and Heart-Mind in China during the Last 150 Years', in M. Feher (ed.), *Fragments for a History of the Human Body, Part Two* (New York: Zone, 1989), pp. 299, 349 n. 10.
12. See M. Kuo, *Intolerable cruelty: marriage, law and society in early twentieth-century China* (Lanham, MD: Rowman & Littlefield, 2012), especially chapter 6, 'Running Away: Cohabitation Litigation and the Reconfiguration of Husband Patriarchy', pp. 139–54.
13. Yeh Wen-hsin, 'Progressive Journalism and Shanghai's Petty Urbanites: Zou Taofen and the *Shenghuo Weekly*', in F. Wakeman, Jr. and Wen-hsin Yeh (eds), *Shanghai Sojourn-*

ers (Berkeley, CA: Institute of East Asian Studies, University of California, 1992), pp. 214–16.

14. 'Qingnian wenti taolunhui, Huijia jiehun ma? Tuoli jiating ma? 青年問題討論會,回家結婚嗎？脱离家庭媽'？[Forum on Issues Concerning Youth: Return Home and Marry? Break Away and Leave Home?]', *Duzhe yuekan* 讀者月刊 [Monata Revuo] 1:3 (1933), pp. 105–7.
15. Yuan Qi 元启, 'Duiyu 'Taohun' de tongqing 对于『逃婚』的同情' [On Sympathy for 'Escape from Marriage'], *Funü zazhi* 妇女杂志 [The Ladies' Journal] 9:4 (1923), pp. 32–5.
16. C. Gilmartin, *Engendering the Chinese Revolution, Radical Women, Communist Politics and Mass Movements in the 1920s* (Berkeley, CA: University of California Press, 1995), pp. 32, 49.
17. Ibid., pp. 32, 35–6.
18. Lao She 老舍, 'Xisheng 犠牲 [Sacrifice]', in Lao She et al., *Xisheng* [Sacrifice] (Shanghai: Shenghuo shudian, 1937), pp. 1–46, on p. 46.
19. 'Spousal cruelty was the most commonly cited grounds for divorce', from 1934 to 1939. K. Bernhardt, 'Women and the law: divorce in the Republican period', in K. Bernhardt, P. C. C. Huang (eds), *Civil law in Qing and Republican China* (Stanford, CA: Stanford University Press, 1994), pp. 200, 187–214.
20. P. C. C. Huang, *Code, custom and legal practice in China: the Qing and the Republic compared* (Stanford, CA: Stanford University Press, 2001), p. 195.
21. M. Kuo, 'Spousal Abuse: Divorce Litigation and the Emergence of Rights Consciousness in Republican China', *Modern China*, 38:5 (2012), pp. 551, 523–58.
22. P. C. C. Huang, *Chinese civil justice, past and present* (New York: Rowman & Littlefield, 2010), p. 24.
23. G. Hershatter, *The Gender of Memory: Rural Women and China's Collective Past* (Berkeley, CA: University of California Press, 2011), p. 109.
24. *Xiehe yiyuan* 協和醫院 [Peking Union Medical College], Case No. 56954, pp. ss1–3. Hereafter cited as, XHYY, 56954, pp. ss1–3. Pseudonyms used for all patients. The 'old-fashioned' woman had 'received no education'; the man was a highly educated 'returned-student' from France, who had grown up in rural Shanxi, 550 miles southwest of Beijing. He excelled in government middle and high schools and his family moved to Beijing, to advance his education. He attended Beijing's French High School (Fawen Xueyuan), graduated from the city's Sino-French University (Zhongfa Daxue) and on scholarship, spent one year of study in France. A friend of his father's, a manager of a Beijing paper shop in Tan'er hutong near Qianmen (前外炭兒胡同), had arranged the marriage.
25. On the habitual predation by warlord soldiers on civilians, see, E. A. McCord, 'Burn, Kill, Rape and Rob: Military Atrocities, Warlordism and Anti-Warlordism in Republican China', in Diana Lary and Stephen MacKinnon (eds), *Scars of War: The Impact of Warfare on Modern China* (Vancouver: UBC Press, 2001), pp. 18–49.
26. 高公庵精神病院.
27. 山西太原第四典獄長. *Shanxi Taiyuan Disi Dianyu Zhang* [Warden of Prison Number Four, Taiyuan, Shanxi].
28. Such as luminary Cai Yuanpei's 1935 disappointment in *Hong Loumeng* character Caiyun, who 'fails to live up to his image of the new woman, the post-May Fourth ideal of an independent woman'; Hu Ying, *Tales of Translation, Composing the New Woman in China, 1898–1918* (Stanford, CA: Stanford University Press, 2000), pp. 63–4.

29. P. Bailey, ''Women Behaving Badly': Crime, Transgressive Behaviours and Gender in Early Twentieth Century' *Nan nü* 8:1 (2006), pp. 160–1, 156–97.
30. J. Judge, 'Talent, Virtue and the Nation: Chinese Nationalisms and Female Subjectivities in the Early Twentieth Century', *American Historical Review* 106:3 (2001), pp. 803, 765–803.
31. G. Hershatter, *Dangerous pleasures: prostitution and modernity in twentieth-century Shanghai* (Berkeley, CA: University of California Press, 1999), p. 224.
32. Judge, 'Talent, Virtue and the Nation', p. 802.
33. G. Hershatter, *The Gender of Memory: Rural Women and China's Collective Past* (Berkeley, CA: University of California Press, 2011), pp. 109–10.
34. Lu Xun 鲁迅, 'Nala zou hou zhenyang 娜拉走后怎样' [What Happens After Nora Leaves Home]', *Funü zazhi* 妇女杂志 [The Ladies' Journal] 10:8 (1924), pp. 1218–22, on p. 1220. On Qiu Jin, see Hu Ying, A. Dooling and K. Torgeson (eds), *Writing Women in Modern China* (New York: Columbia University Press, 1998).
35. D. Strand, *Rickshaw Beijing: City People and Politics in the 1920s* (Berkeley, CA: University of California Press, 1989), p. 84, quoting the 'Rules of Police Work' (*Jingwu guize*).
36. Ibid.
37. S. Borthwick, 'Changing Concepts of the Role of Women from the Late Qing to the May Fourth Period', in D. Pong and E. S. K. Fung (eds), *Ideal and Reality, Social and Political Change in Modern China, 1860–1949* (Lanham, MD: University Press of America, 1985), pp. 71–2.
38. Pan Guangdan's pioneering study analyzes concubine Feng Xiaoqing, who was sold into a wealthy late Ming household of Hangzhou. The principal wife forced Feng Xiaoqing into an isolated residence, where she died in 1612 at age seventeen, evidently of despair. Pan Guangdan, *Feng Xiaoqing xing xinli biantai jiemi* [Uncovering the abnormal sexual psychology of Feng Xiaoqing], commentary by Zhen Xiang and Bo Shi, ed. by Xu Yanjun, 1927 edn (Beijing: Arts and Culture Press, 1990).
39. See S. Glosser, *Chinese Visions of Family and the State, 1915–1953* (Berkeley, CA: University of California Press, 2003)
40. See Chapter Five in this volume, pp. 91–110.
41. J. G. Kerr, *First Report for the Refuge for the Insane in Canton* (n.p., n.p., February, 1898 to August, 1901, inclusive), pp. 24d, 25b.
42. C. C. Selden, 'Conditions in South China in Relation to Insanity', *American Journal of Insanity* 70 (Oct 1913), p. 412.
43. R. M. Ross, 'The Insane in China: Examinations Hints', *Chinese Medical Journal* 34:5 (Sept 1920), pp. 515–16.
44. Ibid., p. 517.
45. J. Lincoln McCartney, 'Neuropsychiatry in China: A Retrospect of Diagnosis', *Chinese Medical* Journal, 40:9 (Sept 1926), p. 836. See Chapter Six in this volume, pp. 111–28.
46. A. H. Woods, 'The Nervous Diseases of the Chinese', *Archives of Neurology and Psychiatry*, 21:3 (March 1929), p. 567.
47. Ibid., p. 569. Woods writes that these 'perversions' served also as contraception.
48. Ross, 'The Insane in China: Examination Hints', p. 516.
49. McCartney, 'Neuropsychiatry in China', p. 836.
50. M. Jaschok, 'Chinese 'Slave' Girls in Yunnan-Fu: Saving (Chinese) Womanhood and (Western) Souls, 1930–1991', in Jaschok and Miers (eds), *Women and Chinese Patriarchy: Submission, Servitude and Escape*, p. 178.

51. Song Chengzhang 宋誠彰, et al. (eds), *Shanghai fengdian zhuanmen yiyuan yuanwu gaiyao* 上海瘋癲專門醫院 [An Outline of the Administration of the Shanghai Special Hospital for the Insane] (Shanghai: *Shanghai fengdian zhuanmen yiyuan*, 1934). (hereafter SFDZMYY or Special Hospital).
52. 'Organization', SFDZMYY, case no. 2.
53. On Du Yuesheng, Huang Jinrong and the Green Gang, see B. G. Martin, *The Shanghai Green Gang: Politics and Organized Crime, 1919–1937* (Berkeley, CA: University of California Press, 1996). The Chairman, Xu Shiying, had managed famine relief for the Nationalist Government and had founded in 1932 the 'Shanghai War Zone Refugee Relief Association'. H. Boorman (ed.), *Biographical Dictionary of Republican China, Volume II* (New York: Columbia University Press, 1967), pp. 140a–143a.
54. E. Showalter, 'Victorian Women and Insanity', in A. Scull (ed.), *Madhouses, Mad-Doctors and Madmen: The Social History of Psychiatry in the Victorian Era* (Philadelphia, PA: University of Pennsylvania Press, 1983), p. 331.
55. SFDZMYY, case no. 1, p. 1.
56. Ibid., case no. 30, p. 114.
57. Ibid., case no. 60–1, p. 229.
58. Ibid., case no. 67, p. 250.
59. Ibid., case no. 15, p. 56.
60. Ibid., case no. 20, p. 74. The sense of enclosure expressed by this patient resonates with the theme of female depression developed by sociologist Pan Guangdan a 1927 study. Pan conducts a word analysis of a late Qing collection of women's poetry, finding that negative expressions of enclosure appeared 1,600 times. See Zhang Jingyuan, *Psychoanalysis in China, literary transformations, 1919–1949* (Ithaca, NY: East Asia Program, Cornell University, 1992).
61. Spitting blood, '*tuxue*' is a colloquialism for intense anger.
62. SFDZMYY, case no. 30, p. 116.
63. Ibid., case no. 64, p. 240. In addition to proven extra-marital affairs, a group of cases represented at the psychiatric hospital were the result of 'suspected affairs' (*yifu you waiyu*); Ibid., case no. 18, p. 68; case no. 29, p. 110; case no. 32, p. 124; case no. 60, p. 228.
64. Ibid., case no. 55, p. 211.
65. Ibid., case no. 15–16, p. 59.
66. The Song period (907–1279 CE) classic, *Good Prescriptions for Women* (*Furen liangfang*), states, 'If her anger is great, the liver will be injured'. C. Furth, 'Blood, Body and Gender, Medical Images of the Female Condition in China', *Chinese Science*, 7 (1986), pp. 51, 43–66.
67. SFDZMYY, case no. 73, p. 271. On 'menstrual regulation' (*tiaojing*) in China's scholarly medical writings, see C. Furth, *A Flourishing Yin: Gender in China's Medical History, 960–1665* (Berkeley, CA: University of California Press, 1999) and Furth, 'Blood, Body and Gender', pp. 44–55.
68. '*Pinfu*' exists in both feminine and masculine forms 姘婦, 姘夫.
69. SFDZMYY, case no. 14, p. 53.
70. Ibid., case no. 72, p. 267. In 1940 Beijing, a wife was promised an inheritance of five *mo* of land. When the time came to pass down the property, her brother interceded and took her share. She suffered mental disturbance for one month. XHYY, 71728, p. 7.
71. SFDZMYY, case no. 20, p. 73.
72. Ibid., case no. 12, p. 44; Ibid., case no. 69, p. 259. *Dianshizhai huabao*, the famous weekly pictorial from the late 1880s, depicts a woman driven mad by husband's disappearance.

Wu Youru, 'Suckling a Baby Corpse' trans. by Don J. Cohn, in 'Selections from the Dianshizhai Pictorial', *Renditions*, 23 (Spring 1985), p. 64.

73. SFDZMYY, case no. 31, p. 117.
74. Ibid., case no. 9, p. 33.
75. Ibid., case no. 68, p. 256; case no. 16, p. 61.
76. C. Furth, 'Concepts of Pregnancy, Childbirth and Infancy in Ch'ing Dynasty China', *Journal of Asian Studies*, 46:1 (February 1987), p. 15. See also Furth, *A Flourishing Yin*, p. 151; Wu Yi-Li, *Reproducing Women, Medicine, Metaphor and Childbirth in Late Imperial China* (Berkeley, CA: University of California Press, 2011).
77. Furth, 'Concepts of Pregnancy', p. 15.
78. SFDZMYY, case no. 19, p. 72. *Bufu shuitu*, or *shuitu bufu*, remains a colloquialism for the discomforts of travel.
79. M. Hanson, *Speaking of Epidemics in Chinese Medicine: Disease and the Geographic Imagination in Late Imperial China* (London and New York: Routledge, 2011).
80. See E. Honig, *Creating Chinese Ethnicity: Subei People in Shanghai, 1850–1980* (New Haven, CT: Yale University Press, 1992)
81. SFDZMYY, case no. 31, p. 120.
82. Ibid., case no. 16, p. 62; case no. 37, p. 143; case no. 71, p. 265.
83. See Hershatter, *Dangerous pleasures*, 1999.
84. C. Hart Westbrook, 'Psychiatry and Mental Hygiene in Shanghai: Historical Sketch', *American Journal of Psychiatry*, 110 (October 1953), p. 301.
85. M. Bullock, *An American Transplant: The Rockefeller Foundation and Peking Union Medical College* (Berkeley, CA: University of California Press, 1980); M. Bullock, *The Oil Prince's Legacy: Rockefeller Philanthropy in China* (Stanford, CA: Stanford University Press, 2011).
86. A. Meyer, 'Objective Psychology or Psychobiology with Subordination of the Medically Useless Contrast of Mental and Physical', *Journal of the American Medical Association*, 65 (1915), pp. 860–3; see S. D. Lamb, *Pathologist of the Mind: Adolf Meyer, Psychobiology and the Phipps Psychiatric Clinic, 1908–1917* (PhD dissertation, The Johns Hopkins University, 2010).
87. N. Diamant, 'China's 'Great Confinement': Missionaries, Municipal Elites and Police in the Establishment of Chinese Mental Hospitals', *Republican China*, 19:1 (1993), pp. 3–50, on pp. 23–30.
88. Ibid., pp. 23–7.
89. On prolonged institutionalization, see E. Goffman, *Asylums: Essays on the Social Situation of Mental Patients and Other Inmates* (New York: Anchor Books, 1959).
90. Diamant, 'China's 'Great Confinement'', p. 30.
91. F. L. K. Hsu (Xu Langguang), 'A Brief Report on the Police Co-operation in Connection with Mental Cases in Peiping' in R. S. Lyman, V. Maeker and P. Liang (eds), *Social and Psychological Studies in Neuropsychiatry in China* (Peking: Henri Vetch and Peking Union Medical College, 1939), p. 202.
92. For an example of the Nationalist (GMD) police imprisoning political suspects in late 1940s Shanghai who were then admitted to asylums, see E. J. Perry, *Patrolling the revolution: worker militias, citizenship and the modern Chinese state* (Lanham, MD: Rowman & Littlefield Publishers, 2005), p. 141.
93. August Vollmer describes 'police work as a scientific struggle against social pathology', in F. Wakeman, Jr., 'Policing Modern Shanghai', *China Quarterly*, 115 (Sept 1988), p.

428; Strand, *Rickshaw Beijing*, 'Policemen as Mediators and Street-Level Bureaucrats', pp. 65–97.

94. XHYY, 50903, p. 5.
95. XHYY, 49925, p. 13.
96. XHYY, 72119, p. ss4.
97. The Pinghan ran between (Bei)Ping and (Wu)Han.
98. XHYY, 72119, p. ss4.
99. XHYY, 72119, pp. ss4–5.
100. XHYY, 72119, p. ss5.
101. XHYY, 72119, p. 17.
102. XHYY, 65010, pp. 6–7.
103. XHYY, 65010, pp. 27–8.
104. XHYY, 76205, p. 5.
105. 'The John G. Kerr Hospital for the Insane – Report for the Years 1922 and 1923', Guangzhou Psychiatric Hospital archives, Guangzhou, China, p. 5.
106. XHYY, 15891.
107. XHYY, 15891:232.
108. XHYY, 15891:73–4.
109. XHYY, 15891:98.
110. XHYY, 15891:153, ss3.
111. Zhang Jingsheng, popular sexologist of the 1920s, was known to urbanites of the time as 'Dr. Sex'. Ding Ling's short story, 'Miss Sophia's Diary' (1927), became a powerful symbol of personal and sexual exploration. See, T. Barlow's translation in T. Barlow and G. J. Bjorge (eds), *I Myself Am A Woman: Selected Writings of Ding Ling* (Boston, MA: Beacon Press, 1989), pp. 49–81. See R. Witke, 'Chastity Cultism', *Transformation of Attitudes Towards Women During the May Fourth Era of Modern China* (PhD dissertation, University of California, 1970), pp. 104–33; C. Leary, 'Intellectual Orthodoxy, the Economy of Knowledge and the Debate over Zhang Jingsheng's Sex Histories', *Republican China*, 18 (1994), pp. 99–137; H. Chiang, 'Epistemic Modernity and the Emergence of Homosexuality in China', *Gender and History*, 22:3 (2010), pp. 629–57.

8 Blowers, Wang, 'Gone With the *West Wind*: The Emergence and Disappearance of Psychotherapeutic Culture in China (1936–68)'

1. Wen-Ji Wang, '*West Wind Monthly* and the Popular Mental Hygiene Discourse in Republican China', *Taiwanese Journal for Studies of Science, Technology and Medicine*, 13 (2011), pp. 15–88. See also G. Blowers, B. T. Cheung and H. Ru, 'Emulation vs. indigenization in the reception of western psychology in republican China: An analysis of the content of Chinese psychology journals (1922–37)', *Journal of the History of the Behavioural Sciences*, 45:1 (2009), pp. 21–33.
2. *Xi Feng* [West Wind], 58 (1941), pp. 357–8.
3. H. Shapiro, 'The View from a Chinese Asylum: Defining Madness in 1930s Beijing' (PhD dissertation, Harvard University, 1995). See also M. Ferguson, *China Medical Board and Peking Union Medical College: A chronicle of fruitful collaboration 1914–1951* (New York: China Medical Board of New York, 1970).

4. R. Fosdick, *The Story of the Rockefeller Foundation*, (London: Odhams, 1952), pp. 128–9, cited in J. Z. Bowers, *Western Medicine in a Chinese Palace: Peking Union Medical College 1917–1951* (New York: Josiah Macy Jr Foundation, c. 1972), p. 194.
5. *West Wind*, 83 (19460, pp. 496–500; Ibid., 60 (1941), pp. 569–72; Ibid., 58 (1941), pp. 353–5.
6. Ibid., 54 (1941), pp. 606–9; Ibid., 56 (1941), pp. 147–52; Ibid., 67 (1944), pp. 30–3; Ibid., 68 (1944), pp. 161–3; Ibid., 73 (1945), pp. 2–7; Ibid., 89 (1946), pp. 474–8; Ibid., 107 (1948), pp. 375–82.
7. Wen-Ji Wang, '*West Wind Monthly* and the Popular Mental Hygiene Discourse in Republican China', pp. 15–88.
8. Halpern Papers, Simon Fraser University Archives, Box 17, File 1.
9. Letter dated 9 May 1939, Ibid.
10. At the outbreak of the Sino Japanese war and the incursion of Japanese troops from Manchuria into Peking, Dai decided to return to America. B. Dai, 'My experience of psychotherapy: some reasons for my relative freedom from fatigue', *Voices: The Art and Science of Psychotherapy*, 15:2 (1979), pp. 26–33. Reprinted in S. Atkins (ed.), *Becoming Fully Human: Writings of Bingham Dai*, Boone, NC: Appalachian State University, Hubbard Center, 1997), pp. 49–54.
11. Dai Letter to Bolton, 11th April 1986 Appalachian State University, Boone, NC, Bingham Dai Papers, Rare Books & Manuscripts, RB.8007.
12. Ding Tsan, 'Talk on Psychological Cultivation', *Mental Cultivation of Youth* (Beijing: Bing Huang Medical Press, 1947), pp. 1–9.
13. See note 6, above, p. 247.
14. Ding Tsan, *Mental Health Essays* (Shanghai: Commerce Publishing House, 1945); Ding Tsan, 'Talk on Psychological Cultivation', pp. 1–9. Note: Bing Ying refers to the year 1926, when a group of young doctors in Peking Union Hospital set up its medical association and named it the Bing Ying Medical Society.
15. Ding Tsan, *Mental Health Essays* (Shanghai: Commerce Publishing House, 1945), p. 114.
16. Ibid.
17. Ding Tsan, Zhao Wanhe and Yao Xiuhua, 'Yao Xiu Ha Investigation of Chinese Children's Behavioral Problems', *West Wind*, 840 (1946), pp. 626–30, cited in Fan Tingwei, *Ding Tsan – Thoughts and Practices in the Period of the Sinicization of Mental Health*, Ding Tsan's 100th Anniversary Special Issue (Nanjing, China: Department of Psychology, Nanjing University, 2010), pp. 114–26.
18. Ibid.
19. Ibid.
20. Ding Tsan, Zhao Wanhe and Yao Xiuhua, 'Psychoanalysis and Medicine: Speech in Medical School of Central University, 1947', in Tang Cimei and Li Xintian (eds), Ding Tsan`s Psychological Corpus (Beijing: People's Education Press, 2009), pp. 230–6; Ding Tsan, *Mental Cultivation of Youth*, p. 238.
21. Ding Tsan, 'I am Psychoanalyst; Talk About Psychological Cultivation', *Psychological Cultivation of Youth* (Beijing: Bing Huang Medical Press, 1947), pp. 1–2.
22. Ibid.
23. Ibid.
24. Fan Tingwei, 'Ding Tsan and his Practice of Psychoanalysis', *Chinese Journal of Medical History*, 40:5 (Sept 2010), pp. 306–10.
25. Bingham Dai, 'Asian Psychoanalysis in China before the Revolution: A Letter From Bingham Dai', *Transcultural Psychiatry*, 21 (1984), pp. 280–3. See also Bingham Dai,

Letter to George Stevenson, 28 August 1941, Rockefeller Archives, CMB collection, Box 92 Folder 655.

26. Ding Tsan, 'The Girl who was Hooked by the Devil' in Tang Ci-mei and Li Xing-tian (eds), *Collection of Psychological Articles of Ding Tsan* (Beijing: People's Education Press, 2009), pp. 161–70.
27. Ding Tsan, 'Life Style in Reality' in Tang Ci-mei and Li Xing-tian, *Collection of Psychological* Articles, pp. 178–85.
28. Zhu Qi, later became an editor of Yi Lin ['Forest of Translation], the top literary journal of translation works in China.
29. Yeh Hsueh and Benyu Guo, 'China' in D. B. Baker (ed.), *Oxford Handbook of the History of Psychology: Global Perspectives (*New York: Oxford University Press, 2012), pp. 81–194.
30. XL Fang, 'Rethinking Huang Jia-yin', *Xin Ming Evening News*, 20 October 1998, B7.
31. Huang Jiayin, *Psychotherapy 300 Cases* (Shanghai: Family Press, 1952), p. 50.
32. Shen Decan, 'Changes to China as a Result of Freud's Theory and Practice' in Shi Qijia and Wolfgang Senf (eds), *Psychotherapy in Dialogue, Psychoanalysis in China* (Hangzhou, China: Hang Zhou Publishing House, 2009), pp. 126–30. See also Li Mengchao, 'The History of Psychotherapy in China', 19 June 2010, at http://psychspace.com/psych/viewnews-2050 [accessed March 2012].
33. Li Mengchao, 'The History of Psychotherapy in China'.
34. Su Zonghua and Huang Jiayin, *The Girl who Thought she was the Queen: A Case Analysis and Therapy of Abnormal Psychology* (Shanghai: Family Publishing House, 1950).
35. Hu Zhiwei, 'What happened to Huang Jia yin and Huang Jia de Brothers', *The Corpus of Hu Zhiwei*, Independent Chinese Pen Center, at http://blog.boxun.com/hero/2007/huzhiweiwenji/85_1.shtml [accessed March 2012].
36. Mang Yan, 'Did One of Our Families Start Psychotherapy Practice in China?', 15 June 2010, at http://blog.sina.com.cn/s/blog_5f07c1960100jqe2.html [accessed March 2012].
37. Tai Nan, *The Life in Ning Xia of an Old Couple from Shanghai, Huang Jia yin and Zhu Qi* at http://blog.sina.com.cn/s/blog_452e534b0100j2ry.html, 2010 [accessed April 2012].
38. L. Rao, 'Left Behind Dream of Shanghai', *Flying Like Wind: The Story of Zhu Wei-heng, Father of Chinese Magnetic Train* (China: China Writers Publishing House, 2009); Nan, *The Life in Ning Xia*.
39. Wang Canfa and He Xinhua, 'Research on the Style of Free Talk in Shen Daily [Shun Pao] in the Period of Huang Jiayin', *Journal of Hubei Social Science*, 1 (2006), pp. 122–3.
40. Yeh Hsueh and Benyu Guo, 'China', p. 101.
41. Li Ming, 'Zan Ding: Founder of Medical Psychology in China', *Protein and Cell*, 3:1 (January 2012), pp. 8–9.
42. 'The History of Nanjing Neuropsychiatric Hospital' at http://www.c-nbh.com/about/lsyg.asp [accessed May 2012].
43. Li Ming, 'Zan Ding: Founder of Medical Psychology in China', pp. 8–9.
44. Xue Pangao and Xiong Weiming, 'Freedom and Intervention: Psychology in China (1949–76)', *Science and Culture Review* (2006) at http://blog.sciencenet.cn/blog-1203335-756315.html [accessed April 2012]. Also, Fu Weinan Ding Zan, 'The Hero in the Smoke of Gunpowder', 2012 at http://blog.sciencenet.cn/blog-1203335-756315.html [accessed April 2012].
45. Ibid.

46. Ding Zongyi, *Ding Tsan and his Academic Record*, Ding Tsan's 100th Anniversary Special Issue (Nanjing, China: Department of Psychology, Nanjing University, 2010), pp. 22–63.
47. Ibid.
48. Yeh Hsueh and Benyu Guo, 'China', pp. 81–124.
49. Xue Pangao and Xiong Weiming, 'Freedom and Intervention'. See also, G. H. Blowers, 'Chen Li: China's elder psychologist', *History of Psychology*, 1 (1998), pp. 310–15.
50. Wang Zucheng, 'Chinese Mental Health's Forerunner – Su Zonghua', *Journal of Shanghai* Psychiatry, 12 (2000), pp. 1–7.
51. Rui Z. *The Saint on the Communion Table – Biography of Lin Zhao* (Taipei: Xiuwei Press, 2006), p. 177.
52. Peng Linfan, *Recollections of My Sister Lin Zhao.*
53. J. Dechu, 'Recollections of a discussion in Shanghai in the 1950s of Adolf Mayer's psychobiology involving Ji Ming's 'Anti-scientific and anti-revolutionary Psychology of Adolf Mayer' and Su Zonghua's 'My reconsideration of Mayer's psychobiology'', *Shanghai Archives of Psychiatry*, 13:1 (2001), at http://d.wanfangdata.com.cn/Periodical_shjsyx200101018.aspx. [accessed May 2012].
54. Wang Zucheng, 'Chinese Mental Health's Forerunner', *Shanghai Archives of Psychiatry*, 12 (2000), pp. 1–7.
55. Ge Minren 'Is this the Scientific Method and Right Direction for Studying Psychology? Asking Psychologists' Advice', *Renmin Ribao*, 28 October 1966.

9 Wu, 'A Charted Epidemic of Trauma: Case Notes at the Psychiatric Department of National Taiwan University Hospital Between 1946 And 1953'

1. According to Charles E. Rosenberg (1989), epidemics start 'at a moment in time, proceed on a stage limited in space and duration, follow a plot line of increasing and revelatory tension, move to a crisis of individual and collective character, then drift toward closure" (p. 2). The epidemic of psychoneurotic trauma described in this chapter partly follows Rosenberg's definitive pattern. It, however, is unique since it nether won public attention, nor did it obtain any official acknowledgement. This chapter is mainly concerned about the ways in which a professional community was mobilized to act out their diagnoses, treatment and care to these patients that incorporate and reaffirm their social values and modes of understanding the phenomena.
2. A. Cambrosio, A. Young and M. Lock, 'Introduction', in A. Cambrosio et al. (eds), *Living and Working with the New Medical Technologies: Intersections of Inquiry* (Cambridge: Cambridge University Press, 2000), pp. 1–16. Also see P. Mühlhäusler, 'Ecolinguistics, Linguisti Diversity, Ecological Diversity', in L. Maffi (ed.), *On Biocultural Diversity: Linking Language, Knowledge and the Environment* (Washington: Smithsonian Institution Press, 2001), pp. 133–44.
3. 'Taiwanese' mainly refers to residents in Taiwan. Most of them are of Chinese decent. After World War II, many of them either claim or are ascribed themselves Taiwanese as a regional or cultural identity resulted from the authoritarian governance of the Nationalist Chinese Party (Kuomintang), social conflices and all other reasons. In this chapter, 'Taiwanese" was also used as an ethnic category in the statistical studies conducted by the NTUH.

4. See M. Foucault and R. Howard, *Madness and Civilization: A History of Insanity in the Age of Reason* (London: Tavistock Publications, 1967). Also see C. E. Rosenberg, 'Towards an Ecology of Knowledge: On Discipline, Context and History', in Alexandra Oleson and John Voss (eds), *The Organization of Knowledge in Modern America, 1860–1920* (Baltimore, MD: Johns Hopkins University Press, 1979).
5. For the discussion about patient's voice, see R. Porter, 'The Patient's View', *Theory and Society,* 14:2 (1985), pp. 175–98.
6. Cambrosio et al., *Living and Working with the New Medical Technologies*, pp. 1–16. Also see L. Fleck, *Genesis and Development of a Scientific Fact*, trans. F. Bradley and T. J. Trenn (Chicago, IL and London: University of Chicago Press, 1979).
7. See N. D. Jewson, 'The Disappearance of the Sick-Man from Medical Cosmology, 1770–1870', *Sociology,* 10:2 (1976), pp. 225–44.
8. See M. Barfoot and A. Beveridge, ''Our most notable inmate': John Willis Mason at the Royal Edinburgh Asylum, 1864–1901', *History of Psychiatry,* IV (1993), pp. 159–208 and A. Beveridge, 'Madness in Victorian Edinburgh: A Study of Patients Admitted to the Royal Edinburgh Asylum under Thomas Clouston, 1873–1908 Part I', *History of Psychiatry,* VI (1995), pp. 21–54.
9. Examples include H. Marland, 'Disappointment and Desolation: Women, Doctors and Interpretations of Puerperal Insanity in the Nineteenth Century', *History of Psychiatry,* 14:3 (2003), pp. 303–20; M. S. Micale and P. F. Lerner, 'Trauma, Psychiatry and History: A Conceptual and Historiographical Introduction', in M. S. Micale and P. F. Lerner (eds), *Traumatic pasts : history, psychiatry and trauma in the modern age, 1870–1930* (Cambridge: Cambridge University Press, 2001), pp. 1–30 and K. E. Williams, 'Hysteria in Seventeenth-Century Case Records and Unpublished Manuscripts', *History of Psychiatry,* I (1990), pp. 383–401.
10. C. Berkenkotter, *Patient Tales: Case Histories and the Uses of Narrative in Psychiatry* (Columbia, SC: The University of South Carolina Press, 2008).
11. See D. Doyle, ''A Fine New Child': The Lafargue Mental Hygiene Clinic and Harlem's African American Communities, 1946–1958', *Journal of the History of Medicine and Allied Sciences,* 64:2 (2008), pp. 173–212.
12. Examples please see L. Barry and C. Coleborne, 'Insanity and Ethnicity in New Zealand: Ma–ori Encounters with the Auckland Mental Hospital, 1860–1900', *History of Psychiatry,* 22:3 (2011), pp. 285–301; W. Ernst, 'Doctor-Patient Interaction in Colonial India: A Case of 'intellectual insanity'', *History of Psychiatry,* I (1990), pp. 207–22; M. Gambino, ''These Strangers Within our Gates': Race, Psychiatry and Mental Illness Among Black Americans at St Elizabeths Hospital in Washington, DC, 1900–40', *History of Psychiatry,* 19:4 (2008), pp. 387–408; E. Jones, S. Rahman and B. Everitt, 'Psychiatric Case Notes: Symptoms of Mental Illness and their Attribution at the Maudsley Hospital, 1924–1935', *History of Psychiatry,* 23:2 (2012), pp. 156–68; S. Ledebur, 'Schreiben und Beschreiben. Zur epistemischen Funktion von psychiatrischen Krankenakten, ihrer Archivierung und deren bersetzung in Fallgeschichten', in *Berichte Zur Wissenschaftsgeschichte,* 34:2 (2011), pp. 102–24; J. Mills, 'The History of Modern Psychiatry in India, 1858–1947', *History of Psychiatry,* XII (2001), pp. 431–58 and S. Wulf, ''The Communication is of course Very Difficult'. The 'insane re-migrants' from America in the Hamburg Asylum Friedrichsberg 1909', *Medizinhistorisches Journal,* 43:3–4 (2008), pp. 231–63.
13. See A. Suzuki, 'A Brain Hospital in Tokyo and its Private and Public Patients, 1926–45', *History of Psychiatry,* 14:3 (2003), pp. 337–60.

14. The content is in the lecture notes given by A. Suzuki, 'Case Histories and the Institutional Demography of a Japanese Psychiatric Hospital in Early 20c Tokyo' (Institute of History and Philology, Academia Sinica, 2011).
15. See P. P. Szto, 'The Accommodation of Insanity in Canton, China, 1857–1935' (PhD Dissertation, University of Pennsylvania, 2002).
16. See K. S. Yip, 'A Historical Review of Mental Health Services in Hong Kong (1841 To 1995)', *Journal of Social Psychiatry,* 44:1 (1998), pp. 46–55.
17. H. Shapiro, 'The View From A Chinese Asylum: Defining Madness in 1930s Peking' (PhD Dissertation, Harvard University, 1995)
18. See J. L. Cox, *Transcultural Psychiatry* (London; Dover, N.H: Croom Helm, 1986).
19. Y. C. Wu and H. W. Teng, 'Tropics, Neurasthenia and Japanese Colonizers: The Psychiatric Discourses in Late Colonial Taiwan', *Taiwan, A Radical Quarterly in Social Studies,* 54 (2004), pp. 61–103. Also see Y. C. Wu, 'Nostalgia and 'Sexual Syndrome': Hypochondriasis and Masculinity in Late Colonial Taiwan', *Journal of Women's and Gender Studies,* 21 (2006), pp. 1–46 and Y. C. Wu, 'Disappearing Anger: The Psychological Experiment on Anger among Formosan Aborigines Conducted by Fujisawa Shigeru in Late Colonial Taiwan', *New History,* 18:2 (2007), pp. 103–55.
20. Chen, Ta, 'The Need of Population Research in China', *Population Studies,* 1:4 (1948), pp. 342–52.
21. See P. Cheung, 'Adult Psychiatric Epidemiology in China in the 80s', *Culture, Medicine and Psychiatry,* 15:4 (1991), pp. 479–96.
22. See C. J. Wong, *Postwar Taiwan in historical perspective* (Studies in Global Chinese affairs, Bethesda, MD: University Press of Maryland, 1998).
23. See S. F. Chen, *Post-War Epidemics: Issues and Institutionalisation of Public Health in Taiwan, 1945–1954* (Taipei: Daw Shiang Publishing, 2000).
24. See H. Cai, *Taiwan in Japan's Empire-Building: An Institutional Approach to Colonial Engineering* (Academia Sinica on East Asia.; London ; New York: Routledge, 2009).
25. See C. K. Chen, *Studies on the Social Status of Taiwanese Doctors under Japanese Rules* (Graduate Institute of History Series, Taipei: National Taiwan Normal University, 1992).
26. To diminish the influence of Taiwanese intellectuals, the Japanese colonial government either prevented Taiwanese from working or minimized the number of Taiwanese staff in most public sectors, including educational institutions. According to the statistics conducted by the adoption committee, among the 600 Taiwanese who worked at Imperial Taihoku University, there was only one professor, Congming Tu, of the Medical School and one higher ranking lecturer, Bosei Lim, at the School of Humanities. Other Taiwanese were mostly administration staff. No Taiwanese worked in the affiliated hospital as operating officers. Thirty-nine Taiwanese clinicians were all assistants (副手). See H. J. Chang, 'The Adoption of Taihoku Imperial University', *National Taiwan University College of Medicine 1945–1950* (Taipei: National Taiwan University Press, 2013). See M. L. Chiu, 'Mind, Body and Illness in a Chinese Medical Tradition' (PhD Dissertation, Harvard University, 1986).
27. See K. M. Lin, 'Traditional Chinese Medical Beliefs and their Relevance for Mental Illness and Psychiatry', in A. Kleinman and T. Y. Lin (eds), *Normal and Abnormal Behavior in Chinese Culture* (Dordrecht, Boston, London: D. Reidel Publishing Company, 1981), pp. 95–111.
28. See T. Y. Lin, *Road to Psychiatry: Across the East and the West* (Taipei: Daw Shiang Publishing, 1994).

29. See T. Y. Lin, 'My Father Bosei Lim', in H. L. Hu (ed.), *Daoyu Ailian* [Love Stories on the Island] (Taipei: Yu-Shan Books, 1995), pp. 1–23.
30. Matsuzawa Hospital (currently Tokyo Metropolitan Matsuzawa Hospital) is the largest and oldest mental hospital in Japan, founded in 1879 and currently assumed the best Japanese authority of psychiatry in the area. Before Tsung-Yi Lin's departure for the entrance examination at Tokyo University, Bosei Lim gave him a calligraphic rendering of a poem written by Wang Yang-ming (王陽明, 1471–1529), a Neo-Confucian philosopher in Ming China.

    I know you search for Utopia.
    Where may it be found?
    Far away in the deep ravines of the Western Mountains.
    The Ancients say the fisherman knows the way.
    Ask not.
    Follow the river,
    Gather flowers as you climb.

    According to Lin's memoir, T. Y. Lin, *Road to Psychiatry: Across the East and the West* (Taipei: Daw Shiang Publishing, 1994), the cultural foundation embedded in Chinese thought provided him the soil for his studies to take root. Wang Yangming's poem not only reflects how difficult it was to pursue the narrow road so seldom traveled; according to Komagome Takeshi, who studied the intellectual history of Bosei Lim, the 'deepest place in the mountains of the West' reflects the experience of the Taiwanese elite, Lin, who was driven to study in the West in search of the possibility of modernity: Komagome Takeshi, 'Colonial Modernity for an Elite Taiwanese, Lim Bo-Seng: The Labyrinth of Cosmopolitanism', in P. H. Liao and D. Wang (eds), *Taiwan under Japanese Colonial Rule, 1895–1945* (New York: Columbia University Press, 2006), pp. 141–59. In 1984, when he published his memoir, gathered from the lecture handouts from a series of invited talks at his *alma mater*, the University of Tokyo, in September 1979, on his experience of international activities, he entitled the book *The Road to Psychiatry: Across East and West*. This, to a considerable degree, represents the composition and structure of his cross-cultural knowledge.
31. Ibid.
32. Ibid.
33. See Lin, *Road to Psychiatry*, pp. 1–24.
34. See W. S. Tseng, *One Life, Three Cultures: The Self-Analysis on Personality Shaped by China, Japan and America* (Taipei: Psychology, 2010).
35. These included surveys of three areas of different urbanization levels from 1946 to 1948 and of three indigenous populations from 1949 to 1952. His research outcomes, published in 1953, became a policy paper and attracted worldwide notice.
36. See Lin, *Road to Psychiatr*, pp. 1–24.
37. Ibid.
38. Ibid.
39. Ibid.
40. For example, Lin's students Wen-Shing Tseng and Ying-Kun Yeh detailed the social context of language change and their identity shift in the early post-war period. Yeh especially mentioned that during this period, lectures at the medical school were given in mixed official Mandarin (*guoyu*, 國語), Taiwanese, Japanese, English and German. See Wen-Shing Tseng, *One Life, Three Cultures: The Self-Analysis on Personality Shaped by China, Japan and America* (Taipei: Psychology, 2010), pp. 56–8 and J. S. Wu, *The*

Pioneer of Taiwanese Psychiatric Care: Biography of Ying-Kun Yeh (Taipei: Psygarden, 2005), p. 88.

41. See Figure 9.1, p. 171.
42. NTUH Psych Dept Case Note, 1945, No. 119.
43. ICD-6 is the first ICD revision published by the WHO to include a section on mental disorders. It was, however, not widely accepted and used when it was first introduced.
44. NTUH Psych Dept Case Note, 1946, In-patient No. 280.
45. NTUH Psych Dept Case Note, 1946, In-patient No. 217.
46. NTUH Psych Dept Case Note, 1947, No. 208.
47. NTUH Psych Dept Case Note, 1947, No. 299.
48. NTUH Psych Dept Case Note, 1948, No. 299.
49. NTUH Psych Dept Case Note, 1946, No. 262.
50. NTUH Psych Dept Case Note, 1949, No. 236.
51. NTUH Psych Dept Case Note, 1946, No. 51.
52. NTUH Psych Dept Case Note, 1946, No. 115.
53. NTUH Psych Dept Case Note, 1946, No. 204.
54. See A. W. Moore, 'Problems of Changing Language Communities: Veterans and Memory Writing in China, Taiwan and Japan', *Modern Asian Studies,* 45:2 (2011), pp. 399–429.
55. See E. Jones and S. Wessely, *Shell Shock to PTSD: Military Psychiatry from 1900 to the Gulf War* (Hove: Psychology Press, 2005).
56. Oxford St Hugh's Head Hospital Archives, Case 10430(486).
57. Oxford St Hugh's Head Hospital Archives, Case 11428(762).
58. Oxford St Hugh's Head Hospital Archives, Freda Newcombe to Dr. Foster, December 21, 1984.
59. Oxford St Hugh's Head Hospital Archives, Case 10813(561).
60. 「空襲了！飛機來了！」「大水來了！」「豚が來了」. Some Taiwanese people called Japanese people 'pigs" to express their hatred towards colonization. Source: NTUH Psych Dept Case Note, 1945, No. 118.
61. NTUH Psych Dept Case Note, 1946, No. 236.
62. See Lin, 'My Father Bosei Lim', pp. 1–23.
63. NTUH Psych Dept Case Note, 1948, No. 291.
64. C. E. Rosenberg, 'What is an Epidemic? AIDS in Historical Perspectives', *Daedalus,* 118:2 (1989), pp. 1–17.
65. Clinical cases being contested zones of various interests have been much discussed by historians of medicine, for example, see J. Matsumura, 'State Propaganda and Mental Disorders: The Issue of Psychiatric Casualties among Japanese Soldiers during the Asia-Pacific War', *Bulletin of the History of Medicine,* 78:4 (2004), pp. 804–35; H. P. Schmiedebach, 'The Mentally Ill Patient Caught betwen the State's Demands and the Professional Insterests of Psychiatrists', in D. Junker (ed.), *Medicine and Modernity* (Washington D.C.: The German Historical Institute, 1997), pp. 99–119; S. Sturdy, 'Knowing Cases: Biomedicine in Edinburgh, 1887–1929', *Social Studies of Science,* 37:5 (2011), pp. 659–89; A. Young, 'A Description of How Ideology Shapes Knowledge of a Mental Disorder (Posttraumatic Stress Disorder)', in S. Lindenbaum and M. Lock (eds), *Knowledge, Power and Practice: The Anthropolgy of Medicine and Everyday Life* (Berkeley, CA: University of California Press, 1993), pp. 108–28.
66. See M. Matsushita, 'Introduction', in M. Matsushita (ed.), *History of Psychiatric Diagnoses: Proceedings of the 16th International Symposium on the Comparative History of*

Medicine – East and West (Tokyo: Ishiyaku EuroAmerica, Inc. Publishers, 1997), pp. iv–viii.

67. See B. Y. Rhi, 'Modes of Psychiatric Diagnosis in Historical Perspective', in Matsushita, *History of Psychiatric Diagnoses*, pp. 27–54.

10 Huang, 'The Emergence of the Psycho-Boom in Contemporary Urban China'

1. For example, see W. Wan, 'Freud Coming into Fashion in China', *Washington Post*, 11 October 2010; D. K. Tatlow, 'Freudians Put China on the Couch', *New York Times*, 28 October 2010; and E. Osnos, 'Meet Dr. Freud: Does Psychoanalysis Have a Future in China?' *New Yorker*, 86:43 (November 2011), pp. 54–63.
2. The psycho-boom could be seen as a new addition to the feverish trends that emerge at various moments in the post-Mao period, including 'Qigong fever' (*qigong re*), 'culture fever' (*wenhua re*), 'stock fever' (*gupiao re*), 'national studies fever' (*guoxue re*) and many others. The term '*xinli re*', which literally means 'psych fever', is in fact not heard very often as people are getting tired of the constant appearance of new 'fevers'. The term 'psycho-boom' is borrowed from G. R. Bach and H. Molter, *Psychoboom: Wege und Abwege Moderner Therapie* [Psycho-Boom: Ways and Byways of Modern Psychotherapy] (Reinbek bei Hamburg: Rowoholt, 1976); and Johann Schülein, 'Psychoanalyse und Psychoboom: Bemerkungen zum Sozialen Sinnkontext Therapeutischer Modelle' [Psychoanalysis and the Psycho-Boom: Remarks on the Social Meaning-Context of Therapeutic Models], *Psyche*, 32:5–6 (1978), pp. 420–40. They used the notion of 'psychoboom' to describe the proliferation of groups and workshops in 1970s Germany, which was largely inspired by various strands of humanistic psychology. The phenomena they depicted in many ways resemble what is happening in urban China, with a notable difference that in China 'training' is often stated as a major objective.
3. Recent ethnographic endeavors have begun to investigate the emergence of psychological subjectivity in China. Important examples include: A. Kleinman et al. (eds), *Deep China: The Moral Life of the Person* (Berkeley, CA: University of California Press, 2011); A. Kipnis (ed), *Chinese Modernity and the Individual Psyche* (New York: Palgrave Macmillan, 2012); and M. H. Hansen and R. Svarverud (eds), *iChina: The Rise of the Individual in Modern Chinese Society* (Copenhagen: NIAS Press, 2010). The transformation of subjectivity, including the deepening of interiority and growing attention on various aspects of the self, is a salient context of the psycho-boom and the psycho-boom is also vigorously shaping this new subjectivity. This is an issue that I will discuss in the future.
4. T. M. Luhrmann, *Of Two Minds: An Anthropologist Looks at American Psychiatry* (New York: Vintage Books, 2001); J. Davies, *The Making of Psychotherapists: An Anthropological Analysis* (London: Karnac Books, 2009).
5. The Ministry of Labor and Social Security was established in 1998, succeeding the former Ministry of Labor. It was again restructured as the Ministry of Human Resources and Social Security in 2008. However, most of the psycho-boom participants still prefer to call it 'Ministry of Labor'. In this article, 'Ministry of Labor' is used as the abbreviation for 'Ministry of Labor and Social Security' or 'Ministry of Human Resources and Social Security'.

6. My observation is that therapists who manage to stay in the field over these years tend to have a considerable growth in numbers of clients, but they account for a relatively small portion of those who tried to engage in psychotherapy practice. Overall, the number of clients seeking psychotherapy treatments might be growing, but the rate should be slower than that of the population pursuing psychotherapy training.
7. This realization emerged as a result of my fieldwork in Beijing and Shanghai. After two months of preliminary research in the summer of 2008, I did twenty-two months of fieldwork from September 2009 through July 2011. I was principally based in Beijing, but I spent three months in total in Shanghai and made quite a few short trips to several other cities. I have maintained close contact with a group of key informants and continued to observe related activities in cyberspace since then.
8. Psychology in China had remained a research discipline based in universities and research institutes until very recently. Its sole practical branch is college counselling, which first emerged in the 1980s. While in the United States and many other Western countries clinical psychologists are an integral part of the psychiatric team, this clinical discipline rarely exists in Chinese hospitals even today.
9. It is noteworthy that the community of counselling psychology in Taiwan chooses a less casual term, '*zishang*' (諮商), as the translation of 'counselling'.
10. Zhao Gengyuan, 'Xinli zixun de jinzhan' [The Progress of Psychological Counselling] in Chen Xueshi and Chen Xiuhua (eds), *Zhongguo xiandai shenjing jingshen bingxue fazhan zhuangkuang* [The Development of Modern Neurology and Psychiatry in China] (Beijing: Zhongguo kexue jishu chubanshe, 1995), pp. 288–95.
11. Chen Peizhang and He Ruichang, 'Zonghe yiyuan de xinli zixun gongzuo' [Psychological Counselling in General Hospitals], *Yiyuan guanli* [Hospital Administration], 10 (1983), pp. 42–3; Zhao Gengyuan et al., 'Zonghe yiyuan kaizhan xinli zixun 100 li xiaojie' [A Brief Summary of One Hundred Psychological Counselling Cases in General Hospitals], *Zhongshan yixueyuan xuebao* [Acta Academiae Medicinae Zhong Shan], 5:3 (1984), pp. 63–6.
12. S.-M. A. Leung, L. Guo and M. P. Lam, 'The Development of Counselling Psychology in Higher Educational Institutions in China: Present Conditions and Needs, Future Challenges', *The Counselling Psychologist*, 28:1 (2000), pp. 81–99.
13. See A. Kleinman, *Social Origins of Distress and Disease: Depression, Neurasthenia and Pain in Modern China* (New Haven, CT: Yale University Press, 1986). Kleinman's collaboration with the leading psychiatric institutions in China – first the Psychiatry Department at Hunan Medical College in the 1980s and then Shanghai Mental Health Center and Peking Medical College's Institute of Mental Health in the 1990s – facilitated the mental health care reform at the turn of the century.
14. M. R. Phillips, H. Liu and Y. Zhang, 'Suicide and Social Change in China', *Culture, Medicine and Psychiatry*, 23:1 (1999), pp. 25–50, M. R. Phillips, X. Li and Y. Zhang, 'Suicide Rates in China, 1995–1999', *Lancet*, 359:9309 (2002), pp. 835–40.
15. S. Lee, 'Estranged Bodies, Simulated Harmony and Misplaced Cultures: Neurasthenia in Contemporary Chinese Society', *Psychosomatic Medicine*, 60:4 (1998), pp. 448–57; S. Lee, 'Diagnosis Postponed: *Shenjing Shuairuo* and the Transformation of Psychiatry in Post-Mao China', *Culture, Medicine and Psychiatry*, 23:3 (1999), pp. 349–80.
16. V. Pearson, *Mental Health Care in China: State Policies, Professional Services and Family Responsibilities* (London: Gaskell, 1995); M. R. Phillips, 'The Transformation of China's Mental Health Services', *The China Journal*, 39 (1998), pp. 1–36.

17. 'Zhongguo jingshen weisheng guihua 2002–10' [National Mental Health Plan 2002–2010], 10 April 2002, at http://wenku.baidu.com/view/77d469150b4e767f5acfce98.html?from=related [accessed 20 August 2013]; 'Guanyu jinyibu jiaqiang jingshen weisheng gongzuo de zhidao yijian' [Proposal on Further Strengthening Mental Health Work], 2 September 2004, at http://www.gov.cn/ztzl/gacjr/content_459454.htm [accessed 20 August 2013]. In the following paragraphs, I will use the National Plan and the Proposal respectively as their abbreviations.
18. Yin Dakui, 'Qixinxieli jiaotashidi quanmian tuijin xinshiji jingshen weisheng gongzuo' [With All the Hearts Together, Stand on Solid Ground and Advance Mental Health Care in the New Century], *China Mental Health Journal*, 16:1 (2002), pp. 4–8.
19. In Chinese, 'psychiatry' is routinely translated as '*jingshen bing xue*' 精神病学 or '*jingshen yixue*' 精神医学 and 'psychology' is translated as '*xinli xue*' 心理学. While in English these terms share the same prefix, 'psych', their Chinese counterparts have different words at their beginnings: one is '*jingshen*' (spirit or essence) and the other is '*xinli*' (mind or heart). Both '*jingshen weisheng*' and '*xinli weisheng*' could stand for 'mental health', but the former is closely associated with psychiatry.
20. For the '686 Project', see J. Liu et al., 'Mental Health System in China: History, Recent Service Reform and Future Challenges', *World Psychiatry*, 10:3 (2011), pp. 210–6; and H. Ma, 'Integration of Hospital and Community Services – the '686 Project' – Is a Crucial Component in the Reform of China's Mental Health Services', *Shanghai Archives of Psychiatry*, 24:3 (2012), pp. 172–4.
21. It is said that only about two thousand people have attained the certificate for psychotherapist. All of them are physicians or nurses. This is a tiny fraction of those who have passed the Ministry of Labor certification.
22. 'Working Committee on National Occupational Classification and Vocational Qualifications', *Zhonghua renmin gongheguo guojia zhiye fenlei dadian* [The People's Republic of China's National Occupational Classification] (Beijing: Zhongguo laodong shehui chubanshe, 1999).
23. How many certificates have been issued remains a mystery since the Ministry of Labor never releases the official statistics. During my fieldwork, I regularly collected the number of certificates circulated in the field from the influential figures in psychiatry or academic psychology. When I began my fieldwork in 2008, the numbers ranged from 80,000 to 160,000. When I was near the end of my fieldwork in 2011, most of the people I knew put their estimates at around 300,000. It is intriguing that 300,000 still seems to be the number everyone refers to, though it must have increased substantially since then.
24. Ministry of Labor and Social Security, *Guojia zhiye biaojun: xinli zhixun shi shixing* [National Vocational Standards: Psychological Counsellor Interim Version] (Beijing: Zhongguo laodong shehui baozhang chubanshe, 2001); Ministry of Labor and Social Security, *Guojia zhiye biaojun: xinli zhixun shi* [National Vocational Standards: Psychological Counsellor] (Beijing: Zhongguo laodong shehui baozhang chubanshe, 2005).
25. The most popular options for such occasions include CCTV's 'Psychological Interviews' and the American TV series, 'In Treatment', in which each episode features a session with a regular patient.
26. Based on the new Labor Law (1995) and Vocational Education Law (1996), the Ministry of Labor composed the National Occupational Classification, in which the skill standards for a full spectrum of occupations were stipulated. They also established a grand system that was largely borrowed from the UK's National Vocational Qualification. The

system was intended to supplement and replace the Workers Skill Level Assessment (*gongren jishu dengji kaohe* 工人技术等级考核) that dated back to the Maoist period.

27. Guo Nianfeng, 'Zhongguo xinli weisheng shiye de xianzhuang yu duice' [The Current Situation and Strategies of China's Mental Health Enterprise], *Health Psychology Journal*, 8:1 (2000), pp. 2–4.
28. Ibid., pp. 3–4.
29. This early history of the Ministry of Labor program is based on the official documents issued by the Ministry of Labor during the early years of the programme. These documents can be accessed at the online database of National Vocational Qualification at http://ms.nvq.net.cn/htm/_zcfw/index_ad43155ab3d076d7d30e19f75dbc4069.html.
30. Huaxia Xinli now offers a wide range of training courses in addition to the Ministry of Labor program. For more information, see its website (http://www.psychcn.com).
31. Huaxia Xinli, 'Xinli zixun de zhiye qianjing' [The Prospects of Psychological Counsellors], at http://www.psychcn.com/hots/psychcn/200601/1170919282.shtml, [accessed 20 March 2013].
32. Ibid.
33. Ibid.
34. Ibid.
35. For example, it is common that physicians and teachers attend the Ministry of Labor program in order to learn something about psychotherapy, which is increasingly perceived as beneficial to their work.
36. The Sino-German Course is widely regarded as the origin of Western psychotherapy in China because many of the prominent figures in the field were members of its first or second cohort. The collaboration between the German therapist Margarete Haaß-Wiesegart and a group of elite psychiatrists and psychologists in China began in the late 1980s, but the first three-year program did not begin until 1997 in Kunming. It then moved its base to Shanghai in 2000 under the auspices of the Shanghai Mental Health Center. Its influence over the psycho-boom is unmatched by other programs, particularly in terms of producing many of the most charismatic 'masters' in the training industry and shaping the popular preference for psychoanalysis or depth psychology. Currently, the Sino-German Course is still the most esteemed destination for psychotherapy training in China. For the most detailed account of this project written by its founders, see F. B. Simon, M. Haaß-Wiesegart and X. Zhao, '*Zhong De Ban*' *oder Wie die Psychotherapie nach China Kam: Geschichte und Analyse eines Interkulturellen Abenteuers* [The Sino-German Course or How Psychotherapy Came to China: History and Analysis of a Cross-Cultural Adventure] (Heidelberg: Carl-Auer-Systeme Verlag, 2011).
37. 'Sohu Hosts Drs. Yang Fengchi and Li Zixun from CCTV's Psychological Interviews', Sohu Health, at http://health.sohu.com/s2006/xinlifangtan, [accessed 20 March 2013]
38. It is widely known that psychotherapy treatments in China rarely exceed three sessions and one-shot consultations may constitute more than half of the cases. This is contradictory to the ideal of psychoanalytic orientation claimed by many therapists.
39. J. Krieger, 'Manufacturing Psychological Understanding: How China's First National Psychotherapy TV Show Teaches Viewers Psychological Narratives of Chinese Family Problems' (PsyD Dissertation, Write Institute, 2009).
40. One of the most popular web-forums is *zhongguo xinli zhiliao shi* 中国心理治疗师 [Chinese Psychotherapists] at www.easemind.com.
41. For a recent article containing a brief discussion on voluntarism in the relief work for the Wenchuan earthquake and its implications for morality in contemporary China, see

Y. Yan, 'The Changing Moral Landscape', in A. Kleinman et al. (eds), Deep China: The Moral Life of the Person (Berkeley and Los Angeles, CA: University of California Press, 2011), pp. 36–77.

42. These scandalous stories receive minimal news coverage, but they are widely known in the psycho-boom circle. For the accounts that revealed this dark side of the voluntarism, see Chen Tongkui, 'Xinli zixun luanqiang daniao' [Psychological Counselling: Shooting in the Dark], *South Reviews*, 13 (June 2008), at http://www.nfcmag.com/article/866.html [accessed 20 August 2013]; and Li Jing, '512 zhounien fansi: fanghuo, fangdao, fang xinli zixun shi' [Reflections on the Anniversary of 512 Earthquake: Be Watchful of Fire, Thieves and Psychological Counsellors], at http://blog.sina.com.cn/s/blog_5f177eb20100dchk.html [accessed 20 August 2013].
43. Leading institutes in various parts of China, including psychiatric hospitals and psychology departments, were assigned to take care of specific locations of the affected region where they sent in their experts periodically. These efforts have made Chengdu, the provincial capital of Sichuan and the major city closest to the affected area, one of the centers of the psycho-boom.
44. Resolution on Certain Major Issues Regarding Building a Socialist Harmonious Society (The Sixth Plenary Session of the 16th Central Committee of the Chinese Communist Party, 2006). 11 October, 2006, at http://cpc.people.com.cn/GB/64093/64094/4932424.html [accessed 20 August 2013].
45. 'Wenchuan dizhen zaihou huifu chongjian tiaoli' [The Regulations on the Wenchuan Earthquake Post-Disaster Rehabilitation and Rebuilding], 9 June 2008, at http://www.gov.cn/zwgk/2008-06/09/content_1010710.htm [accessed 20 August 2013].
46. 'Wenchuan dizhen zaihou huifu chongjian zongti guihua' [The General Planning on the Wenchuan Earthquake Post-Disaster Rehabilitation and Rebuilding], 19 September 2008, at http://www.gov.cn/zwgk/2008-09/23/content_1103686.htm [accessed 20 August 2013].
47. The International Psychoanalytical Association (IPA), founded by Sigmund Freud in 1910, is considered the bastion of the international psychoanalytic movement. In ordinary circumstances, people in most Asian countries need to go broad to the places that have established psychoanalytic institutions to pursue analytic training. IPA set up direct candidate programs in Beijing (2009) and Shanghai (2011) so that selected candidates could complete the training in their home countries.
48. The China-American Psychoanalytic Alliance (CAPA) is possibly the largest (virtual) psychoanalytic association in the world. It has about 400 members, most of whom are analysts recognized by various psychoanalytic institutes in the United States. Founded by Dr. Elise Snyder, it began to provide long-term, Internet-based training programs that include lectures, individual and small group supervision and individual therapy or analysis to students in several major Chinese cities in 2008. For more information, see CAPA's website (www.chinacapa.org) or R. Fishkin et al., 'Psychodynamic Treatment, Training and Supervision Using Internet-Based Technologies', *The Journal of the American Academy of Psychoanalysis and Dynamic Psychiatry*, 39:1 (2011), pp. 155–68.
49. For example, the extremely popular dating contest show *fei cheng wu rao* 非诚勿扰 [If You Are the One] on Jiangsu Satellite TV Channel featured character analyses of its contestants by a few psychologists who quickly became household names.
50. When I began my fieldwork in 2008, most of the therapists I met in Beijing and Shanghai charged 150–300 yuan for a session. The range dramatically rose to 300–500 yuan during 2009–10 and a number of famous therapists could charge as high as 800 or 1000

yuan per hour. The surge of psychotherapy fees occurred in private agencies as the local health authorities imposed rather strict regulations on the pricing of medical treatments in public institutions. A similar trend occurred in tuition fees of training courses, too. While in 2008 a two-or-three-day workshop typically cost 1000–2500 yuan, from 2010 onward such courses would cost 2000–4000 yuan. During this period (from July 2008 to June 2010), the exchange rate stayed around 1 US dollar to 6.80 yuan.

51. M. Ramsey, *Professional and Popular Medicine in France, 1770–1830: The Social World of Medical Practice* (Cambridge; New York: Cambridge University Press, 1988); R. Porter, *Quacks: Fakers and Charlatans in English Medicine* (Stroud, Gloucestershire: Tempus Publishing Inc., 2001).
52. D. A. Palmer, *Qigong Fever: Body, Science and Utopia in China* (New York: Columbia University Press, 2007), p. 14.
53. The business of selling all sorts of paraphernalia that one needs to furnish the therapeutic facility flourishes with the thriving of psychotherapy. Popular products include computerized psychological tests, Sandplay Therapy equipment (sandboxes, sand and toys), biofeedback machines and lounging chairs that can provide maximum relaxation. Some companies offer packages that range from economic options to setting up an entire counselling center.
54. For the English translation of the law, see H. H. Chen et al., 'Mental Health Law of the People's Republic of China (English Translation with Annotations)', *Shanghai Archives of Psychiatry* 24:6 (2012), pp. 305–21.
55. J. Yang, 'Fake Happiness: Counselling, Potentiality and Psycho-Politics in China', *Ethos*, 41:3 (2013), pp. 292–312; J. Yang, 'Peiliao Companion to Chat: Gender, Psychologization and Psychological Labor in China', *Social Analysis*, 57:2, pp. 41–58; J. Yang, 'Song Wennuan, Sending Warmth: Unemployment, New Urban Poverty and the Affective State in China', *Ethnography*, 14:1 (2013), pp. 104–25.

11 Chen, 'Afterword: Reframing Psychiatry in China'

1. A. Kleinman, *Social Origins of Distress and Disease: Depression, Neurasthenia and Pain in Modern China* (New Haven, CT: Yale University Press, 1986).
2. Sing Lee, 'Cultures in Psychiatric Nosology: the CCMD-2-R and International Classification of Mental Disorders', *Culture, Medicine and Psychiatry*, 20:4 (1996), pp. 421–72.
3. M. R. Phillips, S. H. Lu and R. W. Wang, 'Economic Reforms and the Acute Inpatient Care of Patients with Schizophrenia: The Chinese Experience', *American Journal of Psychiatry*, 154:9 (September 1997), pp. 1228–34.
4. M. R. Phillips, Hanhui Chen, K. Diesfeld, Bin Xie, Hui G. Cheng, G. Mellsop and Xiehe Liu, 'China's New Mental Health Law: Reframing Involuntary Treatment', *American Journal of Psychiatry*, 170:6 (June 2013), pp. 588–91.

INDEX

'100 Flowers' period, 153
abnormal psychology, 144
abstinence, sexual, 120
abuse
  of insane by family, 91, 92, 97, 100–1
  of women, 131, 132, 137, 139
Academia Sinica, 155, 163
academic psychology, 201, 202
acclimatization, white, 113, 117, 119
acupuncture, 42, 155
adaptation, failure of, 120–1
adjustment disorders, 12, 176–8
Adler, Alfred, 146, 147
adolescents, 189, 194
Adorno, T., 94, 101
advice, sources of, 210
aetiology, 37, 39, 53, 54, 59, 62, 64–6, 105, 116, 119, 120, 124, 129, 135, 170, 176, 181, 206
affairs, extramarital, 9
aid, for disaster victims, 198
alienation, 122
All-China Women's Federation, 193
altruism, 198
American culture, 152
American Enlightenment, 77, 78
American Presbyterian Board of Foreign Missions (APBFM), 5, 6, 81, 82, 83, 84, 92, 96
American Psychiatric Association, 14, 209
amnesia, tropical, 117
analytical psychology, 119
ancestor worship, 104
Anderson, Warwick, 7–8, 112–13, 114, 120, 124
anger, 3, 4, 38, 39, 43, 45–6, 48, 50–1, 63
'announcing causes', 41–2, 51, 68–9
anonymity, 210
anti-Christian sentiment, 118
anti-depressants, 17
Anti-Rightist movement, 156, 159
anxiety, 121, 183
apathy, 58
apotropaic methods, 57
architecture
  Cantonese, 84–6
  cottage system, 79, 80, 82, 88
  cruciform plan, 75, 76, 79
  and functionality, 77
  Kirkbride plan, 80, 82
  moral, 80
  of psychiatric space, 73–90, 207
  radial plan, 75, 76
  and therapeutic outcome, 71, 74, 79, 80, 87, 90
asthenopia, 119
asylums
  confinement in, 109
  development of Chinese, 5–6, 71, 164, 206–7
  European, 73–6
  police management and use of, 138–9
  police regulations and detention of insane in, 108
  value-systems, 6

Bao, Mr, 4–5, 55, 61, 62, 63–70
Barlow, T., 95
beggars, 139
behavioural problems, 189
behavioural sciences, Western, 13
Beijing
  psychotherapy in, 143, 183, 201

see also Peking
Beijing Police Academy, 132
Beiping Public Security Bureau, 130
Billinghurst, Walter B., 115, 117
biomedical modernity, 8–12
biopolitics
knowledge/power complex of, 93
literature on Chinese, 95–6
blindness, 50
Blowers, Geoffrey, ix, 10, 11, 143–60, 208
body
imbalances, 62, 65
and mind, 22, 39, 54, 60, 70, 205
and spirit, 25, 60
Bond, M. H., 73
Bosei Lim, 165, 166, 167
bourgeois, psychotherapy as, 159, 183
Bou-Yong Rhi, 182
Bowman, Dr Karl, 155
Boxer Rebellion, 114
brain function, 151
breakdowns, white, 114–19, 123, 125, 128
breathing exercises, 23
British Hospital (Shanghai), 121
British Journal of Medicine, 111, 112
British Psychological Society, 121
bromide therapy, 115
Buddhism
chanting of sutras, 57
teachings of, 35
Bumke, Oswald, 169
Bureau of Prisons, 193
business, 123
private, 152

Cadbury, William W., 117
'call of the East', 122, 126
Canton
climate, 87
location, 83
psychiatric space in, 72, 73, 74, 81–90, 96, 164
Canton Hospital, 117
Canton Medical Hospital, 6, 81, 82, 84
Canton System of Trade (1757–1842), 83
capitalism, 152
Cartesian dualism, 205
case histories/notes, 1, 61–2, 66–7, 69, 137, 152–3, 206
National Taiwan University Hospital, 161, 162–3, 169–74, 209
significance of, 162–3
CCMD-3 *see Chinese Classification of Mental Disorders*
celebrity psychologists, 200–1
Center For Disease Control, 200
Central Health Experimental College, 10, 148, 154
certification, of mental health practitioners, 14, 184, 189, 190–2, 196, 203, 209
Ceylon, mental disorders among Westerners in, 111
chaining, of insane, 92, 98, 99, 100–1, 146
Chakrabarty, D., 97
Charles, Sir Richard Havelock, 111, 116
chastity, 141
Chen, Hsiu-fen, ix, 3–4, 37–54, 206
Chen, Mr, 46
Chen, Nancy N., ix, 14, 205–11
Chen Li, 159
Chen Shiyuan, 19
Chen Yi, 165
Cheng Yu-lin, 10–11, 143, 145, 155, 159
Chiang, Howard, ix–x, 1–15
Chiang Kai-shek, 11, 176
childbirth, trauma of, 137
childlessness, shame of, 133
children
at risk, 189
behavioural disorders, 10, 148–9
preference for male, 133
sold in brothels, 134
sold into slavery, 134
China awareness-raising conference (1999), 188
China Central Television (CCTV), 195–6, 199
China Journal of Science and Art, 121
The China Medical Journal, 6, 92, 97, 101, 103, 111, 116–17, 119
China-American Psychoanalytic Alliance, 200
Chinese Academy of Sciences, Institute of Psychology, 155, 192, 200

Chinese American Overseas Scientific
Scholar Association, 155
Chinese Association for Mental Health, 14, 190, 192, 193
Chinese Civil War, 159, 177, 180
Chinese Classification of Mental Disorders (CCMD), 15, 209
Chinese Communist Party, 153, 154, 176
Chinese Democratic League, 153
Chinese Disabled Persons' Federation, 189, 193
Chinese Enlightenment, 8, 94, 141
Chinese Medical Academy of Sciences, 154
Chinese medicine, clinical hybridity of, 5, 15, 208
Chinese Mental Hygiene Society, 10, 11, 145
Chinese Psychological Institute, 10, 143, 148, 155, 156
Chinese Society of Psychotherapists (planned), 150
Chinese Youth Development Center of the Communist Youth League, 193
Chongqing
as centre of scientific research, 10
psychotherapy in, 143, 148, 149
Chongqing College of Social Education, 154
Christianity
and emergence of psychiatric space, 72, 75, 88
missionary discourse in China, 118
Civil Service Examinations, 4, 35, 49, 64, 67
civilization, measures of, 98
clan system, 97
classification, of psychiatric disease, 182, 209
Classified Studies of Dream Interpretations, 19
climate
and tropical neurasthenia, 8, 116, 117, 125, 126
and Western nervous disorders, 115, 119, 121, 127, 128
clinical psychology, 185, 201
collaborative culture, 144
college counselling, 187, 201–2
colonialism
China's role in, 114, 126
colonial identity, 7
concepts of, 93, 113
and dialectic of Enlightenment, 96, 99, 104, 108, 109
feasibility of Western in tropics, 112, 113–14, 117–18, 119, 124
and introduction of psychiatry, 164
of medical missionaries, 95
and neurasthenia, 175–6
and study of non-Western psychiatry, 15
Taiwan breaks away from, 165
and Western breakdowns, 124, 126
common suffering, 180
communication
between doctors and patients, 40, 206
as central element of clinical care, 4
techniques, 51
with women patients, 53
Communism, 88
and marriage, 131, 132
psychotherapy under, 144, 153, 199
Communist Youth League, 193
community building, 'Shanghai model', 157
community-based care, 5
compensation marriage, 130
compulsive disorders, 58
concubines
and heredity, 105, 106
husbands and, 9
indentured servants as, 130
system of, 7, 94, 105, 106, 108, 139–40
wives and, 133–4, 135
confinement, 5, 205
in asylums, 109
domestic, 6–7, 98–9, 101, 108–9, 207
eugenic rationale for, 94
rules on 'preventive', 98
Confucianism
and care of insane, 5
values seen as backward, 8
values and toleration/care of insane, 73, 74, 77
conjugal family, 133
consciousness, 152
cooling drugs, 65
coping strategies, 13
corruption, political, 73, 74, 152
cortical circulation, 117
cost of living, 180

cottage hospitals/structures, 79, 80, 82, 88
counselling, psychological, 13, 14, 153, 154, 159, 184, 185, 186–7, 189, 191–2, 193, 194, 199, 201, 202–3, 209
 centres, 202
 defined as non-medical, 203
 fees for, 194
 training for, 193–5
counter-therapy, emotional, 38, 52, 206
crime, 7, 105, 134
criminal reform farms, 154
Criticism movement, 156, 159
Crozier, Anna, 113, 118, 126
Cruciform Plan, 75, 76, 79
Csordas, Thomas, 68
Culpin, Millais, 115, 120–1, 125, 126, 127, 128
cultural beliefs, 205
cultural modernity, 8–9
cultural psychiatry, 12, 169
Cultural Revolution, 13, 90, 158, 192
 assault on psychology, 156, 183, 187
Curing the Ills of Medicine (Wu Tang), 68
customs, Western respect for Chinese, 123, 125, 126

Dai, Bingham, 10, 108, 147, 149
Daoism, 19, 33
 exorcism, 57
Davies, James, 185
de-institutionalization, 211
deception, 41, 46, 48, 53
dehumanization, of insane, 91, 98, 100–1
delusional disorders, 12
dementia, 14, 189
 female, 133
demons, 18, 59, 100
Department of Health and Social Security (DHSS), 179
depletion, 64, 65, 68, 137
deportment, changes in, 23, 34
depression, 14, 49, 157, 183, 188, 189, 210
 psychogenic, 176, 180
 war termination, 174
Depression era, 138
desertion, within marriage, 131, 135, 136
design
 of John G. Kerr Refuge, 84–90
 of psychiatric space, 71, 72, 75–90
desire, repressed, 120, 121, 122, 150, 151
destitution, 137
developmental psychology, 144
the devil, 150–1
Dewey, John, 165
diagnoses
 analysis of, 161, 162, 163, 181
 colonialism and range of, 164
 time and space factors, 181
 of trauma, 169, 174–82
Diagnostic and Statistical Manual of Mental Disorders (DSM), 14, 58, 178, 209, 210
dialectical materialism, 151, 153
dian, 4, 56, 58, 63, 64, 206
dian-kuang-xian, 58
diet, and nightmares, 17
dignity, 93
Ding Tsan, 10–11, 143, 145, 146, 147–51, 154–6, 159
disasters, 184, 197–200, 201, 209
disease, prevention of, 23
distance-learning, 193
distraction, 41, 45
divorce, 131–2, 140
Dix, Dorothea, 74, 77, 82
doctors, Chinese
 certification system, 14
 engagement with global psychiatry, 209–11
 importance of communication with patients, 40
 language skills, 53
 moralizing by, 67
 relations with patients, 163
 risk to lives of, 52, 144, 159
 status of, 52
 study abroad, 10, 12, 144, 155, 160
 in Taiwan, 165–6
 training in psychoanalysis, 150, 160
 training in psychotherapy, 145, 147, 160
domestic abuse, 131, 139
dreams
 and belief system, 19
 categorization of, 17
 and choice of talisman, 31
 encyclopedias, 1, 2, 15
 exorcism of, 2, 17–36

inauspicious, 22, 31, 33, 35, 36
interpretations of, 18, 19, 22, 35
late Ming understanding/definition of, 21–3
medicalization of, 18
study of, 2–3
see also Forest of Dreams; nightmares
drug therapy, 4
for emotional disorders, 51–2, 53–4
and globalization, 209–10
relative importance in 19th century China, 55, 61, 68, 70, 206
replenishing, 65, 66
speedy synthetic method, 155, 159, 192
Wu Tang's use of, 65–7
DSM *see Diagnostic and Statistical Manual of Mental Disorders*
Du Yuesheng, 134
Dutch East India Company, 112

e meng, 22
earthquakes, 14, 184, 197–200, 201, 209, 211
East Africa, tropical neurasthenia in, 113, 118
eccentricity, 56
economic development
and crisis in mental health, 187
and openness to Western science and technology, 15
and psychotherapy, 13, 183, 184
and public awareness of mental health, 210–11
and stress, 183
education
counselling in, 187, 201–2, 203
mental health programs, 210
reform of, 8
electric shock therapy, 155, 157
emetics, 59, 65, 206
Emmanuel Movement, 119
emotional catharsis, 40, 51
emotional control, loss of, 148
emotional counter-therapy, 38, 52, 206
emotional disorders, 40, 42
as disorders of *qi*, 54
origins of, 42
emotional therapy, 3, 37–54, 107, 209
in clinical encounters, 42–51
labour intensive nature of, 206
less prevalent than drug therapy, 38, 51–4, 206
risks involved in, 52
success of, 38, 53
see also psychotherapy
emotions
Chinese understanding of, 61
Five Intents, 37, 38–9, 47
and health/illness, 3, 37, 38–40, 51, 69, 205
imbalance of, 3, 59, 61, 68
and insanity, 55, 63, 64, 69
seven, 3, 37, 39, 47, 51, 53
and supervenience, 61
therapeutic approaches to disorders of, 3–4, 37–54
emperors, anxieties about health, 35
employment assistance programs (EAPs), 202
energy
blockages of, 205
see also qi
engineering psychology, 200
Enlightenment, 78, 93, 94, 97, 98, 101, 141
colonial dialectic of, 96, 99, 104, 108, 109, 207
epidemiology, 169
eroticism, 106
ethics, medical, 46
ethnic conflicts, 12, 169
ethnic factors, and mental disorders, 181
eugenics, 7, 96, 104, 105, 106, 107, 108
Europe
and development of modern medicine, 15
psychiatric space in, 73–7, 78, 80, 88
exhortation, 5
in treatment of psycho-behavioural pathologies, 55, 67–8
exorcism
Daoist, 57
of dreams and nightmares, 2, 17–36
external causes, 39, 59
extramarital affairs, 135

family, Chinese
- antithesis of modernity, 6, 94, 109
- changing meaning of, 9, 206, 208
- character of, 93–6
- and domestic confinement, 6–7, 98–9, 101
- and emotional therapy, 4, 53
- familial authority, 94
- and hospitalized relatives, 100, 109, 207
- illtreatment of mentally ill relatives, 91, 92, 97, 100–1
- intervention in, 110
- as 'iron cage', 7, 91, 92, 94, 96, 101, 105, 108–10, 207
- missionary view of, 93, 94, 95, 96, 98, 101, 108
- relations with state, 205
- as reproductive machine, 104–5, 109
- responsibility for care of insane, 5, 72, 73, 74, 77, 96, 98–9, 206–7
- restructuring of, 108
- and run away women, 130, 132
- sexual life, 106, 109
- traditional, 94
- unchaining insane from care of, 6–7, 91, 99, 108–9, 207
- and understanding of causes of insanity, 6
- weakening of family ties, 73, 109
- women and conflict with, 135, 136

family patients, 99, 100
Family Publishing House, 151, 152
Fan Tingwei, 149
fear, 3, 38, 39, 44, 49, 175
February 28 Incident (1947), 11, 12, 169, 172, 174–6
feminism, 8, 94, 131
feng, 56, 58
Feng Xiaoqing, 107
Feng Yingkun, Dr, 140
filial piety, 67, 73
Fire
- attribution of madness to, 59, 65–6
- signs of, 65
- treatments for excessive/depleted, 59, 65–6
- *see also* inner Fire

First Beiping Health Centre, 154
'Five Intents', 37, 38–9, 47
'Five Phases', 38–9, 51, 53
'Five Viscera', 38–9
Fong Tsuen district (Canton), 82, 83–4, 86
food
- hygiene, 123
- resources, 180

footbinding, movement against, 8
forced labour, 154, 158
foreign exploitation, 73
forensic psychiatry, 15
Forest of Dreams, 2–3, 17, 18–20
- definition of terms, 21–3
- Dream Exorcism, 17–36
- sections of, 20

Forsyth, David, 125, 126
fortune-telling, 48
Four Treasuries Imperial Library, 19
Franklin, Benjamin, 6, 78
free association, 150
free love, 9
freedom, individual, 93, 94
French Hospital (Beijing), 131
Freud, Sigmund, 2, 125, 147, 149–50
- and anxiety states, 121
- and neurasthenia, 123, 124
- and psychoanalysis, 7–8, 149
- theory of projection and repression, 151
- theory of sexuality, 8, 112, 120

Friends Hospital, 6, 71, 78, 79, 81, 82
fright, 3, 39, 41
frustration, 46, 64, 65
functional psychosis, 172
Funü zazhi (*Ladies' Journal*), 132
Furth, Charlotte, 137

Gamble, Sidney, 130
Gang-of-Four, 156
Gao Lian, 23
Gaogong An Jinshen Bingyuan (Beijing), 131
Ge Hong, 19
gender
- and different treatments, 62
- and emotional therapy, 53
- equality, 8–9
- and madness, 9
- and suicide, 188
- and use of psychiatric services, 181

The General Planning on the Wenchuan Earthquake Post-Disaster Rehabilitation and Rebuilding, 199
gengshen days, 33
German psychiatry, 164, 170
Gesell, Professor, 147
ghosts, 59, 68
'Global Burden of Disease' (World Bank), 188
Global South, 180
globalization, 209–10
GMD (Guomingdang), 11, 134, 154, 156
Goldin, G., 76, 86
Goldstein, Jan, 65
grains, abstention from, 23
Grandier, Father Urbain, 151
Grant, Joanna, 48–9
Green Gang, 134
Gregotti, Vittorio, 73
grief, 3, 39, 50
Grob, Gerald, 79–80
group therapy, 156
Guam, tropical neurasthenia in, 122
Guangzhou, 13
Guidelines to Dreams and Dream Interpretation, 19
Guo, Benyu, 152
Guo Nianfeng, Professor, 192, 193
Guomingdang *see* GMD
gymnastics, 23

Halpern, Fanny, 146–7, 156
Han Chinese, 166
Hangchow Medical Mission, 115
Harper, Donald, 56
Harrison, F. L., 115
Havelock Ellis, Henry, 133
He, Mr, 49
He Dongru, 19–20, 21
He Jiyue, Dr, 91
Head Injury Advice Bureau (DHSS), 179
headaches, 155
  psychogenic, 123–4
health psychology, 159
heart
  disease, 44
  dysfunctions and insanity, 5, 58, 60
  and spirit, 60
heat
  and European constitution, 115, 208
  inner, 4, 5, 59, 61, 63, 64, 65, 206
hebephrenia, 12
Henderson, Edward, 115
herbal medicine
  for nightmares, 33, 34
  prevalence of, 51
hereditary conditions, 7, 104, 105, 108
Hershatter, Gail, 132
hobbyists, and therapists, 202
Hoffmann, Dr J. Allen, 98, 104
holism, 39, 54, 70
Hong Kong, 164
Hongqiao Psychiatric Rehabilitation Hospital (Shanghai), 10, 152, 157
Horkheimer, M., 94, 101
Horney, Karen, 108, 147
hospitality, to sick and strangers, 75
hospitals
  contemporary psychiatric, 210
  differentiation of, 77
  in medieval Europe, 75
  psychiatric, 5–7, 71–90, 92
  in Renaissance Europe, 77
  shift from specialized psychiatric, 211
  war and relocation of, 158
  see also hospitals by name
hotlines, 210
houses of sworn sisters, 130
housing shortages, 74
Hsueh, Yeh, 152
Hua Yuanhua/Hua Tuo, 52
Huang, Hsuan-Ying, x, 13, 14, 183–204, 209
Huang Jiade, 144
Huang Jian-hou, 146
Huang Jiayin, 10, 11, 143, 144, 145, 151–4, 157, 159
Huang Jinrong, 134
Huangzhou University, 187
Huaxia xinli, 14, 193–5
human resources management, 159
humanization, of insane, 97–8, 109
husbands
  death of, 136
  desertion by, 131, 136
  extramarital affairs, 135

taking of concubine by, 135
Hwang, K., 73
hybridity, of Chinese medicine, 5, 15, 208
hypertension, 156
hypnotism, 119
hypochondriasis, 164
hysterics, 176

Ibsen, Henrik, 130, 132
identity
loss of, 122
sense of, 69, 70, 107
ideological education, 187
immigration
and adjustment disorders, 12, 176–8, 181
experiences of, 12, 167, 169, 172, 173, 174
Imperial China
dream and nightmare exorcism in, 17–36
emotional therapy and talking cures in late, 37–54
medical therapies for madness in late, 55–70
Imperial Taihoku University, 165, 166, 169, 170
Imperial Tokyo University, 164, 166, 168
incantations
and dream exorcism, 2, 17, 22, 23, 29, 30, 32, 34
and good sleep, 24
India, mental disorders among Westerners in, 111
indigenous people, hypotheses on personality of, 164
individuality, 107
Industrial Health Research Board, 127
industrialization, 180
inheritance, women's lack of, 135, 136
Inner Canon, 3, 4, 37, 38, 39, 40, 43, 44, 45, 50, 54, 56, 60, 62, 63
inner Fire, 4, 5, 59, 61, 63, 64, 65, 206
inner injury/harm, 42, 68
insanity
causes of, 59, 65
concept of, 4, 5
and eugenics, 104, 105
and institutionalization, 12, 74, 79–80
kinship-based approach to, 72, 73, 77
late 19th-century understanding of, 57
move from religious to secular understanding of, 77
need to separate insane from sane, 78–9, 82
physical and organic bases of, 4
and sexual intercourse, 108
and social disappointment, 4, 64, 65, 69
ties between emotions and, 55, 63, 64, 69
insomnia, 44, 119, 155, 175, 177
Institute of Psychology *see* Chinese Academy of Science; Chinese Psychological Institute
institutionalization, 12, 74, 79–80, 161, 163, 188, 205, 207, 209
intellectuals, persecution of, 159
inter-marriage, middle-class, 7
internal causes, 39, 59
International Classification of Diseases (ICD), 14–15, 175, 177, 179, 209
International Psychoanalytical Association, 200
Internet-based psychotherapy training, 200
Interregnum, 174
'invoking the cause', 68–9
'iron cage(s)', 7, 91, 92, 94, 96, 101, 105, 108–10
isolation review, 158

Japan
defeat and surrender (1945), 165, 169, 174
hands Taiwan back to China, 11
invasion/colonization (1937–45), 10, 88, 143, 148, 149, 150, 154, 156, 158–9, 166
mental disorders among Westerners in, 111, 113
psychiatry in pre-war, 163, 164
and training of Taiwanese physicians, 165–6, 168, 170
Jaschok, M., 130
Jauregg, Julius Wagner, 146
jealousy, 106
Jennings, Michael, 127
Jews, 122
Jiang Qing, 157
Jiangsu Medical University, 147, 156

Jin De-chu, Dr, 158
John G. Kerr Refuge for the Insane (Canton), 6, 7, 71–2, 73, 74, 77, 78, 81–90, 92, 93, 97, 98, 99, 100, 101, 102–3, 104, 133, 140, 164, 207
  building expansion, 88–90
  design, 84–8
  dispensary, 87–8
  location, 85
  mental hygiene campaigns, 105
  photograph of, 86
  plan of, 89
joy, 3, 4, 38, 39, 43, 46, 47–8, 49, 50, 63
Judge, Joan, 132
Jung, Carl C., 119, 121, 149

Kao, J. J., 93
Ke Dashen, 130
Kennedy, Dane, 112, 113, 119
Kerr, Dr. John Glasgow, 5–6, 72, 78–9, 81–8, 90, 92, 96, 97, 98, 99, 133, 164, 207
Kerr, George, 165
Kerr Refuge *see* John G. Kerr Refuge for the Insane
kidneys, 46
  and neurasthenia, 116
kinship-based care, 72, 73, 74, 77
kinship-clan obligation, 73, 97
Kirkbride, Thomas Story, 74, 80–1
Kirkbride Plan, 80, 82
Kleinman, Arthur, 187–8, 208
knowledge, transfer across societies and cultures, 72
Komine Hospital, 163
Korean War, 152
Kraepelin, Emil, 98, 164
Krieger, Josh, 197
kuang, 4, 56, 58, 59, 60, 63, 64, 65, 206
Kuriyama, Shigehisa, 39
Kurosawa, Ryosuke, 168

lagging 'behindness', 8
Lange, Carl and Frederik, 169
language
  in Taiwan, 12, 167, 169–71, 181–2
  Western command of Chinese, 8, 123
Lao She, 131
Laozi, 30, 32
laughing disorders, 49–50, 51
law
  and crimes committed when insane, 57
  marriage and reform of, 131
Le Roy, Jean-Baptiste, 77
'Learning of the Way', 63
Lee, Dr Olga, 146
Lee, Sing, 15, 188
legislation, mental health, 14, 184, 202–3, 209, 210, 211
Lennox, William, 111
Leont'ev, Alexei Nikolaevich, 151
Leung, Seung-Ming, 187
Li Gao, 68
Li Qixing, 49–50, 53
Li Zixun Li, Dr, 196, 197
Liberation era, 90
libido, 8
Lin, Tsung-Yi, 12, 166, 167, 168–9, 170, 175, 177, 178, 180, 182
Lin Peiqin, 42
Lin Rigao, 175
Lin Yu-tang, 144
Lin Zhao, 157–8
literature, and war trauma, 178
Liu Jin, Dr, 91, 200
Liu Lun-ci, 146
Liu Wansu, 4, 63–4
lobotomies, 157
London School of Tropical Medicine, 120, 127
longevity, 23
'loss of face', 73
Loudun, 151
Lu Xun, 132, 134
Luhrmann, Tanya, 185
Luria, Alexander, 151
Lyman, Dr Richard S., 9, 10, 138–9, 141, 145, 147, 149, 156

Ma, Zhiyang, x, 91–110, 207
MacArthur, Douglas, 165
McCartney, James Lincoln, 7, 8, 121–6, 127–8, 133, 134, 208
McNeil, Andrew S., 117
madhouses *see* asylums
madness

19th-century Chinese medical therapies for, 55–70
concept of, 1, 4, 55, 56
considered similar to other illnesses, 55, 60–1, 70
medicalization of, 79
social and moral significance of, 62
somatic element of, 60–1
terms for, 56, 58, 206
magazines, popular, 1, 9–11, 130, 132, 143, 144–5, 147, 149, 152, 158, 160, 210
Mahone, Sloane, 113
Main, David Duncan, 115
Manchuria, 164
mania, 55, 56, 58, 65
mania-depression psychosis, 172
Mann, Horace, 77
Manson-Bahr, Philip, 112
Mao Zedong, 157, 159
Maoist period
attitude to psychological treatments in, 13, 187
political violence during, 187
market economy, transition to, 187
marriage
arranged, 130
avoidance strategies, 129, 130, 140–1
backward customs, 104
changing meaning of, 9
control of, 108
discord in, 9, 135
early, 104
few escape routes, 130–2
men as victims of, 131
psychiatric units as refuge from, 140–1
and psychic disturbance, 132–4
and undesirable offspring, 108
without emotions, 106
women stressed by system of, 129, 207–8
Matsushita, Masaaki, 182
Matsuzawa Hospital (Tokyo), 168
Mawangdui medical manuscripts, 56
Maxwell, John Preston, 116
May Fourth movement, 8
Medical Case Files (Wu Tang), 4, 62
medical examinations, for Westerners, 116
medical facilities, for the insane *see* hospitals, psychiatric
medical psychology, 143, 149
medical thinking, changes in, 56
medicalization
of dreams and nightmares, 18, 205
of madness, 79
of psychotherapy, 202
medication *see* drug therapy
medicine, traditional Chinese, 57, 164, 210
Meiji period, 164, 170
melancholia, 114
meng, 21, 22
menstrual disorders, 9, 129, 137
mental breakdowns, Western, 114–19, 120, 126, 128
Mental Cultivation of Youth (Ding Tsan), 147, 155
mental health
campaigns, 109
reform of care system, 188–9, 202
scholarship on history of Chinese, 1
Mental Health Essays (Ding Tsan), 147–8, 155
Mental Health Law (2013), 184, 202–3, 209, 210, 211
mental hygiene
campaigns, 7, 10, 105, 145, 146, 147
debates about, 208
traditional notions of, 205
Meyer, Adolf, 138, 156, 158
middle class, psychotherapy and emerging, 184, 194, 202
Middle Kingdom, degenerating capability of, 118
mind
and body, 22, 39, 54, 60, 70, 205
medicalization of the, 1, 12
Ming dynasty
dream and nightmare exorcism in late, 17–36, 205
emotional therapy, 46–7
Ministry of Education, 187
Ministry of Health, 13, 14, 187, 189
Ministry of Human Resources and Social Security, 14
Ministry of Labor and Social Security, 14, 184, 185, 186, 189, 195, 200
certification, 190–2, 196, 203
miscarriages, 111

missionaries
  archives, 1
  and care of insane, 5–7, 74, 97–8, 99–100, 104, 108, 206–7
  and Chinese family, 93, 94, 95, 96, 98, 101, 108
  colonialism of, 95
  and command of Chinese language, 8, 123
  and establishment of psychiatry in China, 92, 93
  and government services, 74
  health screening, 116–17
  impact of, 8
  and levels of Chinese insanity, 166
  as medical practitioners, 119, 166, 206
  narrative of self-sacrifice, 118
  need for regular furloughs, 117, 127
  and psychiatric space, 77, 81–90, 92, 96–7
  and psychoanalysis, 106, 107
  and secular charitable obligations, 84
  and tropical neurasthenia, 7–8, 111, 114, 115, 116, 117, 118, 126, 127, 208
  and unchaining of insane from domestic confinement, 6–7, 92, 108–9
mob violence, 116, 118
modernization, 164
monasteries, and care of sick, 75
Moon, Lottie, 114–15
Moore, Aaron William, 178
moral architecture, 80
moral corruption, 34
moral degeneracy, 104, 208
moral education, 187
moral obligation, 73
moral reform, community as means of, 82
moral treatment, 82
moralizing, by Chinese doctors, 67
morphine addiction, 115
moxibustion, 42
mucus, 59, 64, 65, 129, 135
murder, 131
mutilation, 131
mutual aid, 73
Mutual Conquest of the Five Phases, 38–9, 40–1, 42, 43, 45, 47, 52, 53
Nanjing Central Hospital, 11, 155
Nanjing, psychotherapy in, 143
naps, importance of, 117, 123
narcissism, 8, 107, 124
narcoleptics, 17
nation states, 94, 164
National Committee of the Chinese People's Political Consultative Conference (CPPCC), 153
National Conference on Mental Health Care, 188
National Medical College of Shanghai, 138
National Mental Health Plan (2002–12), 13, 188, 189
National Occupational Classification, 190
National Shanghai Medical College, 147, 148, 149, 156
National Taiwan University Hospital (NTUH)
  funding of, 166
  language habit, 12, 169–71, 181–2
  Psychiatry Department, 11, 12, 161, 163, 168–9
  statistical analysis of case notes, 169–74
  trauma diagnoses, 174–82
National Vocational Standards, 190, 191
nationalism, 132
Nationalist government, 10, 134
  and mental health issues, 166
  in Taiwan, 11, 165, 166–7, 172, 174, 176
'Nations for Mental Health' (WHO), 188
natural disasters, 184, 197–200, 201, 209
negative attitudes, 125
Neo-Confucianism, 63
neo-Kraepelinian taxonomy, 15
nervous breakdowns, Western, 114–19, 120, 126, 128
nervous exhaustion, 116
neurasthenia, 111, 115, 117, 118, 119, 125, 148, 155, 175–6, 177, 188, 208
  see also tropical neurasthenia
neuropsychiatry, 129, 145
neuropsychosis, 106
neuroses
  causes of, 124
  and foreign customs and habits, 8, 121–2
  and personality faults, 126
  and repressed desire, 121

traumatic, 178–80
neurotic escapism, 126
neurotic predisposition, 124, 125
neurotransmitters, 59
New Culture Movement, 107
New York Times, 91
New Youth (*Xin Qingnian*), 10, 144
Newcombe, Freda, 179
nightmares
boundary with dreams, 22
contemporary concern over, 206
definition of, 22
detrimental to health, 22, 34
exorcism, 2, 17–36
herbal prescriptions, 33, 34
as indicators of personal failings, 34
nightmare imagery rehearsal therapy, 17
responsibility for, 18
and talismans and incantations, 31–3, 34
see also dreams
non-drug-based interventions, 3
North-China Herald, 119–20, 126
NTUH *see* National Taiwan University Hospital
nuclear family, 94, 107
nunneries, Buddhist, 130

occult, 30
Ohji Brain Hospital, 163
Oldt, Frank, 111, 120, 125, 126
On the Treatise on Causes and Symptons of Various Medical Disorders, 39
opium smoking, 123
Opium Wars, 83
Oriental Magazine (*Dong Fang*), 10, 144
'Oriental Nerves' (McCartney), 121, 122–3
Orientalism, 8
outpatient psychological counselling, 186–7
outreach education programs, 210
over-repletion, 64, 65

Palmer, David, 201
Pan Guangdan, 107, 133
paraphernalia, sale of psychological, 202
Paris Asylum, 92
Parker, Dr Peter, 6, 114
pastoral atmosphere, 84
patients
clinical experience of, 163
language and communication with, 167
negotiations between doctors and, 163
records, 1
voice of, 162
patriarchy, 94, 95, 98, 101, 105, 107, 108
conjugal, 131, 208
patrilineal households, 9, 129, 130, 133, 134
patriotism, 132
pauper lunatics, 134
Pavlov, Ivan, 151
peach wood, 33
Pearson, Veronica, 188
Peking Municipal Psychopathic Hospital, 147
Peking Police Regulations, 108
Peking Union Medical College (PUMC), 105, 108, 111, 133, 145, 147, 149, 150, 156
neuropsychiatric ward, 137–41, 154
Peking University, 187
Pennsylvania Hospital, 6, 71, 78–9, 81
Pennsylvania Hospital for the Insane (PHI), 6, 71, 78, 79–81
pensiveness, 3, 38, 39, 44, 45–6, 48
peptic ulcers, 156
personality, medicalization of, 59
persuasion, importance in treatment of madness, 5, 55, 67–8
pesticides, ingestion of, 188
Pevsner, Nikolaus, 75
pharmaceutical books, 53
pharmaceutical industry, 209
Philadelphia, 77–81
Philippines, tropical neurasthenia in, 111, 112, 120
Phillips, Michael, 188
phlegm, 53, 100
accumulations, 9
physical injury, and trauma, 178–80
Picherella, J., 155
pillows, tiger-shaped, 25
Pinel, Philippe, 92
Pink Pills for Pale People, 115
police
and female madness, 132–3
patients, 99, 100
and Peking asylum, 138–9

and run away women, 130
political decolonization, 11
political disorder, 116, 118
political structure, one-party, 15
polygamy, 7, 104, 105, 106, 133–4, 208
popular culture
psychological health and, 9, 210
and psychotherapy, 183, 195–7, 209
population
control, 108
studies, 164
Porter, Roy, 162
possession, 151
post-disaster conditions, 14, 184, 189, 197–200
post-traumatic stress disorder (PTSD), 198–200
postcolonial period, 12
postpartum madness, 137
poverty, and diagnosis of insanity, 134, 139
prayers, for dream exorcism, 23
PRC (People's Republic of China), 11
'100 Flowers' period, 153
founding of, 151
marriage law, 132
psychotherapy in, 153, 159, 192
science under, 155
severs ties with West, 151, 152
turns towards Soviet Union, 151–2, 159
Presbyterian Mission Hospital (Swatow), 116
Price, G., 111, 116
Principle of Mutual Conquest of the Five Phases, 38–9, 40–1, 42, 43, 45, 47, 52, 53
promiscuity, among colonists, 112
Proposal on Further Strengthening Mental Health Work, 13, 188, 189
prostitution, 7, 105, 132, 137
proto-psychotherapy, 51
Psyche (*Xinli*), 10, 144–5
psychiatric hospitals *see* asylums; hospitals
psychiatric liberation, 91, 96–103
psychiatric space, 5–7, 71–2, 210
emergence of, 73–7, 164, 206–7
and feeling of safety, 86, 87, 88
John G. Kerr Refuge, 81–90, 97
need for, 92, 96
need to separate insane from sane, 78–9, 82
rural location, 84
as sanctuary, 141
in United States, 77–81
see also asylums; hospitals
psychiatry
birth of modern Chinese, 93
birth in West, 92
Chinese, before end of World War II, 163–4
Chinese engagement with global, 209–11
in contemporary China, 91
enhanced public image of, 79
re-institutionalization in Taiwan, 165–7
reframing in China, 205–11
scholarship on history of Chinese, 1, 57
suspension of Chinese in mid-1960s, 164, 165
traditional Chinese, 57, 58
psycho-behavioural pathologies, 4, 55, 57–9, 60, 206
psycho-boom, 13, 14, 183–204, 209
psychoanalysis, 8, 9, 106, 107–8, 119, 147, 149–50, 153
case notes, 162
and neurasthenia, 125
training for, 185, 200
and tropical neurasthenia, 120, 121, 124
and universalization of human experiences, 122
psychobiology, 137–41
psychogenic depression, 176, 180
psychogenic headaches, 123–4
psychogenic reaction, 172, 174–6, 177, 178
psychological aid, 14
psychological counselling *see* counselling, psychological
'Psychological Interviews' ('xinli fangtan') (TV programme), 14, 184, 195–7, 199–200
psychometric testing, 148, 154
psychoneuroses, 112, 120, 121, 123–4, 161, 172, 176, 177
Psychopathic Hospital (Peking), 139
psychopathological mental illness, 167
psychopharmacology, 13, 15, 209

psychophysiology, 158
psychoses, 112, 120, 124, 161, 172, 188, 189
psychosocial needs, 188
psychosocial processes, 156
Psychotherapy 300 Cases (Huang Jiayin), 152–3
psychotherapy
  boom in contemporary urban China, 183–204, 209
  certification for practitioners, 189
  clinics, 202
  in Communist era, 144
  craze as popular movement, 184, 185–6, 203
  definition of, 203
  development in West, 184, 185
  emergence of, 143–6, 158, 208
  fees for, 194, 201
  individualized, 11
  in late Imperial China, 37–54, 119
  in Maoist period, 13, 183
  medicalization of, 202
  political upheaval and disappearance of, 156, 159, 160, 183, 208
  popularity of, 10
  practice of, 146–51, 152–3, 154–6, 157, 158, 159, 160
  recognition of, 14
  resurgence of, 13, 159–60, 183, 186, 187, 192
  state regulation of, 184
  televising, 195–7
  training for, 183, 184, 185–6, 190–2, 193–5, 200, 201–2, 208
  and Wenchuan earthquake, 197–200
public health, 13
  education, 149
pulses, 65, 70
PUMC (Peking Union Medical College), 9, 10
Pure Ones, 30, 32
purgatives, 5, 59, 65–6, 67
purity, 23, 141

qi
  depletion of cardiac, 61
  desecration, 24
  deviant, 59
  effect of emotions on, 3, 53, 63
  emotional disorders as disorders of, 54
  harmful, 24
  movements of, 3, 39, 53
  regulation by drug therapy, 53
  stagnation of, 43, 45
  toxicity of local, 137
Qi, King, 52
'Qigong milieu', 201
Qing dynasty
  creation of psychiatric space in, 72, 73, 77
  loss of grip by, 8, 73
Qiu Jin, 132
Quakers, 79, 80, 82

racial difference
  of psychiatric patients at NTUH, 173, 209
  reinforcement of, 7
racial science, 170
Radcliffe Infirmary (Oxford), 179
Radial Plan, 75, 76
rage, pent-up, 135
rape, 131
rationality
  critiques of, 93
  metamorphosis of value into instrumental, 93–4
  self-alienation of, 94
re-institutionalization, of psychiatry in Taiwan, 11, 161, 163, 165–7
reality, flight from, 124
'Rebuilding the Psychological Home', 200–1
reciprocity, 73
reductionism, 70, 98
Reformation (European), 77
refuges, for marriage escapees, 129
Regulations on the Wenchuan Earthquake Post-Disaster Rehabilitation and Rebuilding, 199
relief work, 184, 198–9, 201
religious fanaticism, 114, 116
religious healing, 119
REM sleep, 17
Renaissance (European), 77
Renli Carpet Factory, 154
replenishing therapy, 65, 66
repression, of desire, 120, 121, 122, 150, 151

Republic of China, 90, 108, 128, 132, 143, 165, 186, 207
Research on Medical Formulas (Wu Kun), 40, 52
restraint, patient, 7, 92, 100–3
Rin Hsien, 12, 163
ritual propriety, 94
ritual treatments, for madness, 57, 67–8
Rockefeller Foundation, 9, 145, 147, 164
Rosenberg, C. E., 181
Ross, Dr Robert, 101, 105, 133–4
Rothman, D. J., 80
Royal Academy of Medicine, 50
Royal Society of Medicine, 125
Rulin waishi (*The Scholars*), 49
rural–urban differences
  in medical care, 15, 91, 210
  in suicide rates, 188
Rush, Dr Benjamin, 78
Russia *see* Soviet Union

St James Hospital (Anking), 119
St Joseph's Asylum (Shanghai), 146
St Mary of Bethlehem (London), 72
salvation, and sanity, 74
sanitary reforms, 116
SARS, 13, 189
Saul, Leon, 147
'saving face', 73
Scattergood, Thomas, 79, 80, 82
schizophrenia, 12, 156, 172, 210
  refractory, 157
segregation, psychiatric, 6, 105
seizure sickness, 56
Selden, Charles, 6, 88, 90, 92, 97, 133, 140
self-care, 210
self-esteem, low, 179
self-harm, 129
self-healing, 17, 18, 23, 35
self-help, 186
selfhood, 205
self-improvement, 144, 210
self-knowledge, 147
self-reflection and examination, 34
self-sacrifice, narrative of, 118
Seven Emotions, 3, 37, 39, 47, 51, 53
sexology, 107
sexual bondage, 130
sexual landscape, 9
sexual life
  Chinese, 105–6, 109
  of colonists, 112
  of missionaries, 120
sexual relations, avoidance of, 140–1
sexuality, Freudian theories of, 8, 112, 120, 123, 124
shamans, 42, 43
Shamian Island (Canton), 93–4
Shanghai
  life for Westerners in, 121, 127
  psychotherapy in, 143, 183
  treatment of neurasthenia in, 115, 117, 121
Shanghai Chief Psychiatric Treatment and Prevention Hospital, 157
Shanghai Medical School, 156
Shanghai Mental Health Promotion Association, 10, 145
Shanghai Municipal Psychiatric Hospital, 157
Shanghai Special Hospital for the Insane, 9, 134–7
Shanghai Translator's Association, 152
Shapiro, Hugh, x, 9, 129–41, 207
shen, 60
Shenghuo (*Life*), 130
Showalter, Elaine, 134
shyness, 125
Sichuan earthquake, 14, 211
Silk Road, 83
Simonis, Fabien, x, 4–5, 55–70, 206
Singapore, Bishop of, 112
Sino-German Course, 195, 196, 200
Sino-Japanese War, 143, 148, 149, 150, 154, 156, 158–9
Sivin, Nathan, 52
slavery, 134
sleep
  artificially induced, 155
  behavioural studies of, 17
  concern over restless, 206
  improved life with improved, 22
  proscriptions for good, 23–5, 205
  techniques, 23
sleepwalkers, 17
Smith, Arthur H., 116

social anxiety, 2–3
social change, rapidity of, 12, 181
social competence
  loss of, 58, 70
  return of, 66, 67
social disappointment, 4, 64, 65, 69
social harmony, 73
social psychiatry, 182
social roles, re-assertion of, 67
social service investigation, 7
social status, and emotional therapy, 52
social suffering, 187–8
social technology transfer, 72, 73, 90, 93
social therapy, 29
social upheaval, in Taiwan, 161
social welfare
  ideology, 74, 90
  organizations, 72
social work, 185
society, Chinese, 122, 125
  values, 205
Song, Miss, 140–1
Song dynasty, 53, 56
sorrow, 3, 38, 39, 47
soul, loss of the, 135
Soviet Union
  ideological turn towards, 11, 15, 151–2, 159
  psychology in, 151–2, 192
speedy synthetic method, 155–6, 159, 192
spells, against nightmares, 18
Spirit
  dysfunction and insanity, 60
  and Heart, 60
  spirit mediums, 48
  spirits, 18, 59, 87
  and clapping the teeth, 23
  and dreams and nightmares, 18, 34
spiritual health, 119
spleen, 44, 45, 46
stasis, 65
sterilization, 104
stimulants, and nightmares, 17
Stockard, J., 130
Stone Mountain Medical Case Histories (1519), 3, 47
stoning, 132
stress, 13, 183
student counselling, 187, 201
Su Zonghua, 10, 11, 143, 145–6, 151, 152, 153, 156–8, 159
suggestion, 119
suicides, 14, 189, 193
  attempted, 129, 140, 193
  demographic features of, 188
  female, and marriage system, 129, 130
  suicidal ideation, 175, 176
Sullivan, Harry Stack, 108, 147
Sun Yikui, 64
supervenience, 59–61
A Survey of Psychiatry (Su Zonghua), 157
Suzuki, Akihito, 163
symbolism
  influence of, 68
  religious, 75
Syuzo, Naka, 168
Szto, Peter, xi, 5–6, 71–90, 93, 207

Ta Chen, 164
Taihoku High School, 166
Taiping upheaval, 114
Taiwan
  ban on Japanese language in, 167
  Chinese immigration in, 12, 167, 169, 172, 173, 174, 176–8
  common suffering in, 180
  during Chinese Civil War, 180
  growth of psychoneurotic patients in, 161
  ill treatment and discrimination of Taiwanese, 166–7
  intellectuals and professionals flee to, 11, 159
  language in, 12, 167, 169–71, 181–2
  living standards in, 180
  Nationalist government in, 11, 65, 66–7, 172, 174, 176
  post-war mental disorder epidemic in, 161, 162, 172–4, 208–9
  psychiatry in pre-war, 164, 166
  re-insitutionalization of psychiatry in, 11–12, 165–7, 168
  trauma in post-war, 167–82
  tropical neurasthenia in, 113, 120, 164
  turmoil in post-war, 167
  white terror, 11, 169, 172

talismans
and dream exorcism, 2, 17, 22, 25–33
examples of, 26–8
function of, 29
talking cures, 3, 107, 153, 195
complementary to drugs, 70
in contemporary urban China, 183
in late Imperial China, 37, 38, 40–2, 45, 51, 52–3, 54, 70
popularity of, 4, 51
Taylor, Harry B., 119, 126
teeth
clapping the, 23, 30
grinding, 148
television talk shows, 1, 14, 184, 195–7, 200–1, 209
Third National Mental Health Care Conference (Beijing, 2001), 13
Thomas Jefferson Medical School (Philadelphia), 78, 81
Thompson, J. D., 76, 86
Thompson, Joseph C., 122
Three-Corpse Gods, 33, 34
Tianjin, Treaty of, 83
To Liang Qichao, 133
Tomes, Nancy, 78, 80
Topley, M., 130
training industry, market-oriented, 184, 193–5
transcultural psychiatry, 163
trauma
epidemic in post-war Taiwan, 12, 161, 167–82, 209
and physical injuries, 178–80
see also post-traumatic stress disorder
traumatic neurosis, 12, 178–80
trials of the insane, 57
tropical amnesia, 117
tropical diseases, 8, 111–12
tropical hygiene, 118, 126
tropical neurasthenia, 7–8, 111–28, 164, 208
tropical psychoanalysis, 125
tropics, mental disorders in, 111
Tseng Wen-Shing, 12
Tu Congming, 165

Uchimura, Yushi, 168–9
Unchaining Movement, 91, 95, 99, 109
unemployment, 181
United Nations Relief and Rehabilitation Administration (UNRA), 11, 155
United States
asylums in, 6, 71, 74, 75, 77–81, 86
Chinese doctors study in, 10, 12, 144, 155
and development of modern medicine, 15
eugenics in, 105
missionaries from, 5–8
philanthropic organizations, 9
psychological counsellors in, 194
uprootedness, 121, 126
urbanization, 74, 180

Vance, Brigid E., xi, 2–3, 17–36, 205, 209
vegetarian halls, 130
venereal disease, 7, 105
verbal communication, 40, 70
Victoria Mental Hospital (Hong Kong), 164
violence
towards women, 131, 132, 137, 139
Western reaction to, 114, 116
virginity, ethos of, 141
viscera
and Five Intents, 38–9
movements of *qi* in the, 3, 39
volunteerism, 198
Vygotsky, Lev, 151

walk-in clinics, 186–7
Wan Tun-mo, 88
Wang, Wen-Ji, xi, 7–8, 9, 111–28, 144, 146
Wang Ansheng, 159
Wang Bing, 63
Wang Ji, 23, 47
Wang Kentang, 54
Wang Xuelai, Shelley, xi, 10, 11, 143–60, 208
war termination depression, 174
warm-factor illnesses/school, 5, 61, 62, 66, 67, 69
Watson, Lord Malcolm, 125
Watson, R. S., 130
web-forums, 197–8

Weber, Hugo, 115
Weber, Max, 93–4
Wei Dexin, 44
Wen Hui Bao, 152
Wen Zhi, 52
Wen-Shing Tseng, 167
Wenchuan earthquake, 184, 197–200, 201, 209
Wenyon, Charles, 96–7, 98, 99
West
  China turns from influence of, 151–2
  culture and lifestyle in, 152
  development of psychotherapy in, 184
  transmission of biomedicine from, 9, 15, 143–4, 158, 160, 163, 164, 195, 208
West Wind (*Xi Feng*), 9–11, 143, 144–6, 147, 149, 152, 158, 160, 208
West Wind Supplement, 144
Westbrook, Hart, 147
Westerners
  breakdowns in China, 111–28, 208
  pressures on, 119–20
White, William A., 121
Whyte, Duncan, 116
Williams, Dr, 115
Wind
  anti-Wind remedies, 59
  attribution of insanity to, 56, 58
  signs of, 65
witches, 48
women
  at risk, 189
  childbirth, 137
  communication with physicians, 53
  and concubinage system, 106
  conflict with family, 135, 136
  destitute, 137
  and divorce, 131–2, 140
  economic rights of, 132, 135, 136
  emancipation of, 9
  emotional disorders, 53
  explanations of disruptive behaviour by, 129
  home environments, 9
  inequality, 132
  and madness, 9, 132–3, 135–7
  marriage and psychic disturbance, 132–4, 207–8
  mental hospitals as refuge for, 9, 139, 140–1, 207–8
  new vision of mental health problems in, 9, 129, 141
  and polygamy/concubines, 133–4
  and psychotherapy training programs, 202
  run away, 130
  sense of failure in domestic role, 135, 136
  stress of marriage system on, 129, 130–2
  and suicide, 188
  treatment in psychiatric hospitals, 134–7
  violence/ abuse towards, 131, 132, 137, 139
Woods, Dr Andrew H., 105–7, 138
work, excess, 119
work-as-therapy, 82
workshops, psychotherapy, 200
World Bank, 188
World Health Organization (WHO), 11, 13, 15, 155, 168, 172, 188, 209
  Social Psychiatry Programme, 182
World War II, 10, 161
  Chinese psychiatry before end of, 163–4
  epidemic of trauma cases in Taiwan after, 167–82, 208–9
  Japanese surrender, 165
  situation in Taiwan after end of, 167–8
worry, 3, 38, 39, 43, 46, 47, 49
wrongdoing, freedom from, 23
Wu, Harry Yi-Jui, xi, 161–82, 208–9
Wu, Yu-Chuan, 113, 120
Wu Jutong *see* Wu Tang
Wu Kun, 39–40, 52, 54
Wu Ruihua, Dr, 193
Wu Tang (Wu Jutong), 4–5, 41–2, 55, 56, 61–70
Wu Zhen, 146

Xi Feng see West Wind
Xian, 13
xian, 58, 206
Xiang, Lady, 43
Xiang Ya Medical School, 156
xin, 60
Xu Shiying, 134

yang
and exorcism, 35
imbalance, 50–1
rebalancing, 67
Yang, Jie, 203
Yang, Mr, 45
Yang, Nianqun, 93
Yang Fengchi, 196–7
Yang Jizhou, 53–4
Yanni, Carla, 80
Yao Wen-yuan, 156, 159
Ye Gui, 61, 69
Ye Tianshi, 50–1, 52, 53
Yellow Emperor's Inner Canon see Inner Canon
Yen, Dr F. C., 138
yin, 50–1
replenishing of, 66, 67
Yin Dakui, 188–9
Yitong (*Comprehensive Medicine*) (Zhang Lu), 61
youth, mental health education for, 147, 148, 149
Yu Ying High School, 154
Yuan Tian, 49
Yushu earthquake, 201

zhan, 21–2, 33
Zhang, Mr, 139–40
Zhang Congzheng, 3, 40–1, 42–5, 46, 49, 51–2
Zhang Fengyi, 19
Zhang Jiebin, 40, 41, 47
Zhang Kan, Professor, 200
Zhang Lu, 61
Zhao Gengyuan, Dr, 186
Zhili–Fengtian Wars, 131
Zhou En Lai, 155
Zhou Xuan, 157
Zhouqu landslide, 201
Zhu Qi, 151
Zhu Xi, 67
Zhu Zhenheng, 3, 4, 45–6, 52, 53, 61, 63–4
Zhuang, Mr, 45
Zou Taofen, 130

For Product Safety Concerns and Information please contact our EU representative GPSR@taylorandfrancis.com Taylor & Francis Verlag GmbH, Kaufingerstraße 24, 80331 München, Germany